POCKET BOOK OF
CRITICAL CARE PHARMACOTHERAPY

POCKET BOOK OF

CRITICAL CARE PHARMACOTHERAPY

Editor

Bart Chernow, M.D., F.A.C.P.

Professor of Medicine
Anesthesia and Critical Care
The Johns Hopkins University
School of Medicine

Physician-in-Chief
Sinai Hospital of Baltimore
Baltimore, Maryland

Editorial Associate

Lisa Daniel Sparks

Material adapted from *The Pharmacologic Approach to the Critically Ill Patient*, Third Edition

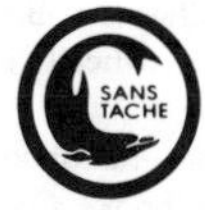

Williams & Wilkins

BALTIMORE • PHILADELPHIA • HONG KONG
LONDON • MUNICH • SYDNEY • TOKYO

A WAVERLY COMPANY

Editor: David C. Retford
Managing Editor: Kathleen Courtney Millet
Production Coordinator: Anne Stewart Seitz
Copy Editor: Klementyna L. Bryte
Designer: Ashley Pound

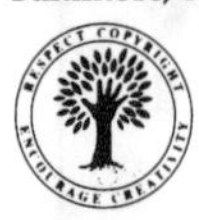

The authors, editor, and publisher have made every effort to provide accurate indications, adverse reactions, and dosage schedules for drugs discussed in this book, but it is possible that they may change. **The reader is urged to review the package information data of the manufacturers of the medications mentioned.**

Printed in the United States of America

Library of Congress Cataloging-in-Publications Data

Pocket book of critical care pharmacotherapy / edited by Bart Chernow; editorial associate, Lisa Daniel Sparks.
p. cm.
"Material adapted from: The pharmacologic approach to the critically ill patient, 3rd edition."
Includes bibliographical references and index.
ISBN 0-683-01535-4
1. Pharmacology—Handbooks, manuals, etc. 2. Critical care medicine—Handbooks, manuals, etc. I. Chernow, Bart. II. Sparks, Lisa Daniel. III. Pharmacologic approach to the critically ill patient. IV. Title: Critical care pharmacotherapy.
[DNLM 1. Pharmacology, Clinical—handbooks. 2. Critical Care—handbooks. 3. Drug Therapy—handbooks. QV 39 P738 1995]
RM301.12.P63 1995
616'.028—dc20
DNLM/DLC 94-37822
for Library of Congress CIP

94 95 96 97 98
1 2 3 4 5 6 7 8 9 10

PREFACE

This pocket manual on critical care pharmacology is intended to be an easy-to-use, portable reference source of value to busy critical care practitioners. It is intended to be a supplement to the large, unabridged text, *The Pharmacologic Approach to the Critically Ill Patient,* Third Edition.

Each chapter contains valuable tables and figures in 12 important subject areas of critical care practice. These tables and figures, and some text, are culled from *The Pharmacologic Approach to the Critically Ill Patient,* Third Edition. A listing of all of the authors whose tables, figures, or texts appear in this manual is found under Contributors.

The chapters are by no means encyclopedic. However, based on my own clinical experience, I know that the material in this manual is *frequently* needed for use at the bedside. The index has been meticulously prepared for easy use.

The complexity of the critically ill patient combined with the multitude of pharmacologic, biochemical, and physiologic variables affecting the patient make it difficult for any practitioner to feel totally at ease in the critical care unit. It is hoped that this pocket manual will ease some of the burden.

Bart Chernow, M.D., F.A.C.P.

CONTRIBUTORS

The following authors contributed material to *The Pharmacologic Approach to the Critically Ill Patient*, Third Edition, from which this book is adapted.

David M. Angaran, M.S., F.C.C.P., F.A.S.H.P.
Professor of Pharmacy
Co-Director, Dubow Family Center for Research in Pharmaceutical Care
University of Florida College of Pharmacy
Gainesville, Florida

Patricia A. Arns, M.D.
Staff Physician in Internal Medicine
Baptist Hospital
Nashville, Tennessee

Frank J. Balestrieri, D.D.S., M.D., F.C.C.P.
Medical Director, Woodburn Surgery Center
Fairfax Hospital
Falls Church, Virginia

Assistant Clinical Professor
Department of Anesthesiology
George Washington University School of Medicine
Washington, DC

Assistant Clinical Professor
Department of Anesthesiology
Bowman Gray School of Medicine
Winston-Salem, North Carolina

Luca M. Bigatello, M.D.
Instructor in Anesthesia
Harvard Medical School

Department of Anesthesia
Massachusetts General Hospital
Boston, Massachusetts

William F. Boyer, M.D.
Assistant Professor
Department of Psychiatry
Emory University
Atlanta, Georgia

Robert A. Branch, M.D.
Professor of Medicine, Pharmacy, Pharmacology and Therapeutics
Director, Center for Clinical Pharmacology
University of Pittsburgh Medical Center
Pittsburgh, Pennsylvania

D. Craig Brater, M.D.
John B. Hickam Professor of Medicine
Chairman, Department of Medicine

Professor of Pharmacology and Toxicology
Chief, Division of Clinical Pharmacology
Indiana University Medical Center
Indianapolis, Indiana

Kenneth D. Burman, M.D., Col., M.C.
Professor of Medicine
Department of Medicine
The Uniformed Services University of the Health Sciences School of Medicine

Director, Section of Endocrinology
Washington Hospital
Washington, DC

Edwin H. Cassem, M.D.
Associate Professor of Psychiatry
Harvard University School of Medicine

Chief, Department of Psychiatry
Massachusetts General Hospital
Boston, Massachusetts

Robert Chasse, M.D.
Clinical Instructor
Section of Pulmonary/Critical Care Medicine
Department of Internal Medicine
Bowman Gray School of Medicine
Wake Forest University
Winston-Salem, North Carolina

Bart Chernow, M.D., F.A.C.P.
Professor of Medicine, Anesthesia, and Critical Care
The Johns Hopkins University School of Medicine

Physician-in-Chief
Sinai Hospital of Baltimore
Baltimore, Maryland

Editor-in-Chief
Critical Care Medicine

Robert Chin, Jr., M.D., F.C.C.P.
Assistant Professor of Medicine
Section of Pulmonary and Critical Care Medicine
Department of Medicine
Bowman Gray School of Medicine
Wake Forest University
Winston-Salem, North Carolina

Robert D. Colucci, Pharm.D., F.C.P., F.C.C.M.
Assistant Director
Clinical Pharmacology, Clinical Research
Schering Plough Research Institute
Kenilworth, New Jersey

David J. Cullen, M.D., M.S.
Professor of Anesthesia
Harvard Medical School

Anesthetist, Department of Anesthesia
Massachusetts General Hospital
Boston, Massachusetts

Harold J. DeMonaco, M.S.
Assistant Professor
MGH Institute of Health Professions

Director, Pharmacy Department
Massachusetts General Hospital
Boston, Massachusetts

Douglas S. DeWitt, Ph.D.
Associate Professor
Department of Anesthesiology
Director, Charles R. Allen Research Laboratories
University of Texas Medical Branch
Galveston, Texas

Michael N. Diringer, M.D.
Assistant Professor of Neurology, Neurosurgery, and Anesthesiology
Director, Neurology/Neurosurgery Intensive Care Unit
Washington University School of Medicine
St. Louis, Missouri

Sudhir K. Dutta, M.D., F.A.C.P.
Professor of Medicine
University of Maryland School of Medicine
Director, Division of Gastroenterology
Sinai Hospital of Baltimore
Baltimore, Maryland

Donald Charles Eagerton, M.D.
Clinical Instructor of Medicine
Division of Endocrinology
Medical University of South Carolina
Charleston, South Carolina

Sherry Fisher, R.N.
Pain Management Coordinator
Department of Anesthesiology
Fairfax Hospital
Falls Church, Virginia

Robert M. Forstot, M.D.
Instructor of Anesthesiology
Division of Cardiothoracic Anesthesia
Department of Anesthesiology
Washington University School of Medicine
St. Louis, Missouri

David W. Fuhs, Pharm.D., M.S.
Assistant Director of Pharmacy
United and Children's Hospitals
St. Paul, Minnesota

Clinical Assistant Professor
Department of Pharmacy Practice
University of Minnesota College of Pharmacy
Minneapolis, Minnesota

Marye H. Godinez, M.D.
Research Associate
The Joseph Stokes Jr. Research Institute
The Children's Hospital of Philadelphia
Philadelphia, Pennsylvania

Rodolfo I. Godinez, M.D., Ph.D.
Associate Professor of Anesthesiology and Pediatrics
University of Pennsylvania School of Medicine

Associate Medical Director, Pediatric Intensive Care Unit
Medical Director, Respiratory Care Services
The Children's Hospital of Philadelphia
Philadelphia, Pennsylvania

John P. Grant, M.D.
Associate Professor of Surgery
Duke University Medical Center
Durham, North Carolina

David J. Greenblatt, M.D.
Professor
Department of Pharmacology and Experimental Therapeutics
Tufts University School of Medicine
Division of Clinical Pharmacology
New England Medical Center Hospital
Boston, Massachusetts

Ake N. A. Grenvik, M.D., Ph.D., F.C.C.M.
Professor of Anesthesiology, Medicine, and Surgery
Director, Multidisciplinary Critical Care Training Program
University of Pittsburgh School of Medicine
Pittsburgh, Pennsylvania

Charles E. Halstenson, Pharm.D., F.C.C.P.
Professor of Pharmacy
University of Minnesota College of Pharmacy

Co-Director, The Drug Evaluation Unit
Minneapolis Medical Research Foundation at Hennepin County Medical Center
Minneapolis, Minnesota

Paul M. Heerdt, M.D., Ph.D.
Associate Professor
Department of Anesthesiology

Assistant Professor
Department of Pharmacology
Cornell University Medical College

Assistant Member
Department of Anesthesiology and Critical Care Medicine
Memorial Sloan-Kettering Cancer Center
New York, New York

Allan S. Jaffe, M.D.
Professor of Medicine
Cardiovascular Division
Washington University School of Medicine
St. Louis, Missouri

Jeffrey S. Kelly, M.D.
Assistant Professor of Anesthesia/Critical Care
Bowman Gray School of Medicine
Department of Anesthesia
Wake Forest University
Winston-Salem, North Carolina

David J. Kramer, M.D.
Assistant Professor of Anesthesiology/Critical Care Medicine
University of Pittsburgh School of Medicine

Co-Director, Liver Transplant ICU Services
University of Pittsburgh Medical Center
Pittsburgh, Pennsylvania

Gregory L. Krauss, M.D.
Assistant Professor
Department of Neurology
The Johns Hopkins University School of Medicine
Baltimore, Maryland

Cheryl A. Kubisty, M.D.
Providence Everett Primary Care
Everett, Washington

C. Raymond Lake, M.D., Ph.D.
Professor and Chairperson
Department of Psychiatry and Behavioral Sciences
University of Kansas School of Medicine
Kansas City, Kansas

Daniel J. Lebovitz, M.D.
Assistant Professor of Pediatrics
Department of Pediatric Critical Care Medicine
Children's Hospital of Oklahoma
Oklahoma City, Oklahoma

Brian Litt, M.D.
Assistant Professor
Departments of Neurology and Medicine
The Johns Hopkins University School of Medicine

Director of Neurophysiology
Division of Neurology
Department of Medicine
Sinai Hospital of Baltimore
Baltimore, Maryland

Drew A. MacGregor, M.D.
Assistant Professor of Anesthesia (Critical Care) and Medicine (Pulmonary/Critical Care)
Department of Anesthesia
Bowman Gray School of Medicine
Wake Forest University
Winston-Salem, North Carolina

J. A. Jeevendra Martyn, M.D., F.F.A.R.C.S.
Professor of Anesthesiology
Harvard Medical School

Director, Clinical Pharmacology
Massachusetts General Hospital

Associate Director of Anesthesia
Shriners Burn Institute
Boston, Massachusetts

Henry Masur, M.D.
Chief, Critical Care Medicine
Clinical Center, National Institutes of Health
Bethesda, Maryland

Professor of Clinical Medicine
George Washington University Medical Center
Washington, DC

Daniel A. Notterman, M.D., F.A.A.P., F.C.C.M.
Associate Professor of Pediatrics, Clinical Pharmacology, and Pediatrics in Surgery
Director, Division of Pediatric Critical Care Medicine
The New York Hospital-Cornell Medical Center
New York, New York

Research Scientist
Department of Molecular Biology
Princeton University
Princeton, New Jersey

Joseph E. Parrillo, M.D.
James B. Herrick Professor of Medicine
Chief, Sections of Cardiology and Critical Care Medicine
Medical Director, Rush Heart Institute
Rush-Presbyterian-St. Luke's Medical Center
Chicago, Illinois

Donald S. Prough, M.D.
Professor and Chairman
Department of Anesthesiology
University of Texas Medical Branch
Galveston, Texas

Russell C. Raphaely, M.D.
Professor of Anesthesia and Pediatrics
University of Pennsylvania School of Medicine

Director of Critical Care Medicine
Department of Anesthesiology/Critical Care Medicine
The Children's Hospital of Philadelphia
Philadelphia, Pennsylvania

Michael D. Reed, Pharm.D., F.C.C.P, F.C.P.
Associate Professor
Department of Pediatrics
Case Western Reserve University School of Medicine
Division of Pediatric Pharmacology and Critical Care
Rainbow Babies and Children's Hospital
Cleveland, Ohio

Alan J. Rosenbloom, M.D.
Assistant Professor of Anesthesiology/Critical Care Medicine
Division of Critical Care Medicine, Department of Anesthesiology
University of Pittsburgh School of Medicine
Pittsburgh, Pennsylvania

Laurence H. Ross, M.D.
Baltimore, Maryland

Anita C. Rudy, Ph.D.
Lecturer
Department of Medicine
Indiana University Medical Center
Indianapolis, Indiana

Pablo F. Ruiz-Ramon, M.D.
Co-Director, Northern California Renal Transplant Program

Department of Medicine
Santa Rosa Memorial Hospital

Clinical Instructor, Community Hospital Residency Program
Santa Rosa, California

Michael Salem, M.D.
Assistant Professor of Surgery and Anesthesia
Director, Surgical Critical Care and Surgical Research
George Washington University Medical Center
Washington, DC

Joseph M. Scavone, M.S., Pharm.D.
Professor and Division Head
Division of Clinical and Administrative Pharmacy
College of Pharmacy
University of Iowa
Iowa City, Iowa

Marissa Seligman, Pharm.D.
Vice President, Academic and Scientific Affairs
SCP Communications, Inc.
New York, New York

Henry J. Silverman, M.D.
Associate Professor of Medicine
Director, Medical Intensive Care Unit
Pulmonary and Critical Care Medicine Division
University of Maryland School of Medicine
Baltimore, Maryland

John C. Somberg, M.D., F.C.P.
Professor of Medicine and Pharmacology
Chief, Division of Clinical Pharmacology and Cardiology
The Chicago Medical School
North Chicago, Illinois

Rajat Sood, M.D.
Fellow in Gastroenterology
Department of Medicine
Henry Ford Hospital
Detroit, Michigan

Wendy L. St. Peter, Pharm.D.
Assistant Professor of Pharmacy
University of Minneapolis College of Pharmacy

Clinical Scientist
The Drug Evaluation Unit
Hennepin County Medical Center
Minneapolis, Minnesota

Keith L. Stein, M.D.
Chief, Critical Care
Department of Anesthesiology/Critical Care Medicine
Mayo Clinic, Jacksonville
Jacksonville, Florida

Barney J. Stern, M.D.
Professor of Neurology
Department of Neurology
Emory University
Atlanta, Georgia

Neelakantan Sunder, M.B.B.S.
Assistant Professor of Anesthesia
Harvard Medical School

Associate Anesthetist, Massachusetts General Hospital
Boston, Massachusetts

Bertil K. J. Wagner, Pharm.D.
Assistant Professor
Department of Pharmacy Practice
Rutgers-The State University of New Jersey
College of Pharmacy

Adjunct Assistant Professor
Department of Surgery and Anesthesia
UMDNJ—Robert Wood Johnson Medical School
Piscataway, New Jersey

Peter J. Wedlund, Ph.D.
Associate Professor of Pharmacology
University of Kentucky College of Pharmacy
Lexington, Kentucky

Howard D. Weiss, M.D.
Assistant Professor of Neurology
The Johns Hopkins University School of Medicine

Division of Neurology
Sinai Hospital of Baltimore
Baltimore, Maryland

Gary P. Zaloga, M.D., F.A.C.P.
Professor of Medicine and Anesthesia/Critical Care Medicine
Head, Section on Critical Care
Department of Anesthesia
Bowman Gray School of Medicine
Wake Forest University
Winston-Salem, North Carolina

Arno L. Zaritsky, M.D.
Associate Professor of Pediatrics
Eastern Virginia Medical School

Co-Director, Pediatric ICU
Children's Hospital of The King's Daughters
Norfolk, Virginia

Michael G. Ziegler, M.D.
Professor of Medicine
Director, Hypertension Services
Program Director, Clinical Research Center
University of California, San Diego Medical Center
San Diego, California

CONTENTS

Preface v

Contributors vii

1 Pharmacokinetics 1

2 Drug Interactions 13

3 Pharmacotherapy in Renal Failure 45

4 Pharmacotherapy in Liver Failure 91

5 Pharmacotherapy in Pulmonary Disease 139

6 Pediatrics 179

7 Special Problems: Sedation, Analgesia, Paralytic Therapy 199

8 Cardiovascular Medications 215

9 Neurologic/Psychiatric Medications 241

10 Gastrointestinal Medications 279

11 Infectious Disease Medications 331

12 Endocrine/Metabolism 371

Index 385

CHAPTER 1

Pharmacokinetics[a]

An important consideration regarding the pharmacologic approach to the critically ill patient is the potential for drug-induced toxicity. This concern is valid in light of the fact that critically ill patients often require multiple medications, often have organ dysfunction, and frequently receive potentially toxic medications with narrow toxic-therapeutic ratios. As a consequence of these characteristics, clinicians must safeguard their patients from adverse drug responses. The best approach to achieve this goal is to:

- Understand the principles of pharmacokinetics and apply these principles in the prescription of drug therapy
- Be diligent to drug-drug interactions
- Adjust the medication dose and the frequency of administration in the setting of organ failure
- Monitor blood drug concentrations when indicated
- Monitor the physiologic and biochemical responses to pharmacologic therapy

When using blood drug concentrations, always remember that the drug concentration in a blood sample merely represents

[a]The material in this chapter was contributed by the following: Tables 1.1, 1.3, 1.6, and 1.7 and Figures 1.1 and 1.2 were part of the contribution by Anita C. Rudy, Ph.D., and D. Craig Brater, M.D., to *The Pharmacologic Approach to the Critically Ill Patient*, Third Edition; Table 1.2 was contributed by Joseph M. Scavone, M.S., Pharm.D.; Tables 1.4 and 1.5 and Figure 1.3 were contributed by Bertil K. J. Wagner, Pharm.D., David M. Angaran, M.S., and David W. Fuhs, M.S., Pharm.D.

a "snapshot" in time. The concentration represents a combination of the rate of appearance of the drug into the blood (absorption), the distribution of the drug between tissues (volume of distribution), and the clearance of the drug from the blood (metabolism, excretion, etc.).

The clinical pharmacologist and clinical pharmacist serve important roles on the ICU team. I encourage you to invite their contribution on clinical rounds and to use their expertise in difficult cases.

In this chapter the tables and figures emphasize certain key issues:

1. The determinants that define the relationship between drug dose, concentration, and response (Fig. 1.1)
2. A glossary of pharmacokinetic terms (Table 1.1)
3. Factors that may alter the pharmacokinetics of drugs (Table 1.2)
4. A clinical illustration of pharmacologic principles using digoxin and lidocaine as examples (Table 1.3)
5. Steps for optimizing drug therapy (Fig. 1.2)
6. The plasma drug concentrations resulting from drugs administered intravenously (Fig. 1.3)
7. Monitoring guidelines and pharmacokinetic issues for drugs commonly used in the ICU (Table 1.4)
8. Examples of alterations in the pharmacodynamics of commonly used medications in critically ill patients (Table 1.5)
9. Drugs with clinically important urine pH-dependent elimination (Table 1.6)
10. Drugs for which resin hemoperfusion has been demonstrated to remove clinically important amounts of drug (Table 1.7)

TABLE 1.1. Glossary of Pharmacokinetic Terms

$t_{1/2}$—Half-life; The amount of time required for the concentration of drug to decrease by ½.
k or ke—Elimination rate constant; determined by the slope of the terminal phase of a plot of the logarithm of the concentration of drug vs. time.
ka—Absorption rate constant.
kr—Elimination rate constant for the renal component of drug elimination.
knr—Elimination rate constant for the nonrenal component of drug elimination.
V_d—Volume of distribution that relates the concentration of drug in the plasma to the amount of drug in the body.
Cl—Clearance; the amount of blood, plasma, or serum from which all drug is removed per unit time.
Cl_r—The component of clearance accounted for by renal elimination.
Cl_{nr}—The component of clearance accounted for by nonrenal elimination.
f_e—Fraction of dose excreted unchanged in the urine.
F—Fraction of the dose that reaches the systemic circulation intact (bioavailability).
δ—Dosing interval; the time between doses.
Cp_{ss}—Average plasma concentration of drug at steady state.
Cp_{max}—The maximum or peak plasma concentration of drug at steady state.
Cp_{min}—The minimum or trough plasma concentration of drug at steady state.

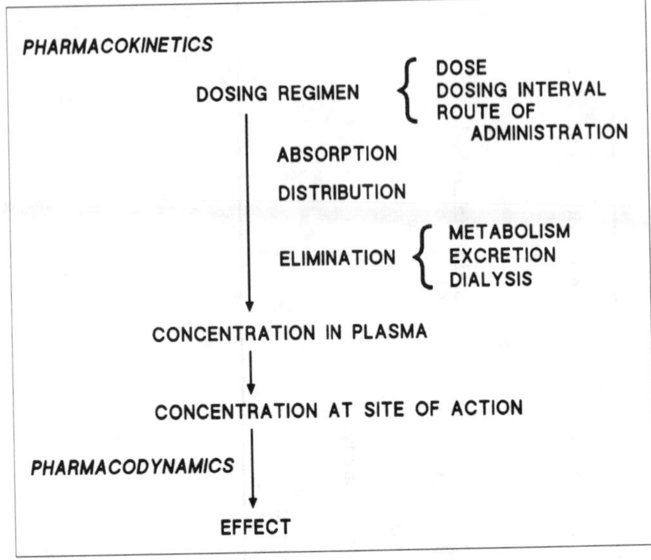

FIGURE 1.1. Schematic representation of the determinants of the relationship between the dose of a drug and the response it elicits.

TABLE 1.2. Factors That Can Affect the Pharmacokinetics of Drugs

Patient Variables
Age
Gender
Body composition
Body weight
Drugs
Nutritional status
Ethanol use
Cigarette smoking
Medical conditions
Congestive heart failure
Kidney disease
Cirrhosis
Hepatitis
Fever
Sepsis
Burns (severe)
Anemia
Shock

TABLE 1.3. Clinical Illustration of Pharmacokinetic Principles

Clinical Setting	*Kinetic Parameter*			*Dose*		*Time to Reach Steady State*
	V_d[a]	*Cl*	$t_{1/2}$	*Loading*	*Maintenance*	
Digoxin in mild-to-moderate renal failure	—	↓	↑	—	↓	↑
Digoxin in end stage renal failure	↓	↓↓	↑	↓	↓↓	↑
Lidocaine in liver disease	—	↓	↑	—	↓	↑
Lidocaine in CHF	↓	↓	—	↓	↓	—

[a] V_d, volume of distribution; Cl, clearance; $t_{1/2}$, half-life; CHF, congestive heart failure.

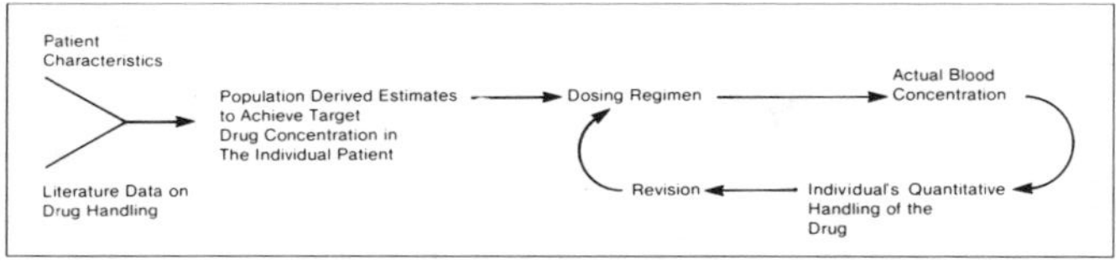

FIGURE 1.2. Steps for optimizing drug therapy to the individual patient.

TABLE 1.4. Pharmacokinetic Parameters of and Monitoring Guidelines for Drugs Commonly Used in the Intensive Care Unit

Drug	*PPB (%)*[a]	*Active Metabolites*	*Elimination*
Antiarrhythmics			
Lidocaine	70	MEGX	Hepatic, metabolite renal
Digoxin	25	None	Renal (60%), hepatic and biliary
Procainamide	16	NAPA	Hepatic, metabolite renal
Anticonvulsants			
Phenytoin	90	None	Hepatic
Valproic acid	93	None	Hepatic
Phenobarbital	51	None	Hepatic
Antihypertensives			
Nitroprusside		Cyanate thiocyanate	Hepatic, metabolite (T) renal
Analgesics and sedatives			
Morphine	35	Morphine-6-glucuronide	Hepatic, metabolite renal
Meperidine	58	Desmethyl-meperidine	Hepatic, metabolite renal
Diazepam	>95	Desmethyl-diazepam	Hepatic
Midazolam	>95	α-hydroxy-midazolam	Hepatic
Lorazepam	93	None	Hepatic
Haloperidol	92	Reduced haloperidol	Hepatic
Propofol	97–99	None	Hepatic
Antiasthmatics			
Theophylline	56	None	Hepatic
Antimicrobials			
Aminoglycosides	<10	None	Renal
Vancomycin	30	None	Renal
Neuromuscular agents			
Pancuronium	30	3-hydroxy-pancuronium	Renal (35%), metabolite renal and bile
Vecuronium	30–90	3-hydroxy-vecuronium, 3-desacetyl-vecuronium	Mostly bile. Renal (20%)
Antiulcer agents			
H_2-receptor blockers	20	None	Renal (65%)

[a] PPB, plasma protein binding; MEGX, monoethylglycylxylidine; DLIS, digoxin-like immunoreactive substance; NAPA, *N*-acetylprocainamide; T, thiocyanate.

Monitoring Guidelines
herapeutic serum concentration 3–6 μg/ml. Initial toxicity with muscle twitching and CNS excitation. Toxicity most common in patients with CHF.
herapeutic serum concentration 0.8–2.5 ng/ml. Monitor ECG (PR prolongation, T wave flattening, ST sloping). DLIS is a problem.
herapeutic serum concentration 4–12 μg/ml. Monitor ECG (QRS prolongation, QT pro- ngation).
herapeutic serum concentration 10–20 μg/ml. Monitor free concentration (1–2 mg/ml) uremic or hypoalbuminemic.
herapeutic serum concentration 30–100 μg/ml
herapeutic serum concentration 10–25 μg/ml
laintain serum thiocyanate concentration <10 mg/dl. Monitor if patient has renal insuffi- iency and is receiving the drug for more than 3 days.
lonitor CNS status. Patients with CHF, cirrhosis, and renal failure are at increased risk r toxicity.
lonitor CNS status. Patients with renal insufficiency are at increased risk for seizures.
void large doses and continuous infusions in patients with liver disease. Rapid injections ill produce apnea and hypotension.
ame as for diazepam. Tolerance is a major problem. Metabolite may accumulate during ng-term infusions.
apid injection will produce apnea and hypotension.
apid injection will produce hypotension. Metabolite accumulation is not a problem with hort-term use.
itrate to desired level of sedation. Monitor blood pressure and cardiac output. For rolonged infusions, monitor lipid profile.
herapeutic serum concentration 5–15 mg/ml. Signs of toxicity include tachycardia and ypertension and seizures.
enal and ototoxicity. Therapeutic peak serum concentration 4–8 mg/ml. Amikacin (20–) μg/ml). Avoid trough concentration above 2 and 4–8 μg/ml, respectively.
herapeutic peak and trough serum concentration 20–40 and <10 μg/ml, respectively.
void high doses and prolonged infusions in patients with renal insufficiency. Monitor vitch response, "train of four."
ame as for pancuronium.
lonitor CNS status. Avoid high doses and prolonged infusions with renal insufficiency. rug interactions (see text).

TABLE 1.5. Alteration of Drug Pharmacodynamics in Critically Ill Patients

Drugs	*Dynamics*	*Disease State*
Antiarrhythmics	Proarrhythmias	CHF[a], ISHD, MI
	Death (?)	Malignant arrhythmias
	CHF	CHF, MI
Dopamine/dobutamine	Worsen DD, wall motion, ABN, increased PCWP, angina, ST changes	CHF, ISHD
	Arrhythmogenic	CHF, ISHD, cardiomyopathy
	Decreased myocardial contractile response, tolerance within 48–72 h	CHF, ISHD, cardiomyopathy
Digoxin	Toxicity, death (?)	CHF, ISHD
	PCWP	CHF, ISHD
β-Blockers	Increased CO or SV	CHF-associated DD, ISHD
	Decreased CO	CHF, ISHD
Calcium channel blockers	Decreased CO	Severe CHF
	Increased CO	ISHD
Vasopressors	Decreased BP response	Sepsis
Dopamine		
Norepinephrine		
Fluids	Blunted CO response	Sepsis/shock, ARDS
Preload challenge		
	Noncardiogenic pulmonary edema	ARDS
Diuretics	Slow onset, decreased diuresis	Shock, ARF, CHF
Furosemide		
Warfarin	Increased PT response	CHF
Nutrition	Increased VO_2, worsening of DO_2/VO_2 match, hypercarbia	Shock, CHF COPD, ARDS
	Fat intolerance	Severe sepsis
Insulin	Hyperglycemia, insulin resistance	DM, stress-induced, sepsis/shock
Vasodilators	Worsening myocardial ischemia	MI, angina, ISHD
Nitroprusside		
	Arterial hypoxemia	ARDS/shock
Nitroglycerin	Increased EF and CO	ISHD, MI

ason	*Therapeutic Alternative*
creased sensitivity, CC-hypoxia, K^+, Mg^{2+}	Use with caution. Monitor serum levels
) MVO_2 balance, LV compliance	DOP > DOB use vasodilators. Avoid HR + SBP > 12,000
creased sensitivity, CC-hypoxia, ISHD, K^+, Mg^{2+}	Avoid or use at lowest possible doses
wn-regulation of β-receptors, DD	Intermittent therapy, use vasodilators
rect toxicity, indirect sympathetic stimulation, CC-ISHD, CC-hypoxia, K^+, Ca^{2+}, Mg^{2+}	Use vasodilators first. Monitor other conditions closely.
tivates sympathetic nervous system. Direct action, vasoconstriction.	Avoid rapid (<10 min) i.v. administration
verses DD, ISHD-induced LV compliance	Unpredictable—use cautiously
creased contractility, β-blockade	Use cautiously and observe
creased contractility	Caution with all, including nifedipine. Monitor carefully.
proves DD	All agents are capable.
Receptor desensitization	Monitor, increase doses.
/ dysfunction, RVF with PAP	Monitor
creased capillary permeability	Use lowest PCWP compatible with best DO_2
creased renal blood flow	Use higher doses cautiously and mannitol and/or dopamine (low doses)
creased metabolism	Use lower doses. Monitor carefully.
erfeeding, VO_2	Moderate caloric input
cess carbohydrate calories, RQ > 1	Decrease carbohydrate, increase fat input
etabolic intolerance	Decrease or discontinue fat input
sulin receptor changes, CC-stress steroids, glucagon, GH, catecholamines	Minimize exogenous glucose
ronary steal, dilates capacitance and resistance vessels, MVO_2 imbalance	Use nitroglycerin
creased pulmonary shunting, dilates pulmonary blood vessels	Monitor. Increase FIO_2.
verses ISHD and DD asynergy, LV compliance	

TABLE 1.5. *(Continued)*

Drugs	*Dynamics*	*Disease State*
H_2 Blockers Cimetidine	Confusion, disorientation	Hepatic/renal failure
	Hypotension/cardiac arrest/ bradyarrhythmias	MI, COPD
ACE inhibitors	First-dose hypotension	CHF

[a] CHF, congestive heart failure; ACE, angiotensin-converting enzyme; ARDS, adu respiratory distress syndrome; ARF, acute renal failure; BP, blood pressure; CC concurrent; CO, cardiac output; COPD, chronic obstructive pulmonary disease; DI diastolic dysfunction; DM, diabetes mellitus; DOB, dobutamine; DOP, dopamin

TABLE 1.6. Drugs with Clinically Important Urine pH-dependent Elimination

Weak acids (alkaline urine increases excretion)
- Phenobarbital
- Salicylates
- Sulfonamide derivatives

Weak bases (acid urine increases excretion)
- Amphetamine
- Ephedrine
- Mexiletine
- Pseudoephedrine
- Quinine
- Tocainide

Reason	Therapeutic Alternative
? increased penetration CSF/CNS blockade	Decrease dose or switch to other agents.
H_2 myocardial blockade with high concentrations	Slow (>15 min. i.v.)
Increased with hyponatremia, high ACE	Start with small dose, e.g., captopril 6.25 mg p.o.

DO_2, oxygen delivery; EF, ejection fraction; GH, growth hormone; HR, heart rate; ISHD, ischemic heart disease; LV, left ventricular; MI, myocardial infarction; MVO_2, myocardial oxygen consumption; RQ, respiratory quotient; PT, prothrombin time; SV, stroke volume; VO_2, total body oxygen consumption.

TABLE 1.7. Drugs for Which Resin Hemoperfusion Has Been Demonstrated to Remove Clinically Important Amounts

Barbiturates
Chloral hydrate (trichloroethanol)[a]
Chloroquine
Digitalis glycosides
Disopyramide
Ethchlorvynol
Glutethimide
Meprobamate
Methaqualone
N-Dexmethylmethsuximide
Phenylbutazone
Salicylate
Theophylline
Tricyclic antidepressants

[a]Trichloroethanol is the active metabolite; the parent, chloral hydrate, is rapidly converted to the metabolite.

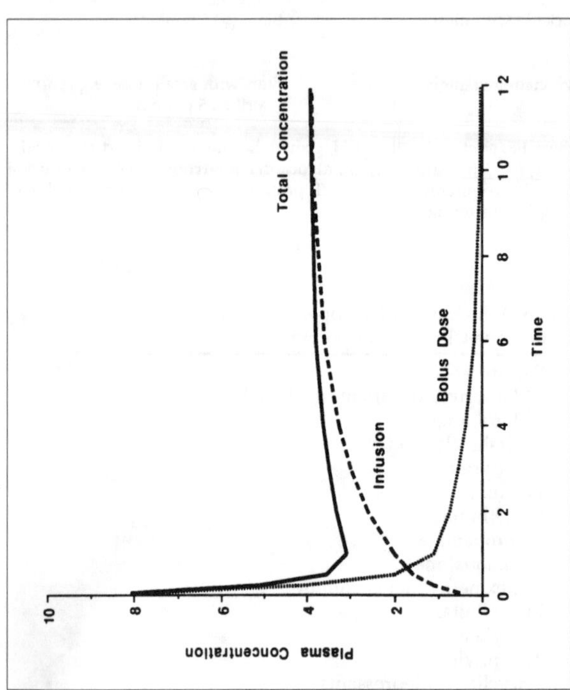

FIGURE 1.3. Plasma drug concentrations resulting from an intravenous bolus dose and infusion.

CHAPTER

2

Drug Interactions[a]

Interactions between medications are common in critically ill patients. It is not unusual for each patient in the intensive care unit to be receiving more than 10 medications! Interactions between medications may take various forms. For example, medications used for cytoprotection of the stomach may alter the absorption of other enterally administered drugs. Other medications may affect protein binding, and as a consequence alter the distribution of other medications within the body. Some medicines may augment or decrease the metabolic ability of organs such as the liver or kidney and may thus prolong or diminish the time span of activity of other administered drugs. Finally, certain medications may alter the ability of some drugs to interface with particular receptors or may limit the physiologic actions of a medicine. Drug interactions may be time-dependent, dose-dependent, or minimal in their actual importance. Other drug interactions may be potentially life-threatening.

Since critically ill patients often require so many medications for different reasons, it may be impossible to avoid drug-drug interactions in each intensive care patient. Clinicians therefore must be cognizant of the potential for a drug interaction and

[a]The material in this chapter was contributed by the following: Tables 2.1–2.7 were contributed by Anita C. Rudy, Ph.D., and D. Craig Brater, M.D.; Table 2.8 was contributed by Alan J. Rosenbloom, M.D., David J. Kramer, M.D., Keith L. Stein, M.D., and Ake N.A. Grenvik, M.D., Ph.D., F.C.C.M.

TABLE 2.1. Types of Drug Interactions

Pharmacokinetic
Absorption
Physicochemical complexing
Changes in gastric pH
Changes in gastrointestinal motility
Effects on gastrointestinal mucosa
Effects on gastrointestinal flora
Changes in first pass effect
Distribution
Protein binding
Elimination
Metabolism
Induction
Inhibition
Excretion
Pharmacodynamic
Receptor (pharmacologic)
Physiologic
Modification of conditions at the site of action
Physicochemical complexing

must analyze the physiologic outcomes from pharmacologic therapy to determine if a clinically relevant drug interaction has occurred. Remember that the patient's physiologic condition may also contribute to an augmentation of a drug interaction or a diminution in this interaction. As an example, if a medication augments liver metabolism of a drug that is hepatically metabolized, but the patient is developing progressive liver failure, the drug interaction is lessened. On the other hand, a medication that increases the circulating concentration of another drug may have an augmented effect as a drug interaction in a patient with progressive renal failure when both medications under discussion are renally metabolized and excreted. Thus, the clinician must be aware not only of these pharmacologic interactions but also must introduce his or her knowledge of the patient's physiology.

In this important chapter, the listings of the various drug-drug interactions are provided. When reviewing your patients' drug therapy, it would be helpful to review the tables listed here:

1. Types of drug interactions (Table 2.1)

2. Medications that affect the absorption of other drugs (Table 2.2)
3. Drugs that displace other medications from protein binding sites (Table 2.3)
4. Drugs that *induce* the metabolism of other drugs (Table 2.4)
5. Drugs that *inhibit* the metabolism of other drugs (Table 2.5)
6. Organic acids actively secreted by the kidney (Table 2.6)
7. Organic bases actively secreted by the kidney (Table 2.7)
8. Drug interactions with cyclosporine (Table 2.8)

TABLE 2.2. Drug Interactions Affecting Absorption

Proposed Mechanism	*Drug Affected*	*Drug Causing Effect*	*Results of Interaction*	*References*
Physicochemical complexing	Atenolol	Antacids	Decreased absorption	1
	Bishydroxycoumarin	Antacids	Increased absorption	2, 3
	Captopril	Antacids	Decreased absorption	1, 4
	Carbamazepine	Activated charcoal	Decreased absorption, increased elimination	5
	Cephalexin	Cholestyramine	Decreased absorption	6
	Chlorothiazide	Cholestyramine	Decreased absorption	7
	Chlorpromazine	Antacids, cimetidine	Decreased absorption	8, 9
	Diflunisal	Antacids	Decreased absorption	10
	Digitoxin	Cholestyramine	Decreased absorption, increased elimination	11, 12
	Digoxin	Activated charcoal	Decreased absorption	13
		Antacids	Decreased absorption	14, 15
		Cholestyramine	Decreased absorption	16
		Kaolin-pectin	Decreased absorption	14, 17
	Isoniazid	Antacids	Decreased absorption	18
	Levodopa	Iron	Decreased absorption	19
	Methyldopa	Iron	Decreased absorption	20
	Penicillamine	Antacids	Decreased absorption	21
	Phenobarbital	Activated charcoal	Decreased absorption, increased elimination	5, 22, 23
	Phenytoin	Activated charcoal	Decreased absorption	13
	Piroxicam	Activated charcoal	Increased elimination	24

	Propranolol	Antacids	Decreased absorption	25
		Cholestyramine	Decreased absorption	26
	Quinine	Activated charcoal	Increased elimination	27, 28
	Quinolone antibiotics	Aluminum or magnesium containing antacids, sucralfate	Decreased absorption	1, 9, 29, 30, 31
	Ranitidine	Antacids	Decreased absorption	32
	Tenoxicam	Activated charcoal	Increased elimination	24
	Tetracyclines	Antacids	Decreased absorption	33, 34
	Theophylline	Activated charcoal	Decreased absorption, increased elimination	35
	Tolbutamide	Activated charcoal	Decreased absorption	36
	Valproate	Activated charcoal	Decreased absorption	36
	Warfarin	Cholestyramine	Decreased absorption, increased elimination	37, 38
Changes in gastric pH	Cimetidine	Antacids	Decreased absorption	39, 40
	Ketoconazole	Antacids, histamine H_2 antagonists, omeprazole	Decreased absorption	41, 42
	Tetracyclines	Cimetidine	Decreased absorption	34
		Sodium bicarbonate	Decreased absorption	33
Changes in gastrointestinal motility				
Increase in motility	Acetaminophen	Metoclopramide	Increased rate of absorption	43
	Chlorothiazide	Metoclopramide	Increased rate of absorption	44
	Cimetidine	Metoclopramide	Decreased absorption	39, 45
	Digoxin	Metoclopramide	Decreased absorption	46

TABLE 2.2. *(Continued)*

Proposed Mechanism	*Drug Affected*	*Drug Causing Effect*	*Results of Interaction*	*References*
	Ethanol	Metoclopramide	Increased rate of absorption	47
	Lithium	Metoclopramide	Increased rate of absorption	48
Decrease in motility	Acetaminophen	Narcotic analgesics	Decreased rate of absorption	49
		Propantheline	Decreased rate of absorption	43
	Benzodiazepines	Antacids	Decreased rate of absorption	50, 51
	Bishydroxycoumarin	Amitriptyline	Increased absorption	52
	Chlorothiazide	Propantheline	Decreased rate of absorption	44
	Digoxin	Propantheline	Increased absorption	53
	Ethanol	Propantheline	Decreased rate of absorption	47
	Isoniazid	Antacids	Decreased rate of absorption	18
	Lithium	Propantheline	Decreased rate of absorption	48
	Phenytoin	Antacids	Decreased rate of absorption	54, 55
	Propranolol	Antacids	Decreased rate of absorption	25
Effects on gastrointestinal mucosa	Aminoglycoside antibiotics	Ethanol	Increased absorption due to mucosal damage	56
	Digoxin	Neomycin	Decreased absorption	57
		Sulfasalazine	Decreased absorption	58
	Furosemide	Phenytoin	Decreased absorption	59
Effects on gastrointestinal flora	Digoxin	Broad spectrum antibiotics	Increased absorption	60
Changes in first-pass metabolism				
Induction	Cyclosporine Felodipine	Anticonvulsants, rifampin	Decreased bioavailability	61

		Anticonvulsants	Decreased bioavailability	62
Inhibition	Bromocriptine	Erythromycin	Increased bioavailability	63
	Cyclosporine	Erythromycin, ketoconazole	Increased bioavailability	61, 64
	Felodipine Imipramine Labetalol Lidocaine Metoprolol Nisoldipine Propranolol Verapamil	Cimetidine	Increased bioavailability	65, 66, 67
	Mercaptopurine	Allopurinol, methotrexate	Increased bioavailability	68, 69

TABLE 2.3. Drug Interactions Due to Displacement from Protein-Binding Sites

Drug Displaced	*Causative Agent*	*References*
Coumarin anticoagulants	Chloral hydrate	70, 71
	Clofibrate	72
	Diazoxide	73
	Ethacrynic acid	73
	Mefenamic acid	73
	Nalidixic acid	73
	Phenylbutazone	74
	Phenytoin	75, 76
	Salicylates	76, 77
Diazepam	Heparin	78
	Valproic acid	79
Phenytoin	Phenylbutazone	80
	Salicylates	77, 81
	Tolbutamide	82
	Valproic acid	83, 84
Tolbutamide	Phenylbutazone	85, 86
	Salicylates	85, 87
Valproic acid	Salicylates	77, 88

TABLE 2.4. Examples of Drugs That Induce the Metabolism of Other Drugs

Drug Induced	*Inducing Agent*	*References*
Acetaminophen	Oral contraceptives	89, 90
Carbamazepine	Phenytoin	91–93
Chloramphenicol	Phenobarbital	94
	Rifampin	95
Chlorpromazine	Phenobarbital	96
Cimetidine	Phenobarbital	97
Clofibrate	Oral contraceptives	89
Clonazepam	Phenytoin	84, 92
Clozapine	Phenytoin	98
Cyclosporin	Anticonvulsants, rifampin	61, 99
Dapsone	Rifampin	100
Diazepam	Phenytoin, rifampin	84, 92, 101
Diflunisal	Oral contraceptives	89
Digoxin	Rifampin	102
Digitoxin	Phenobarbital	103, 104
	Phenytoin	103, 104
	Rifampin	103, 104
Disopyramide	Anticonvulsants	105
Doxycycline	Phenytoin	106
Fluconazole	Rifampin	107, 108
Fludrocortisone	Phenytoin	109
Glucocorticoids	Phenytoin	110, 111
	Rifampin	112

TABLE 2.4. (*Continued*)

Drug Induced	*Inducing Agent*	*References*
Griseofulvin	Phenobarbital	96
Haloperidol	Anticonvulsants, rifampin	113
Lovastatin	Propranolol	114
Meprobamate	Chronic ethanol (prior to hepatic impairment)	115–118
Methadone	Phenytoin	84, 92
Metoprolol	Rifampin	119
Mexiletine	Rifampin	120
Morphine	Oral contraceptives	89
Oral anticoagulants	Carbamazepine	76, 121, 122
	Chronic ethanol	123, 124
	Glutethimide	76, 122
	Griseofulvin	76, 122
	Phenobarbital	76, 122, 124, 125
	Phenytoin	75, 76, 122
	Rifampin	126–128
Oral contraceptives	Anticonvulsants, rifampin	89
Pancuronium	Phenytoin	129
Pefloxacin	Rifampin	130
Pentobarbital	Chronic ethanol	115–118
Phenylbutazone	Phenobarbital	96
Phenytoin	Carbamazepine	92, 93, 121
	Chronic ethanol	115, 117, 131
	Phenobarbital	132–134
	Rifampin	135
	Vigabatrin	136
Pravastatin	Propranolol	114
Quinidine	Phenytoin	137
	Rifampin	138
Salicylate	Oral contraceptives	89
Temazepam	Oral contraceptives	89
Theophylline	Cigarette smoking	139
	Moricizine	140
	Phenobarbital	141
	Phenytoin	142
	Rifampin	143, 144
Tolbutamide	Chronic ethanol	115, 117, 118, 123
	Rifampin	96, 145
Valproic acid	Anticonvulsants	92, 93, 146, 147
Verapamil	Phenobarbital	148

TABLE 2.5. Examples of Drugs That Inhibit the Metabolism of Other Drugs

Drug Causing Inhibition	*Drugs Inhibited*	*References*
Acetaminophen	Fenoldopam	149
Allopurinol	6-Mercaptopurine	69, 150, 151
	Flecainide	152
Amiodarone	Digoxin	153
	Flecainide	153
	Metoprolol	153, 154
	Phenytoin	153, 155–157
	Procainamide	153, 158, 159
	Quinidine	153, 158
	Warfarin	153, 160–162
Bishydroxycoumarin	Tolbutamide	76, 122
Calcium channel antagonists:	Antipyrine	163, 164
	Carbamazepine	165–168
Verapamil > diltiazem ≫	Cyclosporine	166, 168–171
Dihydropyridine	Digitoxin	168
(except nicardipine and	Digoxin	166, 168, 172
nisoldipine)	Doxorubicin	168
	Metoprolol	166, 168, 173
	Prazosin	168
	Propranolol	166, 168, 173, 174
	Quinidine	166, 175
	Theophylline	176, 177

Chloramphenicol	Carbamazepine	92, 178, 179
	Chlorpropamide	178, 179
	Oral anticoagulants	76, 122, 178, 179
	Phenobarbital	178–180
	Phenytoin	92, 93, 178–180
	Tolbutamide	178, 179, 181
Chlorpromazine	Phenytoin	92, 182
	Propranolol	183
Disulfiram	Benzodiazepines	184
	Phenytoin	185, 186
	Theophylline	187
	Warfarin	76, 122, 188
Erythromycin	Alfentanil	189
	Carbamazepine	171, 190, 191
	Cyclosporine	61, 192
	Felodipine	193
	Theophylline	194–198
Ethanol (acute)	Diazepam	199
	Meprobamate	115, 117, 118
	Pentobarbital	115, 117, 118
	Phenytoin	92, 115, 117, 118
	Tolbutamide	115, 181, 200
	Warfarin	76, 115, 122
Flecainide	Dextromethorphan	201
	Propranolol	174

TABLE 2.5. *(Continued)*

Drug Causing Inhibition	*Drugs Inhibited*	*References*
Fluconazole	Chlorpropamide	202
	Glyburide	202
	Glipizide	202
	Phenytoin	202, 203
	Tolbutamide	202
	Warfarin	202
Fluoxetine	Carbamazepine	204
	Diazepam	205
Histamine H_2-antagonists: Cimetidine = etintidine ≫ ranitidine, negligible effect of famotidine, nizatidine, roxatidine	Alprazolam	66
	Amitriptyline	206
	Benzodiazepines	66, 207–213
	Carbamazepine	92, 214
	Chloroquine	215
	Clozapine	216, 217
	Desipramine	218
	Felodipine	219–221
	5-Fluorouracil	150, 222
	Imipramine	66, 223, 224
	Lidocaine	66, 225–227
	Meperidine	66, 228
	Metronidazole	66
	Moricizine	140
	Metoprolol	119, 229

	Nifedipine	66, 230
	Pentoxifylline	231
	Phenytoin	66, 232–236
	Piroxicam	237
	Propranolol	213, 217, 238, 239
	Quinidine	66
	Theophylline	66, 217, 240–246
	Tocainide	247
	Tolbutamide	248
	Triamterene	249
	Warfarin	66, 122, 249a, 250
	Urapidil	251
Isoniazid	Acetaminophen	252
	Carbamazepine	253, 254
	Haloperidol	108
	Phenytoin	92, 255, 256
Ketoconazole	Cyclosporine	61
	Methylprednisolone	257
	Prednisolone	149
	Terfenadine	258
Methylphenidate	Phenobarbital	92, 259
	Phenytoin	92, 259
	Primidone	92, 259
Mexiletine	Theophylline	260, 261
Omeprazole	Diazepam	262–264
	Nifedipine	264
	Phenytoin	262–265
	Warfarin	266

TABLE 2.5. *(Continued)*

Drug Causing Inhibition	*Drugs Inhibited*	*References*
Oral contraceptives	Chlordiazepoxide	89
	Cyclosporine	89
	Diazepam	89, 267
	Imipramine	268
	Metoprolol	119
	Nitrazepam	89
	Oral anticoagulants	76, 122, 269
	Prednisolone	89, 270
	Theophylline	89, 271
Oxyphenbutazone	Phenytoin	237
	Tolbutamide	237
	Warfarin	237
Phenylbutazone	Phenytoin	237
	Tolbutamide	237
	Warfarin	237
Probenecid	Carprofen	237
	Indomethacin	237
	Ketoprofen	237
	Zidovudine	272
Propafenone	Digoxin	273
	Metoprolol	273, 274
	Propranolol	273
	Warfarin	273, 275

Propoxyphene	Carbamazepine	276
	Doxepin	277
	Phenytoin	92, 277
Propranolol	Diazepam	278
	Flecainide	174
	Lidocaine	279, 280
	Nifedipine	166
	Nisoldipine	166
Quinidine	Digitoxin	281
Via inhibition of cytochrome P-450IID6	Digoxin	282
	Desipramine	40
	Imipramine	283
	Propafenone	284
	Propranolol	285
Quinolone antibiotics:	Caffeine	20, 286–288
Enoxacin > ciprofloxacin = pefloxacin; negligible effect of norfloxacin and ofloxacin	Theophylline	20, 286–297
	Warfarin	286, 287, 298
Sulfonamides	Carbamazepine	178, 299
	Phenytoin	92, 178, 299, 300
	Tolbutamide	82, 178, 181, 300
	Warfarin	76, 122, 178, 300
Sulfinpyrazone	Warfarin	301
Tamoxifen	Warfarin	302
Thymidine	5-Fluorouracil	150
Ticlopidine	Theophylline	303
Valproate	Carbamazepine	160, 304

TABLE 2.6. Organic Acids Actively Secreted by the Kidney[a]

Acetazolamide
p-Aminohippurate
Captopril
Cephalosporins (most)
Ciprofloxacin
Dapsone
Dyphylline
Heparin
Loop-acting diuretics
Methotrexate
Nonsteroidal antiinflammatory agents
Penicillins
Probenecid
Salicylates
Sulfonamides
Sulfonylureas
Thiazide diuretics

[a] Data taken from references 20, 77, 150, 288, 305–318.

TABLE 2.7. Organic Bases Actively Secreted by the Kidney[a]

Acecainide (*N*-acetylprocainamide)
Amantadine
Amiloride
Cimetidine
Ethambutol
Flecainide
Mecamylamine
Mepacrine (quinacrine)
Metformin
N-Methylnicotinamide
Procainamide
Pseudoephedrine
Ranitidine
Tetraethylammonium
Triamterene
Trimethoprim

[a] Data from references 66, 319–325.

TABLE 2.8. Drug Interactions with Cyclosporine (CSA)[a]

Increased CSA Levels		*Decreased CSA Levels*	*Enhance CSA Nephrotoxicity*
Ketoconazole	Fluconazole	Phenytoin	Aminoglycosides
Norfloxacin	Metoclopramide	Phenobarbital	Amphotericin B
Erythromycin	Verapamil	Carbamazepine	Trimethoprim
Diltiazem	Nicardipine	Valproic acid	Melphalan
Methylprednisolone	Prednisolone	Nafcillin	Acyclovir
Methyltestosterone	Levonorgestrel	Rifampin	Ganciclovir
Warfarin	Ethanol		Doxorubicin
Imipenem / cilastatin			Digoxin
			Furosemide
			Metolazone
			Indomethacin

[a] Adapted from information appearing in *The New England Journal of Medicine,* Kahan BD: Cyclosporine. *N Engl J Med* 321:1725–1738, 1989; Ptachcinski RJ, Venkataramanan R, Burckart GJ: Clinical pharmacokinetics of cyclosporine. *Clin Pharmacokinet* 11:107–132, 1986; and Rodighiero V: Therapeutic drug monitoring of cyclosporine. Practical applications and limitations. *Clin Pharmacokinet* 16:23–37, 1989; with permission.

REFERENCES

1. Gugler R, Allgayer H: Effects of antacids on the clinical pharmacokinetics of drugs; an update. *Clin Pharmacokinet* 18 (3):210–219, 1990.
2. Akers MA, Lach JL, Fischer LJ: Alterations in the absorption of bishydroxycoumarin by various excipient materials. *J Pharm Sci* 62:391–395, 1973.
3. Ambre JJ, Fisher LJ: Effect of coadministration of aluminum and magnesium hydroxides on absorption of anticoagulants in man. *Clin Pharmacol Ther* 14:231–238, 1973.
4. Duchin KL, McKinstry DN, Cohen AI, Migdalof BH: Pharmacokinetics of captopril in healthy subjects and in patients with cardiovascular diseases. *Clin Pharmacokinet* 14:241–259, 1988.
5. Neuvonen PJ, Elonen E: Effect of activated charcoal on absorption and elimination of phenobarbitone, carbamazepine, and phenylbutazone in man. *Eur J Clin Pharmacol* 17:51–57, 1980.
6. Parsons, RL, Paddock GM: Absorption of two antibacterial drugs, cephalexin and co-trimoxazole in malabsorption syndromes. *J Antimicrob Chemother* 1(suppl):59–67, 1975.
7. Kauffman RE, Azarnoff DL: Effect of colestipol on gastrointestinal absorption of chlorothiazide in man. *Clin Pharmacol Ther* 14:886–889, 1973.
8. Fann WE, Davis JM, Janowsky DS, Sekerke WJ, Schmidt DM: Chlorpromazine: effects of antacids on its gastrointestinal absorption. *J Clin Pharmacol* 13:388–390, 1973.
9. Pinell OC, Fenimore DC, Davis GM, Fann WE: Drug-drug interactions of chlorpromazine and antacids (abstract). *Clin Pharmacol Ther* 23:125, 1978.
10. Verbeeck R, Tjandramaga TB, Mullie A: Effect of aluminum hydroxide on diflunisal absorption. *Br J Clin Pharmacol* 13:519–522, 1979.
11. Caldwell JH, Greenberger NJ: Interruption of the enterohepatic circulation of digitoxin by cholestyramine. I. Protection against lethal digitoxin intoxication. *J Clin Invest* 50:2626–2637, 1971.
12. Carruthers SG, Dujovne CA: Cholestyramine and spironolactone and their combination in digitoxin elimination. *Clin Pharmacol Ther* 27:184–187, 1980.
13. Neuvonen PJ, Elfring SM, Elonen E: Reduction of absorption of digoxin, phenytoin and aspirin by activated charcoal in man. *Eur J Clin Pharmacol* 13:213–218, 1978.
14. Brown DD, Juhl RP: Decreased bioavailability of digoxin due to antacids and kaolin pectin. *N Engl J Med* 295:1034–1037, 1976.
15. Khalil SAH: Bioavailability of digoxin in presence of antacids (letter). *J Pharm Sci* 63:1641–1642, 1974.
16. Brown DD, Juhl RP, Warner SL: Decreased bioavailability of digoxin due to hypocholesterolemia interventions. *Circulation* 58:164–172, 1978.
17. Albert KS, Ayres JW, DiSanto AR, Weidler DI, Sakmar E, Hallmark MR, Stoll RG, Desante KA, Wagner JG: Influence of kaolin-pectin suspension on digoxin bioavailability. *J Pharm Sci* 67:1582–1586, 1978.
18. Hurwitz A, Schlozman DL: Effects of antacids on gastrointestinal absorption of isoniazid in rat and man. *Am Rev Respir Dis* 109:41–47, 1974.
19. Campbell NRC, Hasinoff B: Ferrous sulfate reduces levodopa bioavailability: Chelation as a possible mechanism. *Clin Pharmacol Ther* 45:220–225, 1989.
20. Campoli-Richards DM, Monk JP, Price A, Benfield P, Todd PA, Ward A: Ciprofloxacin: a review of its antibacterial activity, pharmacokinetic properties and therapeutic use. *Drugs* 35:373–447, 1988.
21. Osman MA, Patel RB, Schuna A, Sundstrom WR, Welling PG: Reduction in oral penicillamine absorption by food, antacid and ferrous sulfate. *Clin Pharmacol Ther* 33:465–470, 1983.

22. Berg MJ, Berlinger WG, Goldberg MJ, Spector R, Johnson GF: Acceleration of the body clearance of phenobarbital by oral activated charcoal. *N Engl J Med* 307:642–644, 1982.
23. Levy G: Gastrointestinal clearance of drugs with activated treated charcoal (editorial). *N Engl J Med* 307:676–678, 1982.
24. Guenter TW, Defoin R, Mosberg H: The influence of cholestyramine on the elimination of tenoxicam and piroxicam. *Eur J Clin Pharmacol* 34:283–289, 1988.
25. Dobbs JH, Skoutakis VA, Acchardio SR, Dobbs BR: Effects of aluminum hydroxide on the absorption of propranolol. *Curr Ther Res* 21:877–892, 1977.
26. Hibbard DM, Peters JR, Hunninghake DB: Effects of cholestyramine and colestipol on the plasma concentrations of propranolol. *Br J Clin Pharmacol* 18:337– 342, 1984.
27. Lockey D, Bateman DN: Effect of oral activated charcoal on quinine elimination. *Br J Clin Pharmacol* 27:92–94, 1989.
28. Prescott LF, Hamilton AR, Heyworth R: Treatment of quinine overdosage with repeated oral charcoal. *Br J Clin Pharmacol* 27:95–97, 1989.
29. Garrelts JC, Godley PJ, Peteria JD, Gerlach EH, Yakshe CC: Sucralfate significantly reduces ciprofloxacin concentrations in serum. *Antimicrob Agents Chemother* 34(5):931–933, 1990.
30. Nix DE, Watson WA, Lener ME, Frost RW, Krol G, Goldstein H, Lettieri J, Schentag JJ: Effects of aluminum and magnesium antacids and ranitidine on the absorption of ciprofloxacin. *Clin Pharmacol Ther* 46:700–705, 1989.
31. Parpia SH, Nix DE, Hejmanowski LG, Goldstein HR, Wilton JH, Schentag JJ: Sucralfate reduces the gastrointestinal absorption of norfloxacin. *Antimicrob Agents Chemother* 33(1):99–102, 1989.
32. Mihaly GW, Marino AT, Webster LK, Jones DB, Louis WJ, Smallwood RA: High dose of antacid (Mylanta II) reduces bioavailability of ranitidine. *Br Med J* 285:998–999, 1982.
33. Barr WH, Adir J, Garrettson L: Decrease of tetracycline absorption in man by sodium bicarbonate. *Clin Pharmacol Ther* 12:779–784, 1971.
34. Garty M, Hurwitz A: Effect of cimetidine and antacids on intestinal absorption of tetracycline. *Clin Pharmacol Ther* 28:203–207, 1980.
35. Berlinger WG, Spector R, Goldberg MJ, Johnson GF, Quee CK, Berg MJ: Enhancement of theophylline clearance by oral activated charcoal. *Clin Pharmacol Ther* 33:351–354, 1983.
36. Neuvonen PJ, Kannisto H, Hirvisalo EL: Effect of activated charcoal on absorption of tolbutamide and valproate in man. *Eur J Clin Pharmacol* 24:243–246, 1983.
37. Jahnchen E, Meinertz T, Gilfrich H-J, Kersting F, Groth V: Enhanced elimination of warfarin during treatment with cholestyramine. *Br J Clin Pharmacol* 5:437–440, 1978.
38. Robinson DS, Benjamin DM, McCormack JJ: Interaction of warfarin and nonsystemic gastrointestinal drugs. *Clin Pharmacol Ther* 12:491–495, 1971.
39. Gugler R, Brand M, Somogyi A: Impaired cimetidine absorption by antacids and metoclopramide. *Eur J Clin Pharmacol* 20:225–228, 1981.
40. Steinberg WM, Lewis JH, Katz DM: Antacids inhibit absorption of cimetidine. *N Engl J Med* 307:400–404, 1982.
41. Blum RA, D'Andrea DT, Florentino BM, Wilton JH, Hilligos DM, Gardner MJ, Henry EB, Goldstein H, Schentag JJ: Increased gastric pH and the bioavailability of fluconazole and ketoconazole. *Ann Intern Med* 114(9):755–757, 1991.
42. Levine RR: Factors affecting gastrointestinal absorption of drugs. *Am J Digest Dis* 15:171–188, 1970.
43. Nimmo WS, Heading RC, Tothill P, Prescott LF: Pharmacological evaluation of gastric emptying: effect of propantheline and metoclopramide on paracetamol absorption. *Br Med J* 1:587–589, 1973.

44. Osman MA, Welling PG: Influence of propantheline and metaclopramide on the bioavailability of chlorothiazide. *Curr Ther Res* 34:404–408, 1983.
45. Kanto J, Allonen HJ, Jalonen H, Mantyla R: The effect of metoclopramide and propantheline on the gastrointestinal absorption of cimetidine. *Br J Pharmacol* 11:527–530, 1981.
46. Johnson BF, Bustrack JA, Urbach DR, Hull JH, Marwaha R: Effect of metoclopramide on digoxin absorption from tablets and capsules. *Clin Pharmacol Ther* 36:724–730, 1984.
47. Gibbons DO, Lant AF: Effects of intravenous and oral propantheline and metoclopramide on ethanol absorption. *Clin Pharmacol Ther* 17:578–584, 1975.
48. Cramer JL, Rosser RM, Crane G: Blood levels and management of lithium treatment. *Br Med J* 3:650–654, 1974.
49. Nimmo WS, Heading RC, Wilson J, Tothill P, Prescott LF: Inhibition of gastric emptying and drug absorption by narcotic analgesics. *Br J Clin Pharmacol* 2:502–513, 1975.
50. Greenblatt DH, Allen DA, Maclaughlin DS, Harmatz JS, Shader RJ: Diazepam absorption: effect of antacids and food. *Clin Pharmacol Ther* 24:600–609, 1978.
51. Greenblatt DJ, Shader RI, Harmatz JS, Franke K, Koch-Weser J: Influence of magnesium and aluminum hydroxide mixture on chlordiazepoxide absorption. *Clin Pharmacol Ther* 19:234–239, 1976.
52. Pond SM, Graham GG, Birkett DJ, Wade DN: Effects of tricyclic antidepressants on drug metabolism. *Clin Pharmacol Ther* 18:191–199, 1975.
53. Manninen V, Apajalahti A, Simonen H, Reissel P: Effect of propantheline and metoclopramide on absorption of digoxin. Lancet i:398, 1973.
54. Garnett WR, Carter BL, Bellock JM: Bioavailability of phenytoin administered with antacids. *Ther Drug Monitoring* 1:435–437, 1979.
55. Kulshrestha VK, Thomas M, Wadsworth J, Richens A: Interaction of phenytoin and antacids. *Br J Clin Pharmacol* 6:177–179, 1978.
56. Kitto W: Antibiotics and the ingestion of alcohol. *JAMA* 193:411, 1965.
57. Lindenbaum J, Maulitz RM, Butler VP: Inhibition of digoxin absorption by neomycin. *Gastroenterology* 71:399–404, 1976.
58. Juhl RP, Summers RW, Guillory JK, Blang SM, Cheng RH, Brown DD: Effect of sulfasalazine on digoxin bioavailability. *Clin Pharmacol Ther* 20:387–394, 1976.
59. Fine A, Henderson IS, Morgan DR, Wilstone WJ: Malabsorption of furosemide caused by phenytoin. *Br Med J* 2:1061–1062, 1977.
60. Lindenbaum J, Rund DH, Butler VP, Tse-Eng D, Saha JR: Inactivation of digoxin by the gut flora: reversal by antibiotic therapy. *N Engl J Med* 305:789–794, 1981.
61. Yee GC, McGuire TR: Pharmacokinetic drug interactions with cyclosporin (Part 1). *Clin Pharmacokinet* 19(4):319–332, 1990.
62. Capewell S, Freestone S, Critchley JAJH, Pottage A, Prescott LF: Reduced felodipine bioavailability in patients taking anticonvulsants. *Lancet* ii:480–482, 1988.
63. Nelson MV, Berchou RC, Kareti D, LeWitt PA. Pharmacokinetic evaluation of erythromycin and caffeine administered with bromocriptine. *Clin Pharmacol Ther* 47:694–697, 1990.
64. Gupta SK, Bakran A, Johnson RWG, Rowland M. Cyclosporin-erythromycin interaction in renal transplant patients. *Br J Clin Pharmacol* 27:475–481, 1989.
65. Friedel HA, Sorkin EM: Nisoldipine; a preliminary review of its pharmacodynamic and pharmacokinetic properties, and therapeutic efficacy in the treatment of angina pectoris, hypertension and related cardiovascular disorders. *Drugs* 36:682–731, 1988.
66. Somogyi A, Muirhead M: Pharmacokinetic interactions of cimetidine 1987. *Clin Pharmacokinet* 12:321–366, 1987.

67. van Harten J, van Brummelen P, Lodewijks MTM, Danhof M, Breimer DD: Pharmacokinetics and hemodynamic effects of nisoldipine and its interaction with cimetidine. *Clin Pharmacol Ther* 43:332–341, 1988.
68. Arndt CAS, Balis FM, Lester McCully C, Jeffries SL, Doherty K, Murphy R, Poplack DG: Bioavailability of low-dose vs high-dose 6-mercaptopurine. *Clin Pharmacol Ther* 43:588–591, 1988.
69. Balis FM, Holcenberg JS, Zimm S, Tubergen D, Collins JM, Murphy RF, Gilchrist GS, Hammond D, Poplack DG: The effect of methotrexate on the bioavailability of oral 6-mercaptopurine. *Clin Pharmacol Ther* 41:384–387, 1987.
70. Sellers EM, Koch-Weser J: Potentiation of warfarin-induced hypoprothrombinemia by chloral hydrate. *N Engl J Med* 283:827–831, 1970.
71. Udall JA: Warfarin-chloral hydrate interaction. Pharmacological activity and clinical significance. *Ann Intern Med* 81:341–344, 1974.
72. Bjornsson TD, Meffin PJ, Swezey S, Blaschke TF: Clofibrate displaces warfarin from plasma proteins in man: an example of a pure displacement interaction. *J Pharmacol Exp Ther* 210:316–321, 1979.
73. Sellers EM, Koch-Weser J: Displacement of warfarin from human albumin by diazoxide and ethacrynic, mefenamic, and nalidixic acids. *Clin Pharmacol Ther* 11:524–529, 1970.
74. Aggeler PM, O'Reilly RA, Leong L: Potentiation of anticoagulant effect of warfarin by phenylbutazone. *N Engl J Med* 276:496–501, 1967.
75. Hansen JM, Siersbaek-Nielsen K, Kristensen M, Skovsted L, Christensen LK: Effects of diphenylhydantoin on the metabolism of dicoumarol in man. *Acta Med Scand* 189:15–19, 1971.
76. MacLeod SM, Sellers EM: Pharmacodynamic and pharmacokinetic drug interactions with coumarin anticoagulants. *Drugs* 11:461–470, 1976.
77. Miners JO: Drug interactions involving aspirin (acetylsalicylic acid) and salicylic acid. *Clin Pharmacokinet* 17(5):327–344, 1989.
78. Routledge PA, Kitchell BB, Bjornsson TD, Skinner T, Linnoila M, Shand DG: Diazepam and N-desmethyldiazepam redistribution after heparin. *Clin Pharmacol Ther* 27:528–532, 1980.
79. Dhillon S, Richens A: Serum protein binding of diazepam and its displacement by valproic acid in vitro. *Br J Clin Pharmacol* 12:591–592, 1981.
80. Neuvonen PJ, Lehtovaara R, Bardy A, Elonen E: Antipyrine analgesics in patients on antiepileptic drug therapy. *Eur J Clin Pharmacol* 15:263–268, 1979.
81. Fraser DG, Ludden TM, Evans RP, Sutherland EW: Displacement of phenytoin from plasma binding sites by salicylate. *Clin Pharmacol Ther* 27:165–169, 1980.
82. Pedersen AK, Jackobsen P, Kampmann JP, Hansen JM: Clinical pharmacokinetics and potentially important drug interactions of sulphinpyrazone. *Clin Pharmacokinet* 7:42–56, 1982.
83. Mattson RH, Cramer JA, Williamson PC, Novelly RA: Valproic acid in epilepsy: clinical and pharmacological effects. *Ann Neurol* 3:20–25, 1978.
84. Perucca E, Hebdige S, Gatti G, Leccini S, Frigo BM, Crema A: Interaction between phenytoin and valproic acid: plasma protein binding and metabolic effects. *Clin Pharmacol Ther* 28:779–789, 1980.
85. Koch-Weser J, Sellers EM: Binding of drugs to serum albumin. *N Engl J Med* 294:311–316, 526–531, 1976.
86. Pond SM, Birkett DJ, Wade DN: Mechanisms of inhibition of tolbutamide metabolism: phenylbutazone, oxyphenbutazone, sulfaphenazole. *Clin Pharmacol Ther* 22:573–579, 1978.
87. Wishinsky N, Glasser EJ, Peakal S: Protein interactions of sulfonylurea compounds. *Diabetes* 2 (suppl):18–25, 1962.

88. Orr JM, Abott FS, Farrell K, Ferguson S, Sheppard L, Godolphin W: Interaction between valproic acid and aspirin in epileptic children: serum protein binding and metabolic effects. *Clin Pharmacol Ther* 31:642–649, 1982.
89. Back DJ, Orme ML'E: Pharmacokinetic drug interactions with oral contraceptives. *Clin Pharmacokinet* 18(6):472–484, 1990.
90. Mitchell MC, Hanew T, Meredith CG, Schenker S: Effects of oral contraceptive steroids on acetaminophen metabolism and elimination. *Clin Pharmacol Ther* 34:48–53, 1983.
91. Christiansen J, Dam M: Influence of phenobarbital and diphenylhydantoin on plasma carbamazepine levels in patients with epilepsy. *Acta Neurol Scand* 49:543–546, 1973.
92. Garrettson LK, Perel JM, Dayton PG: Methylphenidate interaction with both anticonvulsants and ethyl discoumacetate. *JAMA* 207:2053–2056, 1969.
93. Perucca E, Richens A: Drug interactions with phenytoin. *Drugs* 21:120–137, 1981.
94. Windorfer A Jr, Pringshein W: Studies on the concentration of chloramphenicol in the serum and cerebrospinal fluid of neonates, infants and small children. Reciprocal reactions between chloramphenicol, penicillin and phenobarbitone. *Eur J Pediatr* 124:129–138, 1977.
95. Prober CG: Effect of rifampin on chloramphenicol levels. *N Engl J Med* 312:788–789, 1985.
96. Burns JJ, Conney AH: Enzyme stimulation and inhibition in the metabolism of drugs. *Proc R Soc Med* 58:955–960, 1965.
97. Somogyi A, Theilscher S, Gugler R: Influence of phenobarbital treatment on cimetidine kinetics. *Eur J Clin Pharmacol* 19:343–347, 1981.
98. Miller DD. Effect of phenytoin on plasma clozapine concentrations in two patients. *J Clin Psychiatry* 52:23–25, 1991.
99. Freeman DJ, Laupacis A, Keown PA, Stiller CR, Carruthers SC: Evaluation of cyclosporin—phenytoin interaction with observations on cyclosporin metabolites. *Br J Clin Pharmacol* 18:887–893, 1984.
100. Zuidema J, Hilbers-Modderman ESM, Merkus FWHM: Clinical pharmacokinetics of dapsone. *Clin Pharmacokinet* 11:299–315, 1986.
101. Ohnhaus EE, Brockmeyer N, Dylewicz P, Habicht H: The effect of antipyrine and rifampin on the metabolism of diazepam. *Clin Pharmacol Ther* 42:148–156, 1987.
102. Gault H, Longerich L, Dawe M, Fine A: Digoxin-rifampin interaction. *Clin Pharmacol Ther* 35:750–754, 1984.
103. Binnion PF: Drug interaction with digitalis glycosides. *Drugs* 15:369–380, 1978.
104. Solomon HM, Abrams WB: Interactions between digitoxin and other drugs in man. *Am Heart J* 83:277–280, 1972.
105. Kapil RP, Axelson JE, Mansfield IL, Edward DJ, McErlane B, Mason MA, Lalka D, Kerr CR: Disopyramid pharmacokinetics and metabolism: effect of inducers. *Br J Clin Pharmacol* 24:781–791, 1987.
106. Penttila O, Neuvonen PJ, Aho K, Lehtovarra R: Interaction between doxycycline and some antiepileptic drugs. *Br Med J* 2:470–472, 1974.
107. Apseloff G, Hilligoss DM, Gardner MJ, Henry EB, Inskeep PB, Gerber N, Lazar JD: Induction of fluconazole metabolism by rifampin: *in vivo* study in humans. *J Clin Pharmacol* 31(4):358–361, 1991.
108. Lazar JD, Wilner KD: Drug interactions with fluconazole. *Rev Infect Dis* 12(3):S327–S333, 1990.
109. Keilholz U, Guthrie GP Jr: Case report: adverse effect of phenytoin on mineralocorticoid replacement with fludrocortisone in adrenal insufficiency. *Am J Med Sci* 291:280–283, 1986.
110. Gambertoglio JH, Holford NHG, Kapusnik JE, Nishikawa R, Saltiel M, Stanik-Lizak P, Birnbaum JL, Hau T, Amend WJC Jr: Disposition of total and unbound

prednisolone in renal transplant patients receiving anticonvulsants. *Kidney Int* 25:119–123, 1984.

111. Petereit LB, Meikle AW: Effectiveness of prednisolone during phenytoin therapy. *Clin Pharmacol Ther* 22:912–916, 1977.
112. Bergrem H, Refvem OK: Altered prednisolone pharmacokinetics in patients treated with rifampicin. *Acta Med Scand* 213:339–343, 1983.
113. Froemming JS, Francis Lam YW, Jann MW, Davis CM: Pharmacokinetics of haloperidol. *Clin Pharmacokinet* 17(6):396–423, 1989.
114. Pan HY, Triscari J, DeVault AR, Smith SA, Wang-Iverson D, Swanson BN, Willard DA. Pharmacokinetic interaction between propranolol and the HMG-CoA reductase inhibitors pravastatin and lovastatin. *Br J Clin Pharmacol* 31:665–670, 1991.
115. Linnoila M, Mattila MJ, Kitchell BS: Drug interactions with alcohol. *Drugs* 18:229–311, 1979.
116. Misra PS, Leferve A, Ishii H, Rubin E, Lieber CS: Increase of ethanol, meprobamate and pentobarbital metabolism after chronic ethanol administration in man and rats. *Am J Med* 51:346–351, 1971.
117. Seixas FA: Alcohol and its drug interactions. *Ann Intern Med* 83:86–92, 1975.
118. Sellers EM, Holloway MR: Drug kinetics and alcohol ingestion. *Clin Pharmacokinet* 3:440–452, 1978.
119. Benfield P, Clissold SP, Brogden RN: Metoprolol: an updated review of its pharmacodynamic and pharmacokinetic properties, and therapeutic efficacy, in hypertension, ischaemic heart disease and related cardiovascular disorders. *Drugs* 31:376–429, 1986.
120. Pentikainen PJ, Koivula IH, Hiltunen HA: Effect of rifampicin treatment on the kinetics of mexiletine. *Eur J Clin Pharmacol* 23:261–266, 1982.
121. Hansen JM, Siersbaek-Nielsen K, Skovsted L: Carbamazepine-induced acceleration of diphenylhydantoin and warfarin metabolism in man. *Clin Pharmacol Ther* 12:539–543, 1971.
122. Koch-Weser J, Sellers EM: Drug interactions with coumarin anticoagulants. *N Engl J Med* 285:487–498, 547–558, 1971.
123. Kater RMH, Roggin G, Tobon F, Zieve P, Iber FL: Increased rate of clearance of drugs from the circulation of alcoholics. *Am J Med Sci* 258:35–39, 1969.
124. Serlin MJ, Breckenridge AM: Drug interactions with warfarin. *Drugs* 25:610–620, 1983.
125. Day MD: Effect of sympathomimetic amines on the blocking action of guanethidine, bretylium, xylocholine. *Br J Pharmacol* 18:421–439, 1962.
126. O'Reilly RA: Interaction of chronic daily warfarin therapy and rifampin. *Ann Intern Med* 83:506–508, 1975.
127. O'Reilly RA: Interaction of sodium warfarin and rifampin. *Ann Intern Med* 81:337–340, 1974.
128. Romankiewicz JA, Ehrman M: Rifampin and warfarin: a drug interaction. *Ann Intern Med* 82:224–225, 1975.
129. Liberman BA, Norman P, Hardy BG: Pancuronium-phenytoin interaction: a case of decreased duration of neuromuscular blockade. *Intern J Clin Pharmacol Ther Toxicol* 26(8):P371–374, 1988.
130. Humbert G, Brumpt I, Montay G, Le Liboux A, Frydman A, Borsa-Lebas F, Moore N: Influence of rifampin on the pharmacokinetics of pefloxacin. *Clin Pharmacol Ther* 50:682–687, 1991.
131. Sandor P, Sellers EM, Dumbrell M, Klouw V: Effect of short and long term alcohol use on phenytoin kinetics in chronic alcoholics. *Clin Pharmacol Ther* 30:390–397, 1981.
132. Buchanan RA, Heffelfinger JC, Weiss CF: The effect of phenobarbital on diphenylhydantoin metabolism in children. *Pediatrics* 43:114–116, 1969.

133. Cucinell SA, Conney AH, Sansur M, Burns JJ: Drug interaction in man. I. Lowering effect of phenobarbital on plasma levels of bishydroxycoumarin (Dicumarol) and diphenylhydantoin (Dilantin). *Clin Pharmacol Ther* 6:420–429, 1965.
134. Kutt H, Haynes J, Verebely K, McDowell F: The effect of phenobarbital on plasma diphenylhydantoin level and metabolism in man and in rat liver microsomes. *Neurology* 19:611–616, 1969.
135. Kay L, Kampmann JP, Svendsen TL, Vergman B, Hansen JE, Skovsted L, Kristensen M: Influence of rifampicin and isoniazid on the kinetics of phenytoin. *Br J Clin Pharmacol* 20:323–326, 1985.
136. Rimmer EM, Richens A: Interaction between vigabatrin and phenytoin. *Br J Clin Pharmacol* 27:27S–33S, 1989.
137. Data JL, Wilkinson GR, Nies AS: Interaction of quinidine with anticonvulsant drugs. *N Engl J Med* 294:699–702, 1976.
138. Twun-Barima Y, Carruthers SG: Quinidine-rifampin interaction. N Engl J Med 304:1466–1469, 1981.
139. Grygiel JJ, Brikett DJ: Cigarette smoking and theophylline clearance and metabolism. *Clin Pharmacol Ther* 30:491–496, 1981.
140. Fitton A, Buckley MMT: Moricine; a review of its pharmacological properties, and therapeutic efficacy in cardiac arrhythmias. *Drugs* 40(1):138–167, 1990.
141. Landay RA, Gonzalez MA, Taylor JC: Effect of phenobarbital on theophylline disposition. *J Allerg Clin Immunol* 62:27–29, 1978.
142. Miller M, Cosgriff J, Kwong T, Morken DA: Influence of phenytoin on theophylline clearance. *Clin Pharmacol Ther* 35:666–669, 1984.
143. Boyce EG, Dukes GE, Rollins DE, Sudds TW: The effect of rifampin on theophylline kinetics. *J Clin Pharmacol* 26:696–699, 1986.
144. Robson RA, Miners JO, Wing LMH, Birkett DJ: Theophylline-rifampin interaction: non-selective induction of theophylline metabolic pathways. *Br J Clin Pharmacol* 18:445–448, 1984.
145. Zilly W, Breimer DD, Richter E: Induction of drug metabolism in man after rifampin treatment measured by increased hexobarbital and tolbutamide clearance. *Eur J Clin Pharmacol* 9:219–227, 1975.
146. Panesar SK, Orr JM, Farrell K, Burton RW, Kassahun K, Abbott FS: The effect of carbamazepine on valproic acid disposition in adult volunteers. *Br J Clin Pharmacol* 27:323–328, 1989.
147. Sackellares JC, Sato S, Dreifuss FE, Penry JK: Reduction of steady state valproate levels by other antiepileptic drugs. *Epilepsia* 22:437–441, 1981.
148. Rutledge DR, Pieper JA, Mirvis DM: Effects of chronic phenobarbital on verapamil disposition in humans. *J Pharmacol Exp Ther* 246(1):7–13, 1988.
149. Zürcher RM, Frey BM, Frey FJ: Impact of ketoconazole on the metabolism of prednisolone. *Clin Pharmacol Ther* 45:366–372, 1989.
150. Balis FM: Pharmacokinetic drug interactions of commonly used anticancer drugs. *Clin Pharmacokinet* 11:223–235, 1986.
151. Murrell GAC, Rapeport WG: Clinical pharmacokinetics of allopurinol. *Clin Pharmacokinet* 11:343–353, 1986.
152. Shea P, Lal R, Kim SS, Schechtman K, Ruffy R: Flecainide and amiodarone interaction. *J Am Coll Cardiol* 7:1127–1130, 1986.
153. Lesko LJ: Pharmacokinetic drug interactions with amiodarone. *Clin Pharmacokinet* 17(2):130–140, 1989.
154. Leor J, Levartowsky D, Sharon C, Farfel Z: Amiodarone and β-adrenergic blockers: an interaction with metoprolol but not with atenolol. *Am Heart J* 116(1):206–207, 1988.
155. Gore JM, Haffajee CI, Alpert JS: Interaction of amiodarone and diphenylhydantoin. *Am J Cardiol* 54:1145, 1984.

156. McGovern B, Geer VR, LaRaia PJ, Garan H, Ruskin JN: Possible interaction between amiodarone and phenytoin. *Ann Intern Med* 101:650–651, 1984.
157. Nolan PE, Marcus FI, Hoyer GL, Bliss M, Gear K: Pharmacokinetic interaction between intravenous phenytoin and amiodarone in healthy volunteers. *Clin Pharmacol Ther* 46:43–50, 1989.
158. Saal AK, Werner JA, Greene HL, Sears GK, Graham EL: Effect of amiodarone on serum quinidine and procainamide levels. *Am J Cardiol* 53:1264–1267, 1984.
159. Windle J, Prystowsky EN, Miles WM, Heger JJ: Pharmacokinetic and electrophysiologic interactions of amiodarone and procainamide. *Clin Pharmacol Ther* 41:603–610, 1987.
160. Kerin NZ, Blevins RD, Goldman L, Faitel K, Rubenfire M: The incidence, magnitude, and time course of the amiodarone-warfarin interaction. *Arch Intern Med* 148:1779–1781, 1988.
161. O'Reilly RA, Trager WF, Rettie AE, Goulart DA: Interaction of amiodarone with racemic warfarin and its separated enantiomorphs in humans. *Clin Pharmacol Ther* 42:290–294, 1987.
162. Watt AH, Stephens MR, Buss DC, Routledge PA: Amiodarone reduces plasma warfarin clearance in man. *Br J Clin Pharmacol* 20:707–709, 1985.
163. Bauer LA, Stenwall M, Horn JR, Davis R, Opheim K, Greene L: Changes in antipyrine and indocyanine green kinetics during nifedipine, verapamil, and diltiazem therapy. *Clin Pharmacol Ther* 40:239–242, 1986.
164. Carrum G, Egan JM, Abernethy DR: Diltiazem treatment impairs hepatic drug oxidation: studies of antipyrine. *Clin Pharmacol Ther* 40:140–143, 1986.
165. Brodie MJ, MacPhee GJA: Carbamazepine neurotoxicity precipitated by diltiazem. *Br Med J* 292:1170–1171, 1986.
166. Kirch W, Kleinbloesem CH, Belz GG: Drug interactions with calcium antagonists. *Pharmacol Ther* 45:109–136, 1990.
167. Macphee GJA, Thompson GG, McInnes GT, Brodie MJ: Verapamil potentiates carbamazepine neurotoxicity: a clinically important inhibitory interaction. *Lancet* 1:700–703, 1986.
168. Schlanz KD, Myre SA, Bottorff MB: Pharmacokinetic interactions with calcium channel antagonists (Part I). *Clin Pharmacokinet* 21 (5):344–356, 1991.
169. Brockmöller J, Neumayer HH, Wagner K, Weber W, Heinemeyer G, Kewitz H, Roots I: Pharmacokinetic interaction between cyclosporin and diltiazem. *Eur J Clin Pharmacol* 38:237–242, 1990.
170. Maggio TG, Bartels DW: Increased cyclosporine blood concentrations due to verapamil administration. *Drug Intell Clin Pharmacol* 22:705–707, 1988.
171. Wroblewski BA, Singer WD, Whyte J: Carbamazepine-erythromycin interaction. *JAMA* 255:1165–1167, 1986.
172. Hedman A, Angelin B, Arvidsson A, Beck O, Dahlqvist R, Nilsson B, Olsson M, Schench-Gustafsson K: Digoxin-verapamil interaction: reduction of biliary but not renal digoxin clearance in humans. *Clin Pharmacol Ther* 49:256–262, 1991.
173. Tateishi T, Nakashima H, Shitou T, Kumagai Y, Ohashi K, Hosoda S, Ebihara A: Effect of diltiazem on the pharmacokinetics of propranolol, metoprolol and atenolol. *Eur J Clin Pharmacol* 36:67–70, 1989.
174. Holtzman JL, Kvam DC, Berry DA, Mottonen L, Borrell G, Harrison LI, Conard GJ: The pharmacodynamic and pharmacokinetic interaction of flecainide acetate with propranolol: effects on cardiac function and drug clearance. *Eur J Clin Pharmacol* 33:97–99, 1987.
175. Edwards DJ, Lavoie R, Beckman H, Blevins R, Rubenfire M: The effect of coadministration of verapamil on the pharmacokinetics and metabolism of quinidine. *Clin Pharmacol Ther* 41:68–73, 1987.
176. Nafziger AN, May JJ, Bertino JS: Inhibition of theophylline elimination by diltiazem therapy. *J Clin Pharmacol* 27(11):862–865, 1987.

177. Sirmans SM, Pieper JA, Lalonde RL, Smith DG, Self TH: Effect of calcium channel blockers on theophylline disposition. *Clin Pharmacol Ther* 44:29–34, 1988.
178. Bint AJ, Burtt I: Adverse antibiotic drug interaction. *Drugs* 20:57–68, 1980.
179. Christensen LK, Skovested L: Inhibition of drug metabolism by chloramphenicol. *Lancet* 2:1397–1399, 1969.
180. Koup JR, Gilbaldi M, McNamara P, Hilligoss DM, Colburn WA, Bruck E: Interaction of chloramphenicol with phenytoin and phenobarbital. *Clin Pharmacol Ther* 24:571–575, 1978.
181. Prescott LF: Pharmacokinetic drug interactions. *Lancet* 2:1239–1243, 1969.
182. Vincent FM: Phenothiazine-induced phenytoin intoxication (letter). *Ann Intern Med* 93:56–57, 1980.
183. Vestal RE, Kornhauser DM, Hollifield JW, Shand DG: Inhibition of propranolol metabolism by chlorpromazine. *Clin Pharmacol Ther* 25:19–24, 1979.
184. MacLeod SM, Sellers EM, Giles HG, Billings BJ, Martin PR, Greenblatt DJ, Marshman JA: Interaction of disulfiram with benzodiazepines. *Clin Pharmacol Ther* 24:583–589, 1978.
185. Kiorboe E: Phenytoin intoxication during treatment with Antabuse (disulfiram). *Epilepsia* 7:246–249, 1966.
186. Olesen OV: Disulfiram (Antabuse[R]) as inhibitor of phenytoin metabolism. *Acta Pharmacol Toxicol* 24:317–322, 1966.
187. Loi CM, Day JD, Jue SG, Bush ED, Costello P, Dewey LV, Vestal RE: Dose-dependent inhibition of theophylline metabolism by disulfiram in recovering alcoholics. *Clin Pharmacol Ther* 45:476–486, 1989.
188. O'Reilly RA: Interaction of sodium warfarin and disulfiram (Antabuse[R]) in man. *Ann Intern Med* 78:73–76, 1973.
189. Bartkowski RR, Goldberg ME, Larijani GE, Boerner T: Inhibition of alfentanil metabolism by erythromcycin. *Clin Pharmacol Ther* 46:99–102, 1989.
190. Miles MV, Tennison MB: Erythromycin effects on multiple-dose carbamazepine kinetics. *Ther Drug Monit* 11:47–52, 1989.
191. Wong YY, Ludden TM, Bell RD: Effect of erythromycin on carbamazepine kinetics. *Clin Pharmacol Ther* 33:460–464, 1983.
192. Martell R, Heinrichs D, Stiller CR, Jenner M, Keown PA, Dupre J: The effects of erythromycin in patients treated with cyclosporine. *Ann Intern Med* 104:660–661, 1986.
193. Liedholm H, Nordin G: Erythromycin-felodipine interaction. *Ann Pharmacother* 25:1007–1008, 1991.
194. Branigan TA, Robbin RA, Cady WJ, Nickols JG, Ueda CT: The effects of erythromycin on the absorption and disposition kinetics of theophylline. *Eur J Clin Pharmacol* 21:115–120, 1981.
195. May DC, Jarboe CH, Ellenburg DT, Roe EJ, Karibo J: The effects of erythromycin on theophylline elimination in normal males. *J Clin Pharmacol* 22:125–130, 1982.
196. Paulsen O, Höglund P, Nilsson LG, Bengtsson HI: The interaction of erythromycin with theophylline. *Eur J Clin Pharmacol* 32:493–498, 1987.
197. Renton KW, Gray JD, Hung OR: Depression of theophylline elimination by erythromycin. *Clin Pharmacol Ther* 30:422–426, 1981.
198. Richer C, Mathieu M, Bah H, Thuillex C, Duroux P, Giudicelli J-F: Theophylline kinetics and ventilatory flow in bronchial asthma and chronic airflow obstruction: influence of erythromycin. *Clin Pharmacol Ther* 31:579–586, 1982.
199. MacLeod SM, Giles HG, Patzalek G, Thiessen JJ, Sellers EM: Diazepam actions and plasma concentrations following ethanol ingestion. *Eur J Clin Pharmacol* 11:346–349, 1977.
200. Carulli N, Manenti F, Gallo M, Salvioli GF: Alcohol-drugs interaction in man: alcohol and tolbutamide. *Eur J Clin Invest* 1:421–424, 1971.

201. Haefeli WE, Bargetzi MJ, Follath F, Meyer UA: Potent inhibition of cytochrome P450IID$_6$ (Debrisoquin 4-hydroxylase) by flecainide *in vitro* and *in vivo*. *J Cardiovasc Pharmacol* 15:776–779, 1990.
202. Grant SM, Clissold SP: Fluconazole: a review of its pharmacodynamic and pharmacokinetic properties, and therapeutic potential in superficial and systemic mycoses. *Drugs* 39(6):877–916, 1990.
203. Blum RA, Wilton JH, Hilligoss DM, Gardner MJ, Henry EB, Harrison NJ, Schentag JJ: Effect of fluconazole on the disposition of phenytoin. *Clin Pharmacol Ther* 49:420–425, 1991.
204. Grimsley SR, Jann MW, Carter JG, D'Mello AP, D'Souza MJ: Increased carbamazepine plasma concentrations after fluoxetine coadministration. *Clin Pharmacol Ther* 50:10–15, 1991.
205. Lejonc JL, Gusmini D, Brochard P: Isoniazid and reaction to cheese (letter). *Ann Intern Med* 91:793, 1979.
206. Curry SH, DeVane CL, Wolfe MM: Cimetidine interaction with amitriptyline. *Eur J Clin Pharmacol* 29:429–433, 1985.
207. Desmond PV, Patwardhan RV, Schenker S, Speeg KV: Short term ethanol administration impairs the elimination of chlordiazepoxide in man. *Eur J Clin Pharmacol* 18:275–278, 1980.
208. Greenblatt DJ, Duhme DW, Allen MD, Koch-Weser J: Clinical toxicity of furosemide in hospitalized patients. *Am Heart J* 94:6–13, 1977.
209. Klotz U, Reimann IW: Delayed clearance of diazepam due to cimetidine. *N Engl J Med* 304:1012–1014, 1980.
210. Ochs HR, Greenblatt DJ, Friedman H, Burstein ES, Locniskar A, Harmatz JS, Shader RI: Bromazepam pharmacokinetics: influence of age, gender, oral contraceptives, cimetidine, and propranol. *Clin Pharmacol Ther* 41:562–570, 1987.
211. Ochs HR, Greenblatt DJ, Gugler R: Cimetidine impairs nitrazepam clearance. *Clin Pharmacol Ther* 34:227–230, 1983.
212. Ruffolo RL, Thompson JF, Segal JL: Diazepam-cimetidine drug interaction: a clinically significant effect. *South Med J* 74:1075–1078, 1981.
213. Somogyi A, Gugler R: Drug interactions with cimetidine. *Clin Pharmacokinet* 7:23–41, 1982.
214. Macphee GJA, Thompson GG, Scobie G, Agnew E, Park BK, Murray T, McColl KEL, Brodie MJ: Effects of cimetidine on carbamazepine auto- and hetero-induction in man. *Br J Clin Pharmacol* 18:411–419, 1984.
215. Ette EI, Brown-Awala EA, Essien EE: Chloroquine elimination in humans: effect of low-dose cimetidine. *J Clin Pharmacol* 27:813–816, 1987.
216. Szymanski S, Lieberman JA, Picou D, Masiar S, Cooper T: A case report of cimetidine-induced clozapine toxicity. *J Clin Psychiatry* 52:21–22, 1991.
217. Labs RA: Interaction of roxatidine acetate with antacids, food and other drugs. *Drugs* 35(3):82–89, 1988.
218. Steiner E, Spina E: Differences in the inhibitory effect of cimetidine on desipramine metabolism between rapid and slow debrisoquin hydroxylators. *Clin Pharmacol Ther* 42:278–282, 1987.
219. Dunselman PHJM, Edgar B: Felodipine clinical pharmacokinetics. *Clin Pharmacokinet* 21(6):418–430, 1991.
220. Edgar B, Lundborg P, Regårdh CG: Clinical pharmacokinetics of felodipine: A summary. *Drugs* 34(3):16–27, 1987.
221. Saltiel E, Ellrodt AG, Monk JP, Langley MS: Felodipine: a review of its pharmacodynamic and pharmacokinetic properties, and therapeutic use in hypertension. *Drugs* 36:387–428, 1988.
222. Harvey VJ, Slevin ML, Dilloway MR, Clark PI, Johnston A, Lant AF: The influence of cimetidine on the pharmacokinetics of 5-fluorouracil. *Br J Clin Pharmacol* 18:421–430, 1984.

223. Abernethy DR, Greenblatt DJ, Shader RI: Imipramine-cimetidine interaction: impairment of clearance and enhanced absolute bioavailability. *J Pharmacol Exp Ther* 229:702–705, 1984.
224. Henaver SA, Hollister LE: Cimetidine interaction with imipramine and nortriptyline. *Clin Pharmacol Ther* 35:183–187, 1984.
225. Bauer LA, Edwards AD, Randolph FP: Cimetidine-induced decrease in lidocaine metabolism. *Am Heart J* 108:413–414, 1984.
226. Feely J, Wilkinson GR, McAllister CB, Wood AJJ: Increased toxicity and reduced clearance of lidocaine by cimetidine. *Ann Intern Med* 96:592–594, 1982.
227. Wing LMH, Miners JO, Birkett DJ, Fornander T, Lillywhite K, Wanwimolruk S: Lidocaine disposition—sex differences and effects of cimetidine. *Clin Pharmacol Ther* 35:695–701, 1984.
228. Guay DRP, Meatherall RC, Chalmers JL, Grahame GR: Cimetidine alters pethidine disposition in man. *Br J Clin Pharmacol* 18:907–914, 1984.
229. Toon S, Davidson EM, Garstang FM, Batra H, Bowes RJ, Rowland M: The racemic metoprolol H_2-antagonist interaction. *Clin Pharmacol Ther* 43:283–289, 1988.
230. Schwartz JB, Upton RA, Lin ET, Williams RL, Benet LZ: Effect of cimetidine or ranitidine administration on nifedipine pharmacokinetics and pharmacodynamics. *Clin Pharmacol Ther* 43:673–680, 1988.
231. Mauro VF, Mauro LS, Hageman JH: Alteration of pentoxifylline pharmacokinetics by cimetidine. *J Clin Pharmacol* 28:649–654, 1988.
232. Algozzine GJ, Stewart RB, Springer PK: Decreased clearance of phenytoin with cimetidine (letter). *Ann Intern Med* 95:244–245, 1981.
233. Hetzel DJ, Bochner F, Hallpike F, Shearman DJC, Hann CS: Cimetidine interaction with phenytoin. *Br Med J* 282:1512, 1981.
234. Neuvonen PJ, Tokola RA, Kaste M: Cimetidine-phenytoin interactions: effect on serum phenytoin concentration and antipyrine test in man. *Eur J Clin Pharmacol* 21:215–220, 1981.
235. Salem RB, Breland BD, Mishra SK, Jordan JE: Effect of cimetidine on phenytoin serum levels. *Epilepsia* 24:284–288, 1983.
236. Sambol NC, Upton RA, Chremos AN, Lin ET, Williams RL: A comparison of the influence of famotidine and cimetidine on phenytoin elimination and hepatic blood flow. *Br J Clin Pharmacol* 27:83–87, 1989.
237. Verbeeck RK: Pharmacokinetic drug interactions with nonsteroidal anti-inflammatory drugs. *Clin Pharmacokinet* 19(1):44–66, 1990.
238. Feely J, Wilkinson GR, Wood AJJ: Reduction of liver blood flow and propranolol metabolism by cimetidine. *N Engl J Med* 304:692–695, 1981.
239. Huang SM, Weintraub HS, Marriott TB, Marinan B, Abels R: Etintidine-propranolol interaction study in humans. *J Pharmacokinet Biopharm* 15(6):557–568, 1987.
240. Boehningh W: Effect of cimetidine and ranitidine on plasma theophylline in patients with chronic obstructive airways disease treated with theophylline and corticosteroids. *Eur J Clin Pharmacol* 38:43–45, 1990.
241. Campbell MA, Plachetka JR, Jackson JE, Moon JF, Finley PR: Cimetidine decreases theophylline clearance. *Ann Intern Med* 95:68–69, 1981.
242. Cluxton RJ, Rivera JO, Ritschel WA, Pesce AJ, Hanenson IB: Cimetidine-theophylline interaction (letter). *Ann Intern Med* 96:684, 1982.
243. Jackson JE, Powell JR, Wandell M, Bentley J, Dorr R: Cimetidine decreases theophylline clearance. *Am Rev Respir Dis* 123:615–617, 1981.
244. Powell JR, Rogers JF, Wargin WA, Cross RE, Eshelman FN: Inhibition of theophylline clearance by cimetidine but not ranitidine. *Arch Intern Med* 144:484–486, 1984.
245. Reitberg DP, Bernhard H, Schentag JJ: Alteration of theophylline clearance and half-life by cimetidine in normal volunteers. *Ann Intern Med* 95:582–586, 1981.

246. Vestal RE, Cusack BJ, Mercer GD, Dawson GW, Park BK: Aging and drug interactions. I. Effect of cimetidine and smoking on the oxidation of theophylline and cortisol in healthy men. *J Pharmacol Exp Ther* 241:488–499, 1987.
247. North DS, Mattern AL, Kapil RP, Lalonde RL: The effect of histamine-2 receptor antagonists on tocainide pharmacokinetics. *J Clin Pharmacol* 28:640–643, 1988.
248. Cate EW, Rogers JF, Powell JR: Inhibition of tolbutamide elimination by cimetidine but not ranitidine. *J Clin Pharmacol* 26:372–377, 1986.
249. Muirhead MR, Somogyi AA, Rolan PE, Bochner F: Effect of cimetidine on renal and hepatic drug elimination: studies with triamterene. *Clin Pharmacol Ther* 40:400–407, 1986.
249a. O'Reilly RA: Comparative interaction of cimetidine and ranitidine with racemic warfarin in man. *Arch Intern Med* 144:989–991, 1984.
250. Toon S, Hopkins KJ, Garstang FM, Rowland M: Comparative effects of ranitidine and cimetidine on the pharmacokinetics and pharmacodynamics of warfarin in man. *Eur J Clin Pharmacol* 32:165–172, 1987.
251. Kirsten R, Nelson K, Steinijans VW, Zech K, Haerlin R: Clinical pharmacokinetics of urapidil. *Clin Pharmacokinet* 14:129–140, 1988.
252. Murphy R, Swartz R, Watkins PB: Severe acetaminophen toxicity in a patient receiving isoniazid. *Ann Intern Med* 113(10):799–800, 1990.
253. Valsalan VC, Cooper GL: Carbamazepine intoxication caused by interaction with isoniazid. *Br Med J* 285:261–262, 1982.
254. Wright JM, Stokes EF, Sweeny VP: Isoniazid-induced carbamazepine toxicity and vice versa: a double drug interaction. *N Engl J Med* 307:1325–1327, 1982.
255. Kutt H, Verebely K, McDowell F: Inhibition of diphenylhydantoin metabolism in rats and in rat liver microsomes by antitubercular drugs. *Neurology* 18:706–710, 1968.
256. Murray FJ: Outbreak of unexpected reactions among epileptics taking isoniazid. *Am Rev Respir Dis* 86:729–732, 1962.
257. Kandrotas RJ, Slaughter RL, Brass C, Jusko WJ: Ketoconazole effects on methylprednisolone disposition and their joint suppression of endogenous cortisol. *Clin Pharmacol Ther* 42:465–470, 1987.
258. Monahan BP, Ferguson CL, Killeavy ES, Lloyd BK, Troy J, Cantilena LR: Torsades de pointes occurring in association with terfenadine use. *JAMA* 264(21):2788–2790, 1990.
259. Perucca E: Pharmacokinetic interactions with antiepileptic drugs. *Clin Pharmacokinet* 7:57–84, 1982.
260. Hurwitz A, Vacek JL, Botteron GW, Sztern MI, Hughes EM, Jayaraj A: Mexiletine effects on theophylline disposition. *Clin Pharmacol Ther* 50:299–307, 1991.
261. Loi CM, Wei X, Vestal RE: Inhibition of theophylline metabolism by mexiletine in young male and female nonsmokers. *Clin Pharmacol Ther* 49:571–580, 1991.
262. Andersson T: Omeprazole drug interaction studies. *Clin Pharmacokinet* 21(3):195–212, 1991.
263. Gugler R, Jensen JC: Omeprazole inhibits oxidative drug metabolism: studies with diazepam and phenytoin *in vivo* and 7-ethoxycoumarin *in vitro*. *Gastroenterol* 89:1235–1241, 1985.
264. Howden CW: Clinical pharmacology of omeprazole. *Clin Pharmacokinet* 20(1):38–49, 1991.
265. Prichard PJ, Walt RP, Kitchingman GK, Somerville KW, Langman MJS, Williams J, Richens A: Oral phenytoin pharmacokinetics during omeprazole therapy. *Br J Clin Pharmacol* 24:543–545, 1987.
266. Sutfin T, Balmer K, Boström H, Eriksson S, Höglund P, Paulsen O: Stereoselective interaction of omeprazole with warfarin in healthy men. *Ther Drug Monit* 11:176–184, 1989.

267. Abernethy DR, Greenblatt DJ, Divoll M, Arendt R, Ochs HR, Shader RI: Impairment of diazepam metabolism by low-dose estrogen-containing oral-contraceptive steroids. *N Engl J Med* 306:791–792, 1982.
268. Abernethy DR, Greenblatt DJ, Shader RI: Imipramine disposition in users of oral contraceptive steroids. *Clin Pharmacol Ther* 35:792–797, 1984.
269. DeTeresa E, Vera A, Ortigosa J, Pulpon LA, Arus AP, DeArtaza M: Interaction between anticoagulants and contraceptives: an unsuspected finding. *Br Med J* 2:1260–1261, 1979.
270. Legler UF, Benet LZ: Marked alterations in dose-dependent prednisolone kinetics in women taking oral contraceptives. *Clin Pharmacol Ther* 39:425–429, 1986.
271. Tornatore KM, Kanarkowski R, McCarthy TL, Gardner MJ, Yurchak AM, Jusko WJ: Effect of chronic oral contraceptive steroids on theophylline disposition. *Eur J Clin Pharmacol* 23:129–134, 1982.
272. de Miranda P, Good SS, Yarchoan R, Thomas RV, Blum MR, Myers CE, Broder S: Alteration of zidovudine pharmacokinetics by probenecid in patients with AIDS or AIDS-related complex. *Clin Pharmacol* 46:494–500, 1989.
273. Hii JTY, Duff HJ, Burgess ED: Clinical pharmacokinetics of propafenone. *Clin Pharmacokinet* 21(1):1–10, 1991.
274. Wagner F, Kalusche D, Trenk D, Jähnchen E, Roskamm H: Drug interaction between propafenone and metoprolol. *Br J Clin Pharmacol* 24:213–220, 1987.
275. Kates RE, Yee YG, Kirsten EB: Interaction between warfarin and propafenone in healthy volunteer subjects. *Clin Pharmacol Ther* 42:305–311, 1987.
276. Dam M, Kristensen B, Hansen BS, Christiansen J: Interaction between carbamazepine and propoxyphene in man. *Acta Neurol Scand* 56:602–607, 1977.
277. Abernethy DR, Greenblatt DJ, Steel K, Shader RI: Impairment of hepatic drug oxidation by propoxyphene. *Ann Intern Med* 97:223–224, 1982.
278. Ochs HR, Greenblatt DJ, Verburg-Ochs B: Propranolol interactions with diazepam, lorazepam, and alprazolam. *Clin Pharmacol Ther* 36:451–455, 1984.
279. Branch RA, Shand DG, Wilkinson GR, Nies AS: The reduction of lidocaine clearance by dl–propranolol: An example of hemodynamic drug interaction. *J Pharmacol Exp Ther* 184:515–519, 1973.
280. Ochs HR, Carstens G, Greenblatt DJ: Reduction in lidocaine clearance during continuous infusion and by coadministration of propranolol. *N Engl J Med* 303:373–377, 1980.
281. Kuhlmann J, Dohrmann M, Marcin S: Effects of quinidine on pharmacokinetics and pharmacodynamics of digitoxin achieving steady-state conditions. *Clin Pharmacol Ther* 39:288–294, 1986.
282. Hedman A, Angelin B, Arvidsson A, Dahlqvist R, Nilsson B: Interactions in the renal and biliary elimination of digoxin: stereoselective difference between quinine and quinidine. *Clin Pharmacol Ther* 47:20–26, 1990.
283. Brosen K, Gram LF: Quinidine inhibits the 2-hydroxylation of imipramine and desipramine but not the demethylation of imipramine. *Eur J Clin Pharmacol* 37:155–160, 1989.
284. Funck-Brentano C, Kroemer HK, Pavlou H, Woosley RL, Roden DM: Genetically-determined interaction between propafenone and low dose quinidine: role of active metabolites in modulating net drug effect. *Br J Clin Pharmacol* 27:435–444, 1989.
285. Zhou HH, Anthony LB, Roden DM, Wood AJJ: Quinidine reduces clearance of (+)-propranolol more than (−)-propranolol through marked reduction in 4-hydroxylation. *Clin Pharmacol Ther* 47:686–693, 1990.
286. Edwards DJ, Bowles SK, Svensson CK, Rybak MJ: Inhibition of drug metabolism by quinolone antibiotics. *Clin Pharmacokinet* 15:194–204, 1988.
287. Henwood JM, Monk JP: Enoxacin: a review of its antibacterial activity, pharmacokinetic properties and therapeutic use. *Drugs* 36:32–66, 1988.

288. Vance-Bryan K, Guay DRP, Rotschafer JC: Clinical pharmacokinetics of ciprofloxacin. *Clin Pharmacokinet* 19(6):434–461, 1990.
289. Beckmann J, Elsaßer W, Gundert-Remy U, Hertrampf R: Enoxacin—a potent inhibitor of theophylline metabolism. *Eur J Clin Pharmacol* 33:227–230, 1987.
290. Bowles SK, Popovski Z, Rybak MJ, Beckman HB, Edwards DJ: Effect of norfloxacin on theophylline pharmacokinetics at steady state. *Antimicrob Agents Chemother* 32(4):510–512, 1988.
291. Raoof S, Wollschlager C, Khan FA: Ciprofloxacin increases serum levels of theophylline. *Am J Med* 82(4A):115–118, 1987.
292. Rogge MC, Solomon WR, Sedman AJ, Welling PG, Koup JR, Wagner JG: The theophylline-enoxacin interaction: II. Changes in the disposition of theophylline and its metabolites during intermittent administration of enoxacin. *Clin Pharmacol Ther* 46:420–428, 1989.
293. Rogge MC, Solomon WR, Sedman AJ, Welling PG, Toothaker RD, Wagner JG: The theophylline-enoxacin interaction. I. Effect of enoxacin dose size on theophylline disposition. *Clin Pharmacol Ther* 44:579–587, 1988.
294. Sano M, Kawakatus K, Ohkita C, Yamamoto I, Takeyama M, Yamashina H, Goto M: Effects of enoxacin, of loxacin and norfloxacin on theophylline disposition in humans. *Eur J Clin Pharmacol* 35:161–165, 1988.
295. Schwartz J, Jauregui L, Lettieri J, Bachmann K: Impact of ciprofloxacin on theophylline clearance and steady-state concentrations in serum. *Antimicrob Agents Chemother* 32(1)75–77, 1988.
296. Takagi K, Hasegawa T, Yamaki K, Suzuki R, Watanabe T, Satake T: Interaction between theophylline and enoxacin. *Intern J Clin Pharmacol Ther Toxicol* 26(6):288–292, 1988.
297. Wijnands WJA, Vree TB, Baars AM, van Herwaarden CLA: Steady-state kinetics of the quinolone derivatives ofloxacin, enoxacin, ciprofloxacin and pefloxacin during maintenance treatment with theophylline. *Drugs* 34(1):159–169, 1987.
298. Toon S, Hopkins KJ, Garstang FM, Aarons L, Sedman A, Rowland M: Enoxacin-warfarin interaction: pharmacokinetic and stereochemical aspects. *Clin Pharmacol Ther* 42:33–41, 1987.
299. Kabins SA: Interactions among antibiotics and other drugs. *JAMA* 219:206–212, 1972.
300. Lumholtz B, Siersbaek-Nielsen K, Skovsted L, Kampmann J, Hensen JM: Sulfamethizole-induced inhibition of diphenylhydantoin, tolbutamide, and warfarin metabolism. *Clin Pharmacol Ther* 17:731–734, 1975.
301. Toon S, Low LK, Gibaldi M, Trager WF, O'Reilly RA, Motley CH, Goulart DA: The warfarin-sulfinpyrazone interaction: stereochemical considerations. *Clin Pharmacol Ther* 39:15–24, 1986.
302. Lodwick R, McConkey B, Brown AM: Life threatening interaction between tamoxifen and warfarin. *Br Med J* 295:1141, 1987.
303. Colli A, Buccino G, Cocciolo M, Parravicini R, Elli GM, Scaltrini G: Ticlopidine-theophylline interaction. *Clin Pharmacol Ther* 41:358–362, 1987.
304. Macphee GJA, Mitchell JR, Wiseman L, McLellan AR, Park BK, McInnes GT, Brodie MJ: Effect of sodium valproate on carbamazepine disposition and psychomotor profile in man. *Br J Clin Pharmacol* 25:59–66, 1988.
305. Aherne GW, Piall E, Marks V, Mould G, White WF: Prolongation and enhancement of serum methotrexate concentrations by probenecid. *Br Med J* 1:1097–1099, 1978.
306. Baber N, Halliday L, Sibeon R, Littler T, Orme ML'E: The interaction between indomethacin and probenecid. A clinical and pharmacokinetic study. *Clin Pharmacol Ther* 24:298–306, 1978.
307. Griffith RS, Black HR, Brier GL, Wolny JD: Effect of probenecid on the blood levels and urinary excretion of cefamandole. *Antimicrob Agents Chemother* 11:809–812, 1977.

308. Kampmann J, Hansen JM, Siersbaek-Nielsen K, Laursen H: Effect of some drugs on penicillin half-life in blood. *Clin Pharmacol Ther* 13:516–519, 1972.
309. Lee BL, Medina I, Benowitz NL, Jacob P, Wofsy CB, Mills J: Dapsone, trimethoprim, and sulfamethoxazole plasma levels during treatment of pneumocystis pneumonia in patients with the acquired immunodeficiency syndrome (AIDS): evidence of drug interactions. *Ann Intern Med* 110:606–611, 1989.
310. May CD, Jarboe CH: Inhibition of clearance of dyphylline by probenecid (letter). *N Engl J Med* 304:791, 1981.
311. Ng HWK, Macfarlane AW, Graham RM, Verbov JL: Near fatal drug interactions with methotrexate given for psoriasis. *Br Med J* 295:752, 1987.
312. Nierenberg DW: Competitive inhibition of methotrexate in kidney slices by nonsteroidal anti-inflammatory drugs. *J Pharmacol Exp Ther* 226:1–6, 1983.
313. Perel JM, Dayton PG, Snell MM, Yu TF, Gutman AB: Studies of interactions among drugs in man at the renal level: probenecid and sulfinpyrazone. *Clin Pharmacol Ther* 10:834–840, 1969.
314. Rose HJ, Pruitt AW, Dayton PG, McNay JL: Relationship of urinary furosemide excretion rate to natriuretic effect in experimental azotemia. *J Pharmacol Exp Ther* 199:490–497, 1976.
315. Rose HJ, Pruitt AW, McNay J: Effect of experimental azotemia on renal clearance of furosemide in the dog. *J Pharmacol Exp Ther* 196:238–247, 1976.
316. Sanchez G: Enhancement of heparin effect by probenecid (letter). *N Engl J Med* 292:48, 1975.
317. Sweeney KR, Chapron DJ, Brandt JL, Gomolin IH, Feig PU, Kramer PA: Toxic interaction between acetazolamide and salicylate: case reports and a pharmacokinetic explanation. *Clin Pharmacol Ther* 40:518–524, 1986.
318. Wesseling H, Mols-Thurkow I: Interaction of diphenylhydantoin (DPH) and tolbutamide in man. *Eur J Clin Pharmacol* 8:75–78, 1975.
319. Christian CD, Meredith CG, Speeg KV: Cimetidine inhibits renal procainamide clearance. *Clin Pharmacol Ther* 36:221–227, 1984.
320. Hughes B, Dyer JE, Schwartz AB: Increased procainamide plasma concentrations caused by quinidine: a new drug interaction. *Am Heart J* 114(4;1):908–909, 1987.
321. Kosoglou T, Rocci ML, Vlasses PH: Trimethoprim alters the disposition of procainamide and *N*-acetylprocainamide. *Clin Pharmacol Ther* 44:467–477, 1988.
322. Peters L: Renal tubular excretion of organic bases. *Pharmacol Rev* 12:1–35, 1960.
323. Rennick BR: Renal tubule transport of organic cations. *Am J Physiol* 240:F83–F89, 1981.
324. Somogyi A, Bochner F: Dose and concentration dependent effect of ranitidine on procainamide disposition and renal clearance in man. *Br J Clin Pharmacol* 18:175–181, 1984.
325. Somogyi A, McLean A, Heinzow B: Cimetidine-procainamide pharmacokinetic interaction in man: evidence of competition for tubular secretion of basic drugs. *Eur J Clin Pharmacol* 25:339–345, 1983.

CHAPTER 3

Pharmacotherapy in Renal Failure[a]

Renal failure is a common occurrence in critically ill patients. The frequency of this important problem is reflected in the plethora of conditions that may lead to failure of this important organ system. Patients may require critical care as a consequence of hypovolemia, diminished cardiac function, alterations in vascular biology, primary renal diseases, vasculitis, hypotension, allergic reactions, intratubular deposition or obstruction, or post-renal obstructive problems. All of these conditions may contribute to the development of acute renal failure.

Since many medications and their metabolites are either metabolized and / or excreted by the kidneys, this common problem of acute and chronic renal failure in acutely ill patients is of paramount importance in our consideration of the pharmacologic approach to critical illness. We may assess the patient's renal function in a number of ways. Certainly, measurement of hourly urine output, the determination of the circulating urea nitrogen and creatinine concentrations, and importantly, the measurement of the creatinine clearance provide the clinician

[a]The material in this chapter was contributed by the following: Tables 3.1–3.3, 3.5, 3.6, and 3.9 were contributed by Wendy L. St. Peter, Pharm.D., and Charles E. Halstenson, Pharm.D., F.C.C.P.; Table 3.4 was contributed by Bertil K. J. Wagner, Pharm.D., David M. Angaran, M.S., F.C.C.P., F.A.S.H.P., and David W. Fuhs, M.S., Pharm.D.; Tables 3.7 and 3.8 were contributed by Robert Chasse, M.D.

with indices of how well the kidneys may perform in handling medications. In addition to the potential loss of metabolic and excretory function, renal failure also contributes to the development of electrolyte, acid-based, vascular volume, nutritional, and even hematologic problems.

The critical care practitioner cannot possibly memorize the specific methods of adjustment for each and every medication in patients with renal dysfunction both with or without renal replacement therapy. For this reason, it is imperative to utilize therapeutic drug monitoring, in addition to reference sources such as those listed in this chapter in order to best predict the proper adjustment of medication dosing and the frequency of medication administration. Of all of the chapters in this book, it is the opinion of this author that the chapters on pharmacotherapy in renal failure and pharamcotherapy in liver failure will be of the greatest use to the reader.

Since many medications and their metabolites are handled and excreted by the kidneys, a knowledge of how to adjust pharmacotherapy in the setting of renal failure is requisite. In addition, since we now have a number of forms of renal replacement therapy, a reference source of which therapy removes what drug is helpful. This chapter provides such useful information as:

1. Methods to estimate a patient's creatinine clearance (Table 3.1)
2. Effect of renal failure on volume of distribution of various drugs (Table 3.2)
3. Reported bioavailability of various antimicrobials after intraperitoneal administration in subjects with or without peritonitis (Table 3.3)
4. How to adjust commonly used medications based on creatinine clearance (Table 3.4)
5. Agents used in the treatment of acute renal failure (Table 3.5)
6. How to adjust medications in renal failure (Table 3.6)
7. Diuretic classes (Table 3.7)
8. Thiazide diuretics (Table 3.8)
9. Agents used in the treatment of hyperkalemia (Table 3.9)

TABLE 3.1. Equations for Creatinine Clearance Estimation[a]

Cockcroft and Gault (1)	
Male	$CL_{CR} = \dfrac{(140 - \text{age})\ \text{Wt}}{72 \cdot \text{Scr}}$
Female	$CL_{CR} = CL_{CR}\ \text{male} \cdot 0.85$
Mawer et al. (2)	
Male	$CL_{CR} = \dfrac{\text{Wt}\ [29.3 - (0.203 \cdot \text{Age})]\ [1 - (0.03 \cdot \text{Scr})]}{72 \cdot \text{Scr}}$
Female	$CL_{CR} = \dfrac{\text{Wt}\ [25.3 - (0.174 \cdot \text{Age})]\ [1 - (0.03 \cdot \text{Scr})]}{14.4 \cdot \text{Scr}}$

[a] Age is in years; Wt is actual body weight in kilograms; Scr is serum creatinine concentration.

TABLE 3.2. Effect of Renal Failure on Volume of Distribution (V_d) of Various Drugs[a]

Increased V_d	Decreased V_d
Amikacin	Chloramphenicol
Azlocillin	Digoxin
Bretyllium	Ethambutol
Cefazolin	Methicillin
Cefonicid	Pindolol
Cefoxitin	
Cefuroxime	
Clofibrate	
Cloxacillin	
Dicloxacillin	
Erythromycin	
Furosemide	
Gentamicin	
Isoniazid	
Moxalactam	
Naproxen	
Phenytoin	
Sulfamethopyrazine	
Trimethoprim	
Vancomycin	

[a] Adapted from Matzke GR, Frye RF: Drug dosing in patients with impaired renal function. In DiPiro JT, Talbert RL, Hayes PE, Yee GC, Matzke GR, Posey LM (eds): *Pharmacotherapy: A Pathophysiologic Approach.* Appleton & Lange, Norwalk, CT, pp 750–763, 1993.

TABLE 3.3. Reported Bioavailability of Various Antimicrobials after Intraperitoneal Administration in Subjects with or without Peritonitis[a]

Drug	*Dose*	*Dwell Time (h)*	*Bioavailability (%)*
Aminoglycosides			
Amikacin	7.5 mg/kg	5	53 ± 14
Gentamicin	100 mg	6	49 ± 15
	1 mg/kg	6	84
	7.5 mg/kg	6	69
		6	85[b]
Tobramycin	2 mg/kg	6	73 ± 10
	1.5 mg/kg	4	52
	100 mg	6	85
Streptomycin	200 mg	6	75[b]
Cephalosporins			
Cefamandol	1000 mg	6	72 ± 13
	1000 mg	6	71 ± 10
	1000 mg	6	71 ± 10
Cefazolin	1000 mg	6	88[b]
	10 mg/kg	4	74
Cefoperazone	1000 mg	10	95 ± 12
	2000 mg	6	61
Cefotaxime	1000 mg	4	59 ± 6
	1000 mg	4	59 ± 5
	2000 mg	6	75 ± 21
	500 mg	5	61[c]
Cefoxitin	50 mg/liter	6	71
Ceftizoxime	500 mg	6	78 ± 4
Ceftriaxone	2000 mg	5	74
	1000 mg	4	44 ± 13
Cefuroxime	500 mg	5	70
Moxalactam	1000 mg	4	57 ± 16
Miscellaneous			
Acyclovir	1000 mg	4	61 ± 10
Ampicillin/ sulbactam	2000 mg	6	60
	1000 mg	6	80
Aztreonam	2000 mg	6	92[b]
	1000 mg	8	91
Ciprofloxacin	5 mg/kg	4	84
	25 mg/liter	4	66

TABLE 3.3. *(Continued)*

Drug	*Dose*	*Dwell Time (h)*	*Bioavailability (%)*
Fluconazole	50 mg	6	87 ± 5
	150 mg	6	88 ± 4
Impipenem/ cilastatin	500 mg	6	79 ± 8
Piperacillin	1000 mg	6	83 ± 5[b]
	1000 mg	6	68 ± 9
Trimethoprim-sulfamethoxazole	320 mg (trimethoprim)	4	84
	1600 mg (sulfamethoxazole)		66
Vancomycin	30 mg/kg	6	52 ± 20
		?	91 ± 10[b]
	1000 mg	6	54 ± 17
	1000 mg	6	73 ± 11
	10 mg/kg	4	65
	37.5 mg/liter	3	70[a]
			39

[a] Compiled from Refs. 3–10.
[b] With peritonitis.
[c] In pediatric patients.

TABLE 3.4. Drug Dosage Adjustment in Renal Failure[a]

Drug	*Half-life*		*Method of Adjustment*	*Adjustment Based on Creatinine Clearance*			*Supplement for Dialysis*[c]
	Normal	*ESRD*[b]		*>50*	*10–50*	*<10*	
Acyclovir	2.5	20	I (D)[d]	8	24	24 (50%)	Yes (H)
Aminoglycosides	2	30	I	8–12	12–18	24–48	Yes (H, P)
Cimetidine	1.8	3.5	I	6	8	12	No
Digoxin	24–36	72–96	D	100%	25–75%	10–25%	No (H, P)
Cephalosporins[e]	1–2	18–36	I	6–8	8–12	24–48	Yes (H, P)
Cefoperazone	1.8	2.1	I		None		Yes (H)
Ceftriaxone	7	12	I		None		No (H)
Cephalosporins[f]	1–2	2–20	I	6–8	8–12	24–48	Yes (H)
Flucytosine	4	75–200	I (D)	6	12–24	24 (50%)	Yes (H)
Nafcillin	0.5	1.2			None		No (H)
Penicillin G	0.5	6–20	I	6–8	8–12	12	Yes (H), no (P)
Piperacillin	1	3–5	I	4–6	6–8	8	Yes (H)
Procainamide	3.5	11–20	I	4	6–12	12–24	Yes (H)
Ranitidine	2.2	8.7	I		12	24	Yes (H)
Ticarcillin	1	16	I	8–12	12–24	24–48	Yes (H, P)
Vancomycin	6	240	I	24–72	72–240	240	No (H, P)

[a] From Mann HJ, Fuhs DW, Cerra FB: Pharmacokinetics and pharmacodynamics in critically ill patients. *World J Surg* 11:210–217, 1987. Used with permission of the publisher.
[b] ESRD, end-stage renal disease.
[c] H, hemodialysis; P, peritoneal dialysis.
[d] I, interval extension; D, dose reduction.
[e] First and second generation cephalosporins.
[f] Other third generation cephalosporins.

TABLE 3.5. Agents Used in the Treatment of Acute Renal Failure[a,b]

Agent	*Dosage*	*Special Considerations*
Mannitol (20%)	25 g i.v. (as a 15–25% solution) over 5–10 min. May repeat in 1 h if no response. If urine output follows, mannitol can be continued as an intermittent infusion or as a continuous infusion. Maximum daily dosage: 100–200 g.	Monitor urine output and serum electrolytes to avoid fluid and electrolyte imbalances, particularly fluid overload. Hemodialysis is indicated for fluid overload and hyperosmolality.
Furosemide	100 mg i.v.; if no response within 1 h, 200 mg i.v.; if no response within 1 h, 400 mg i.v.. Maximum suggested dose: 500–1000 mg	Monitor for fluid and electrolyte disturbances; rate should not exceed 4 mg/min as hearing loss may result if infused too rapidly.
Dopamine	1–5 μg/kg/min	Monitor urine output

[a] Adapted from Heim-Duthoy KL, Kalil RSN, Kasiske BL: Acute renal failure. In DiPiro JT, Talbert RL, Hayes PE, Yee GC, Matzke GR, Posey LM (eds): *Pharmacotherapy: A Pathophysiologic Approach.* Appleton-Lange, Norwalk, CT, 1993, pp 660–672.

[b] Agents may expect beneficial effect when used within 24 hours following the onset of oliguria.

TABLE 3.6. Drugs Commonly Used in Intensive Care Unit Patients: Dosage Adjustments in Various Degrees of Renal Function and with Dialytic Therapies[a]

THERAPEUTIC CATEGORY / ***Drug Class*** / *Drug*	V_d[b] *(liter/kg)* *Normal*	$t_{1/2}\beta$ *(hr)* CL_{CR} *(ml/min)* >50	$t_{1/2}\beta$ *(hr)* CL_{CR} *(ml/min)* <10	*PPB (%)* *Normal*	*fe (%)*
ANTIMICROBIAL AGENTS					
Aminoglycosides					
Dosage should be individualized using patient-specific parameters calculated from plasma concentrations. Initial dose should be based on population-based V_d; V_d is higher in edematous states, ESRD, ascites. Ototoxic, nephrotoxic potential.					
Amikacin	0.20	1.8	31.6	<5	87
Gentamicin	0.27	2.7	41.8	0–25	81
Concomitant penicillin therapy may decrease gentamicin levels.					
Netilmicin	0.22	3.3	37.6	<5	72
May be less ototoxic.					
Streptomycin	0.24	2.6	61.9	34	67–91
Tobramycin	0.25	2.1	58.1	<5	74–93
Concomitant penicillin therapy may decrease tobramycin levels.					
Antitubercular agents					
Ethambutol	3.02	11.3	10.3	25	62–79
Optic neuritis with decreased visual acuity.					
Isoniazid	0.71	2.3	4.3	4–30	3–11 h
Hepatotoxic; Dosages applicable to oral and i.v. dosing; isoniazid acetylator phenotype is major determinant of CL; absorption reduced with concomitant use of aluminum antacids; maximum dose: 300 mg q24h; usual dose should be given after HD.					
Pyrazinamide	0.74	9.5	25.6	<5	1–5
Hepatotoxic; active metabolite with prolonged $t_{1/2}$ in ESRD; maximum dose: 2 g; usual dose should be given after HD.					
Rifampin	0.96	3.3	11.0	57–90	9
Hepatotoxic; concomitant administration of aluminum antacids decreases absorption; PPB % affected by method of quantification; maximum dose 600 mg.					
β-lactamase inhibitors					
These agents are dosed in combination with β-lactam antibiotics.					
Clavulanic acid	0.20	1.1	4.0	22	48
Sulbactam	0.26	1.1	15.2	38	84

Dose for patients with CL_{CR} = >50 ml/min	Adjustment for Renal Failure			Removed Significantly by			
	Method	CL_{CR} = 10–50 ml/min	CL_{CR} = <10 ml/min	HD	PD	CAVH/ CVVH	CAVHD/ CVVHD
Individualize	D or I	Individualize	Individualize	Yes	Yes	Yes	Yes
Individualize	D or I	Individualize	Individualize	Yes	Yes	Yes	Yes
Individualize	D, I	Individualize	Individualize	Yes	Yes	Yes	Yes
Individualize	D, I	Individualize	Individualize	Yes	Yes	Yes	Yes
Individualize	D, I	Individualize	Individualize	Yes	Yes	Yes	Yes
15 mg/kg q24h	D, I	75–100%	5%	No	No	No	No
5 mg/kg q24h	D	100%	100%	Yes	No	No	?
15–30 mg/kg q24h	I	Unknown	q48h	Yes	ND	ND	ND
10 mg/kg q24h	D	100%	100%	No	No	No	No
100 mg q4–6h	NA	NA	NA	Yes	ND	ND	ND
1g q6h	NA	NA	NA	Yes	ND	ND	ND

TABLE 3.6. (*Continued*)

THERAPEUTIC CATEGORY / *Drug Class* / *Drug*	V_d^b (liter/kg) Normal	$t_{1/2}\beta$ (hr) CL_{CR} (ml/min) >50	<10	PPB (%) Normal	fe (%)
Carbapenem and monobactam					
Aztreonam	0.25	1.8	7.5	56	64
Imipenem	0.28	1.0	3.4	20	49
Commercially available product contains equal amounts of cilastatin; post antibiotic effect exhibited.					
Cephalosporins					
Cefamandole	0.20	0.9	9.5	70	54
MTT side chain may prolong PT (INR); vitamin K reverses effect					
Cefazolin	0.11	2.2	32.5	84	75
HD: give 1–2 g after HD.					
Cefmenoxime	0.30	1.4	10.6	43–75	74
Displays concentration dependent PPB.					
Cefmetazole	0.18	1.4	20.8	85	85
MTT side chain may prolong PT (INR), vitamin K reverses effect.					
Cefonicid	0.14	4.9	62.3	97	88
Displays concentration-dependent PPB.					
Cefoperazone	0.22	1.8	3.7	89	27
MTT side chain may prolong PT (INR), vitamin K reverses effect, some active metabolites.					
Cefotaxime	0.25	1.1	3.1	40	52
Active metabolite with prolonged $t_{1/2}$ in ESRD.					
Cefotetan	0.15	3.7	16.5	90	72
MTT side chain may prolong PT (INR); vitamin K reverses effect.					
Cefoxitin	0.13	0.6	11.6	73	80
Interferes with serum creatinine determination with Jaffé method.					
Ceftazidime	0.22	2.0	23.0	17	84
1 g q24h in CAPD.					
Ceftizoxime	0.37	1.7	27.1	28	87
Ceftriaxone	0.11	6.1	14.7	83–95	46
Displays concentration-dependent PPB.					
Cefuroxime (parenteral)	0.18	1.6	13.7	33	95
Cephalothin	0.23	0.4	3.1	65	52/6
Active metabolite with prolonged $t_{1/2}$ in ESRD.					
Moxolactam	0.24	2.3	19.5	59	78
May inactivate gentamicin or tobramycin secondary to complexation. MTT side chain may prolong PT (INR); vitamin K reverses effect.					

Dose for patients with CL_{CR} = >50 ml/min	Adjustment for Renal Failure			Removed Significantly by			
	Method	CL_{CR} = 10–50 ml/min	CL_{CR} = <10 ml/min	HD	PD	CAVH/CVVH	CAVHD/CVVHD
1–2 g q6–8h	D, I	0.5–1 g q8h	0.5–1 g q12h	Yes	No	ND	ND
0.25–1 g q6h	D, I	0.25–0.5 g q6–8h	0.25–0.5 g q12h	Yes	No	No	No
1–2 g q6h	I	q8–12h	q24h	Yes	No	No	Yes
1–2 g q6–8h	D, I	q12–24h	1 g q48h	Yes	No	ND	ND
1 g q4–6h	I	q6–12h	q24h	Yes	No	ND	ND
2 g q6–8h	I	q12–24h	q48h	Yes	No	ND	ND
1–2 g q24h	D, I	0.5–1 g q24–48h	0.25–0.5 g q48h	No	No	No	No
1–2 g q12h	D	100%	100%	No	No	No	No
1–2 g q6–8h	I	q8–12h	q24h	Yes	No	No	No
1–2 g q12h	D, I	q12–24h	0.5–1 g q24h	?	ND	ND	ND
1–2 g q6h	I	q8–12h	q24h	Yes	No	No	Yes
1–2 g q8h	I	q12–24h	q48h	Yes	Yes	Yes	Yes
1–2 g q8h	I	q12–24h	q48h	Yes	No	ND	ND
1–2 g q24h	D	100%	100%	?	No	No	No
0.75–1.5 g q8h	D, I	q8–24h	1 g q24h	Yes	Yes	Yes	Yes
0.5–2 g q4–6h	I	q6–8h	q12h	?	No	ND	ND
1–2 g q8h	D, I	1g q12–24h	1 g q24–48h	Yes	No	Yes	Yes

TABLE 3.6. *(Continued)*

THERAPEUTIC CATEGORY **Drug Class** Drug	$V_d{}^b$ (liter/kg) Normal	$t_{1/2}\beta$ (hr) CL_{CR} (ml/min) >50	<10	PPB (%) Normal	fe (%)
Fluoroquinolones					
Aluminum, calcium and magnesium antacids, sucralfate, iron supplements have been shown to decrease bioavailability of oral quinolones by complexation reaction; quinolones are metabolized to active metabolites.					
Ciprofloxacin-parenteral	2.59	4.6	7.9	20–40	51
Ofloxacin	1.55	5.6	32.5	30	71
CAVHD/CVVHD: 0.1 g q8h.					
Glycopeptides					
Dosage should be individualized using patient-specific parameters calculated from plasma concentrations. Initial dose should be based on population-based V_d.					
Vancomycin	0.58	5.7	139.1	55	ND
Not removed significantly by conventional hemodialyzers; removed significantly with high flux hemodialyzer. Dosage should be individualized using patient-specific parameters calculated from plasma concentrations. Initial dose should be based on population-based V. CAPD: CL may be enhanced in peritonitis.					
Macrolides					
Azithromycin	ND	10–14	ND	12–50	5–12
Displays concentration-dependent PPB.					
Clarithromycin	ND	4–11	ND	ND	ND
Active metabolites; exhibits dose-dependent pharmacokinetics.					
Erythromycin (parenteral)	0.83	1.8	3.2	80–90	5–17
Ototoxicity associated with high doses in renal failure.					
Penicillins					
Ureido penicillins (mezlocillin, piperacillin, and ticarcillin) are associated with abnormal bleeding times which may be more pronounced in renal failure. HD: give dose for CL_{CR} <10 after HD.					
Ampicillin-parenteral	0.29	1.2	19.0	18–28	81
Methicillin	0.36	0.3	4.0	40	80
Mezlocillin	0.23	1.1	2.6	16–40	49
Sodium 1.7 mEq/g; exhibits dose-dependent pharmacokinetics.					

Dose for patients with CL_{CR} = >50 ml/min	Adjustment for Renal Failure			Removed Significantly by			
	Method	CL_{CR} = 10–50 ml/min	CL_{CR} = <10 ml/min	HD	PD	CAVH/ CVVH	CAVHD/ CVVHD
0.2–0.4 g q4–12h	D	75–100%	50%	No	No	No	No
0.4 g q12h	D, I	0.2–0.4 g q24h	0.1–0.2 g q24h	No	No	No	Yes
Individualize	D, I	Individualize	Individualize	No/Yes	Yes	Yes	Yes
0.25–0.5 g q24h	ND	ND	ND	?	ND	ND	ND
0.25–0.5 g q12h	ND	ND	ND	ND	ND	ND	ND
0.5–1 g q6h	D	100%	50%	No	ND	No	No
1–2 g q6h	D, I	0.5 g q6–8h	0.5–1 g q12h	Yes	Yes	No	Yes
1–2 g q4–6h	D, I	q6–8h	0.5–1 g q8–12h	No	ND	ND	ND
2–4 g q4–6h	D, I	q4–6h	1–2 g q6h	No	No	No	No

TABLE 3.6. *(Continued)*

THERAPEUTIC CATEGORY **Drug Class** *Drug*	V_d[b] (liter/kg) Normal	$t_{1/2}\beta$ (hr) CL_{CR} (ml/min) >50	<10	PPB (%) Normal	fe (%)
Nafcillin	1.06	1.4	2.1	87	27/8
Oxacillin (parenteral)	ND	0.4	0.8	93	39
Penicillin G	ND	0.6	4.1	52	ND
HD: give dose for CL_{CR} <10 after HD.					
Piperacillin	0.23	1.0	2.8	16	45–80
Sodium 1.9 mEq/g; may inactivate gentamicin or tobramycin secondary to complexation; displays dose-dependent pharmacokinetics. HD: give dose for CL_{CR} <10 after HD.					
Ticarcillin	0.16	1.2	8.9	35	81
Sodium 5.2 mEq/g; may inactivate gentamicin or tobramycin secondary to complexation; HD: give dose for CL_{CR} <10 after HD.					
Tetracyclines					
Doxycycline	0.58	17.3	22.8	88	50/72
Minocycline	0.99	15.5	20.1	76	12/48
May cause dose-related antianabolic effects					
Tetracycline	ND	6.2	63.4	56	70/96
Antianabolic effect with increase in BUN; avoid in CL_{CR} <30 ml/min; PPB derived from nonhuman data.					
Miscellaneous					
Chloramphenicol succinate	0.40	0.6	1.5	53	24
Dosage should be individualized using patient-specific parameters calculated from plasma concentrations. Initial dose should be based on population-based *V*.					
Cilastatin	0.24	0.9	11.6	44	65
Renal dehydropeptidase inhibitor administered with imipenem; accumulates in renal failure; no apparent toxicity.					
Clindamycin (parenteral)	1.10	2.4	3.1	94	5
Metronidazole	0.70	7.0	8.3	0–20	17
Active metabolite with prolonged $t_{1/2}$ in renal failure					
Pentamidine	55.70	29.0	73–118	69	4–29
Displays dose-dependent pharmacokinetics in both normal and renally impaired patients.					

Dose for patients with CL_{CR} = >50 ml/min	*Adjustment for Renal Failure*			*Removed Significantly by*			
	Method	*CL_{CR} = 10–50 ml/min*	*CL_{CR} = <10 ml/min*	*HD*	*PD*	*CAVH/ CVVH*	*CAVHD/ CVVHD*
1–2 g q4–6h	D	100%	100%	No	ND	ND	ND
1–2 g q4–6h	D	100%	50%	No	No	No	No
2–3 mU q4–6h	D, I	1–1.5 mU q4–6h	1 mU q8h	Yes	ND	ND	ND
3–4 g q6h	D, I	2–4 g q6h	2–3 q8h	Yes	No	No	Yes
3 g q6h	D, I	2 g q6–8h	2 g q12h	Yes	Yes	ND	ND
0.1 g q12h	D	100%	100%	No	No	No	No
0.1 g q12h	D	100%	100%	No	ND	ND	ND
0.25–0.5 g q12h	I	q12–24h	Avoid	No	ND	?	?
Individualize	D, I	Individualize 100%	Individualize 100%	?	No	ND	ND
0.25–1 g q6h	NA	NA	NA	Yes	No	ND	ND
0.9 g q8h	D	100%	100%	No	No	No	No
0.5 g q8h	D	100%	100%	Yes	No	No	No
3–4 mg/kg q24h	I	100%	100%	No	ND	ND	ND

TABLE 3.6. *(Continued)*

THERAPEUTIC CATEGORY *Drug Class* *Drug*	V_d[b] *(liter/kg)* *Normal*	$t_{1/2}\beta$ *(hr)* CL_{CR} *(ml/min)* >50	<10	*PPB (%)* *Normal*	*fe (%)*
Sulfamethoxazole (parenteral) i.v. trimethoprim/sulfamethoxazole is available only as a combination product. Decreased PPB in renal failure; slightly active metabolites with prolonged $t_{1/2}$ in renal insufficiency.	0.27	10.6	22.0	62	9
Trimethoprim (parenteral) i.v. trimethoprim/sulfamethoxazole is available only as a combination product. Inhibits tubular secretion of creatinine; falsely high readings for serum creatinine may result but GFR not affected.	1.26	12.5	27.1	70	56
ANTIFUNGAL AGENTS					
Amphotericin B Nephrotoxic; renal tubular acidosis, magnesium and potassium wasting; initial $t_{1/2}$ ~ 24–48 h; terminal $t_{1/2}$ > 15 days.	4	24–48	24–48	90	<5
Fluconazole $t_{1/2}$ 98–125 h in patients with mean CL_{CR} 13–14 ml/min; HD: 0.2 g after each HD	0.7	31.6	ND	12	73
Flucytosine (5-fluorocytosine) Dosage should be individualized using patient-specific parameters calculated from plasma concentrations. Bone marrow toxicity may be enhanced in renal failure.	0.6	3–6	75–200	<10	90
Intraconazole	Large	21	25	99	Low
Ketoconazole	1.9–3.6	2–3	2–3	84–99	13
ANTIVIRAL AGENTS					
Acyclovir (parenteral) ESRD patients more susceptible to neurotoxicity, rapid i.v. infusion can cause decreased CL_{CR} and acute renal failure.	0.7	2.1–3.8	20	15–30	40–70
Ganciclovir Neutropenia, HD: 1.25 mg/kg q24h, give after HD.	0.47	3–6	30–48.3	1–2	90–100
Antihypertensive agents: Blood pressure response best guide to dose and interval.					
ANTIHYPERTENSIVE AND CARDIOVASCULAR AGENTS					
Antihypertensive agents: Blood pressure response best guide to dose and interval.					

Dose for patients with CL_{CR} = >50 ml/min	Adjustment for Renal Failure			Removed Significantly by			
	Method	CL_{CR} = 10–50 ml/min	CL_{CR} = <10 ml/min	HD	PD	CAVH/CVVH	CAVHD/CVVHD
0.8 g q12h	I	q12–24h	q24h	Yes	No	No	No
0.16 g q12h	I	q12–24h	q24h	Yes	No	No	No
0.5–1 mg/kg q24h	D	100%	100%	No	No	No	No
0.100–0.400 g q24h	I	q24–48h	q48–72h	Yes	Yes	Yes	Yes
Individualize	D, I	Individualize	Individualize	Yes	Yes	Yes	Yes
200 mg q12–24h	D	100%	50–100%	No	ND	No	No
200–400 mg q24h	D	100%	100%	No	ND	ND	ND
5–10 mg/kg q8h	D, I	q12–24h	2.5–5.0 mg/kg q24h	Yes	No	ND	ND
2.5–5 mg/kg q12h	D, I	1.25–2.5 mg/kg q24h	1.25 mg/kg q48h	Yes	ND	ND	Yes

TABLE 3.6. *(Continued)*

THERAPEUTIC CATEGORY / ***Drug Class*** / *Drug*	V_d[b] *(liter/kg)* *Normal*	$t_{1/2}\beta$ *(hr)* CL_{CR} *(ml/min)* >50	<10	*PPB (%)* *Normal*	*fe (%)*
Adrenergic modulators					
Clonidine	3–6	6–23	39–42	20–40	45
Transdermal system effective in ESRD up to dose of 0.12 mg/24 h.					
Doxazosin	1–1.7	9.5–12.5	13	98	<5
Renal patients may be sensitive to small doses.					
Guanabenz	10–12	12–14	ND	90	<5
Methyldopa	0.5	1.5–6	6–16	<15	25–40
Active metabolites with long half-life.					
Prazosin	0.6–0.8	2–3	2–3	97	<5
Renal patients should be titrated starting with low doses.					
Terazosin	0.2–0.4	9–12	8–12	90–94	10–15
Angiotensin-converting enzyme inhibitors					
Hypotensive effects magnified by natriuretic agents or sodium depletion. Can cause hyperkalemia or metabolic acidosis. Acute renal dysfunction with bilateral renal artery stenosis, sodium depletion. Dry cough in 5–10%. Anaphylactoid reactions reported with concurrent angiotensin-converting enzyme inhibitors and polyacrylonitrile dialyzers.					
Captopril	0.7–0.8	1.9	21–32	25–30	30–40
Enalapril	ND	11–24	34–60	50–60	43
Prodrug converted to active moiety.					
Lisinopril	1.3–1.5	30	40–50	0–10	?
Ramipril	~1.3	5–8	15–35	55–70	20–50
Prodrug converted to active moiety.					
Benazepril	0.2	25	>24	95	20
Prodrug converted to active moiety.					
Fosinopril	0.2	12	20	95	10–15
Prodrug converted to active moiety. Only ACE inhibitor with significant amount of hepatic elimination.					
Quinapril	ND	2.3	12.1	>90	37–50.9
Prodrug converted to active moiety; decreased conversion of quinapril to active moiety in renal failure.					

Dose for patients with CL_{CR} = >50 ml/min	*Adjustment for Renal Failure*			*Removed Significantly by*			
	Method	*CL_{CR} = 10–50 ml/min*	*CL_{CR} = <10 ml/min*	*HD*	*PD*	*CAVH/CVVH*	*CAVHD/CVVHD*
0.1–0.6 mg bid	D	100%	100%	No	No	No	No
1–15 mg/d	D	100%	100%	No	No	ND	ND
8–16 mg bid	D	100%	100%	ND	ND	ND	ND
250–500 mg tid	I	q8–12h	q12–24h	Yes	No	ND	ND
1–15 mg bid	D	100%	100%	No	No	No	No
1–20 mg/d	D	100%	100%	ND	ND	ND	ND
25 mg q8–12h	D, I	50–75% q12h	50% q24h	Yes	No	No	No
5–40 mg q24h	D	75–100%	50%	Yes	No	No	No
10–40 mg q24h	D	50–75%	25–50%	Yes	No	ND	ND
2.5–20 mg q24h	D	50–75%	25–50%	Yes	No	No	No
10–40 mg q24h	D	100%	50%	No	No	No	No
10–40 mg q24h	D	100%	100%	No	No	No	No
10–80 mg q24h	D	50%	25%	No	No	No	No

TABLE 3.6. *(Continued)*

THERAPEUTIC CATEGORY *Drug Class* *Drug*	V_d[b] *(liter/kg)* *Normal*	$t_{1/2}\beta$ *(hr)* CL_{CR} *(ml/min)* *>50*	*<10*	*PPB (%)* *Normal*	*fe (%)*
β-Blockers					
Hyperkalemia in ESRD.					
Acebutolol	1.2	7–9	7	20	55
Active metabolites with long half-life.					
Atenolol	1.1	6.7	15–35	2	>90
Accumulates in ESRD.					
Carteolol	3.5–4.5	5.7	30–40	15	55–65
Esmolol	1–1.5	7–15 min	7–15 min	55	<2
Inactive metabolite accumulates. *See manufacturer's guidelines for titration regimen; stated dose is maintenance infusion.					
Labetalol	5.6	3–9	3–9	50	<5
Metoprolol	5.5	3.5	2.4–4.5	8	5
Nadolol	1.9	19	45	28	90
Penbutolol	ND	22	24	>95	<10
Pindolol	1.2	2.5–4	3–4	50	40
Propranolol	2.8	2–6	1–6	93	<5
Increased bioavailability in RF secondary to decreased first-pass metabolism.					
Sotalol	1.3	7.5–15	56	<1	60
Timolol	1.7	2.7	4	60	15
Vasodilators					
Diazoxide	0.2–0.3	17–31	30–60	>90	50
Hydralazine	0.5–0.9	2–4.5	7–16	87	12–14
Acetylator status determines rate of hepatic metabolism.					
Isosorbide	1.5–4	0.15–0.5	4	72	10–20
Active metabolites with long half-life; need nitrate-free interval of 10–12 h for continued effect.					
Minoxidil	2–3	2.8–4.2	2.8–4.2	0	15–20
Nitroglycerin	2–3	2–4 min	2–4 min	ND	<1
Nitroprusside	0.2	<10 min	<10 min	0	<10
Toxic metabolite, thiocyanate accumulates in RF and may cause seizures, coma. Thiocyanate is hemodialyzable. Measure thiocyanate levels after 48 h of high-dose therapy.					
CARDIOVASCULAR DRUGS					
Antiarrhythmic agents					
Hepatic metabolism of encainide, flecainide, and propafene is genetically determined.					
Amiodarone	70–140	14–120 d	14–120 d	96	<5
Active metabolite.					

Dose for patients with CL_{CR} = >50 ml/min	Adjustment for Renal Failure			Removed Significantly by			
	Method	CL_{CR} = 10–50 ml/min	CL_{CR} = <10 ml/min	HD	PD	CAVH/CVVH	CAVHD/CVVHD
400–800 mg qd or bid	D	50%	30–50%	No	No	ND	ND
50–100 mg qd	D, I	25–50 mg q48h	25 mg q48h	Yes	No	Yes	Yes
2.5–10 mg/d	D	50%	25%	ND	No	ND	ND
*50–200 µg/kg/min by infusion	D	100%	100%	No	No	ND	ND
200–600 mg bid	D	100%	100%	No	No	No	No
50–200 mg bid	D	100%	100%	Yes	No	No	No
80–120 mg qd	D	50%	25%	Yes	No	No	Yes
10–40 mg qd	D	100%	100%	No	No	ND	ND
10–30 mg bid	D	100%	100%	No	No	No	No
80–160 mg bid	D	100%	75–100%	No	No	No	No
160 mg qd	D	30%	15–30%	Yes	ND	Yes	Yes
10–20 mg bid	D	100%	100%	No	No	No	No
150–300 mg bolus	D	100%	100%	No	No	ND	ND
20–40 mg q6–8h	D	100%	100%	No	No	No	No
10–40 mg tid	D	100%	100%	No	No	No	No
5–30 mg bid	D	100%	100%	No	No	ND	ND
Many methods and routes of dosing	D	100%	100%	No	No	No	No
0.25–8 µg/kg/min by infusion, titrate	D	100%	100%	No	No	ND	ND
800–1600 mg load, 200–600 mg/d	D	100%	100%	No	No	No	No

TABLE 3.6. (*Continued*)

THERAPEUTIC CATEGORY / ***Drug Class*** / *Drug*	V_d^b (liter/kg) Normal	$t_{1/2}\beta$ (hr) CL_{CR} (ml/min) >50	<10	PPB (%) Normal	*fe* (%)
Bretylium	8.2	6–13.6	32–105	6	75
Disopyramide	0.8–2.6	5–8	10–18	54–81	35–65
Active metabolite; PPB dose-dependent. V_d decreased in ESRD.					
Encainide	2–2.7	3–9	1.5–9	75–81	5–60
Active metabolites which accumulate in RF.					
Flecainide	8.4–9.5	12–19.5	19–26	52	10–40
Excretion enhanced in acid urine.					
Lidocaine	1.3–2.2	2–2.2	1.3–3	60–66	10
Mexiletine	5.5–6.6	8–13	16	70–75	10
Increased renal excretion in acid urine.					
N-Acetylprocainamide	1.5–1.7	6–8	42–70	10–20	80
Redose by monitoring plasma levels. Hemofiltration useful in poisoning.					
Procainamide (parenteral)	2.2	2.5–4.9	5.3–14	15	50–60
Redose by monitoring plasma level. Half-life and *fe* (%) acetylator phenotype-dependent. Active metabolite is *N*-acetylprocainamide. Hemofiltration useful in poisoning. V_d unchanged in RF.					
Propafenone	3	2–3	2–3	>95	<1
Half-life acetylator phenotype dependent.					
Quinidine sulfate	2–3.5	6	4–14	70–95	20
Active metabolite. Excretion enhanced by acid urine. Hemodialysis useful in poisoning. Redose by monitoring plasma levels.					
Tocainide	3.2	14	22–27	10–20	10–40
Excretion decreased in alkaline urine.					
Calcium channel blockers					
Amlodipine	21	35–50	50	>95	<10
Diltiazem (oral, parenteral)	3–5	2–8	3.5	98	<10
Active metabolites. Continuous infusion can be used.					
Felodipine	9–7	10–14	21	99	<1
Isradipine	3–4	8–12	10–11	96	<5
Nicardipine	1–1.5	5	5–7	98–99	<5
Nifedipine	1.4	4–5.5	5–7	97	<5
PPB decreased in ESRD.					

Dose for patients with CL_{CR} = >50 ml/min	Adjustment for Renal Failure: Method	CL_{CR} = 10–50 ml/min	CL_{CR} = <10 ml/min	Removed Significantly by: HD	PD	CAVH/ CVVH	CAVHD/ CVVHD
5–30 mg/kg load, 5–10 mg q6h or 1–2 mg/min infusion	D	25–50%	25%	No	No	No	No
100–200 mg q6h	I	q12–24h	q24h	?	No	ND	ND
25 mg q8h to 50 mg q6h	D	75–100%	50%	No	ND	ND	ND
100–200 mg q12h	D	100%	50–75%	No	No	No	No
50 mg over 2 min, repeat q5 min × 3, then 1–4 mg/min	D	100%	100%	No	No	No	No
100–300 mg q6–12h	D	100%	100%	No	No	No	No
500 mg q6–8h	D, I	Individualize	Individualize	Yes	No	?	No
Load: 12–17 mg/kg MD: Individualize	D, I	Load: 100% MD: Individualize	Load: 100% MD: Individualize	Yes	No	No	No
150–300 mg q8h	D	100%	100%	No	No	No	No
Initial: 10–15 mg/kg/d divided q6h	D	100% Individualize	100% Individualize	Yes	No	No	No
400–600 mg q8h	D	100%	50%	Yes	No	Yes	Yes
5–10 mg/d	D	100%	100%	No	No	ND	ND
60–120 mg q8h 20–25 mg	D	100%	100%	No	No	No	No
5–20 mg q24h	D	100%	100%	No	No	ND	ND
2.5–5 mg bid	D	100%	100%	No	No	ND	ND
20–30 mg bid-tid	D	100%	100%	No	No	ND	ND
10–30 mg q8h	D	100%	100%	No	No	No	No

TABLE 3.6. *(Continued)*

THERAPEUTIC CATEGORY / ***Drug Class*** / *Drug*	V_d[b] *(liter/kg) Normal*	$t_{1/2}\beta$ *(hr)* CL_{CR} *(ml/min)* >50	<10	*PPB (%) Normal*	*fe (%)*
Nimodipine	0.9–2.3	1–2.8	22*	98	<1
*Age-related hepatic impairment may be responsible for prolonged $t_{1/2}$ reported in renal insufficiency patients.					
Nitrendipine	6.6	4.6	3.3–5.8	99	<1
Verapamil (oral, parenteral)	3–6	3–7	2.4–4	83–93	<10
Active metabolites.					
Cardiac glycosides					
Digitoxin	0.6	144–200	210	94	20–25
8–10% converted to digoxin					
Digoxin	5–8	36–44	80–120	20–30	76–85
V_d and total body clearance decreased in ESRD. Decrease loading dose by 30–50% in ESRD.					
Various digoxin assays overestimate serum levels in uremia. Bioavailability of oral tablets only 65– 75%.					
Diuretics					
Thiazide diuretics generally ineffective alone in CL_{CR} <30 ml/min but show synergism when administered with loop diuretics in renal failure.					
Amiloride	5–5.2	6–8	10–144	30–40	50
Increased risk of hyperkalemia in renal insufficiency and with concomitant ACE inhibitors.					
Bumetanide	0.2–0.5	1.2–1.5	1.5	96	33
Doses higher than 2 mg may be necessary in ESRD or ARF. Maximum daily dose: 20 mg; oral and i.v. dose identical.					
Chlorothiazide (parenteral)	0.2	0.75–2	Increased	95	>95
Chlorthalidone	3.9	44–80	ND	76–90	50
Ethacrynic acid (parenteral)	0.1	2–4	ND	90	20
Higher incidence of ototoxicity than with furosemide or bumetanide; increased ototoxicity risk with low GFR.					
Furosemide (parenteral)	0.07–0.2	0.5–1.1	2–4	95	67
Ototoxicity with rapid infusions; doses of 100–1000 mg may be necessary in ESRD or ARF; oral bioavailability only 40–60%.					
Hydrochlorothiazide	0.83	2.5	12–20	64	>95
Indapamide	0.3–1.3	14–18	14–18	76–79	<5
Ineffective in ESRD.					

Dose for patients with CL_{CR} = >50 ml/min	*Adjustment for Renal Failure*			*Removed Significantly by*			
	Method	*CL_{CR} = 10–50 ml/min*	*CL_{CR} = <10 ml/min*	*HD*	*PD*	*CAVH/ CVVH*	*CAVHD/ CVVHD*
60 mg q4h	D	100%	?	No	No	ND	ND
20 mg bid	D	100%	100%	No	No	No	No
80–120 mg q8h	D	100%	100%	No	No	No	No
5–10 mg							
0.1–0.2 mg/d	D	100%	100%	No	No	No	No
10–15 μg/kg load, 0.25–0.5 mg/d	D, I	25–75% q24–48h	25% q48h	No	No	No	No
5–10 mg q24h	D	50%	Avoid	NA	NA	NA	NA
1–2 mg q8–12h	D	100%	100%	No	No	No	No
0.5–1 g q12–24h	D	100%	Avoid	No	ND	No	No
25 mg/d	I	q24h	Avoid	ND	ND	ND	ND
50 mg prn	I	100%	Avoid	No	ND	No	No
40–80 mg q12h	D	100%	100%	No	No	No	No
25–50 mg qd	D	100%	Avoid	No	ND	No	No
2.5 mg/d	D	100%	Avoid	ND	ND	ND	ND

TABLE 3.6. *(Continued)*

THERAPEUTIC CATEGORY / ***Drug Class*** / *Drug*	*V_d^b (liter/kg) Normal*	*$t_{1/2}\beta$ (hr) CL_{CR} (ml/min)*		*PPB (%) Normal*	*fe (%)*
		>50	*<10*		
Metolazone	1.6	4–20	ND	95	70
High doses effective alone in ESRD; smaller doses synergistic with loop diuretics in ESRD.					
Spironolactone	ND	10–35	10–35	98	20–30
Usually ineffective with GFR <30 ml/min. Active metabolite with long half-life; hyperkalemia.					
Triamterene	2.2–3.7	2–12	10	40–70	4–10
Usually ineffective with GFR <30 ml/min; hyperkalemia.					
Miscellaneous cardiac drugs					
Amrinone	1.3–1.6	2.6–8.3	ND	20–40	10–40
Dobutamine	0.25	2 min	ND	ND	<10
Dopamine	ND	2 min	ND	ND	Small
Increases renal blood flow at doses between 0.5 and 2 μg/kg/min.					
Milrinone	0.25–0.35	1	1.5–3	70	80–85
Norepinephrine	ND	min	ND	ND	Negligible
SEDATIVES, HYPNOTICS, DRUGS USED IN PSYCHIATRY					
Barbiturates					
Charcoal hemoperfusion and hemodialysis more effective than peritoneal dialysis for overdose.					
Pentobarbital (parenteral)	1	35–50	35–50	60–70	<1
PPB decreased in ESRD.					
Phenobarbital	0.6	60–150	117–160	40–60	25
PPB decreases in hypoalbuminemia. Monitor plasma levels; alkalinization of urine increases excretion.					
Secobarbital (parenteral)	1.5–2.5	20–35	ND	44	5
Thiopental	1–1.5	4	6–18	72–86	<1
Benzodiazepines					
Alprazolam	0.9–1.3	9.5–19	9.5–19	70–80	20
Active metabolite; does not accumulate in ESRD; PPB decreased in ESRD, HD, and CAPD—patients show enhanced sensitivity to some pharmacodynamic effects.					
Clonazepam	1.5–4.5	18–50	18–50	86	<1

Dose for patients with CL_{CR} = >50 ml/min	Adjustment for Renal Failure			Removed Significantly by			
	Method	CL_{CR} = 10–50 ml/min	CL_{CR} = <10 ml/min	HD	PD	CAVH/CVVH	CAVHD/CVVHD
5–10 mg/d	D	100%	100%	No	No	No	No
100–200 mg qd	D	50%	Avoid	No	ND	No	No
50–100 mg q12h	D	100%	Avoid	ND	ND	ND	ND
0.75 mg/kg load, 5–10 μg/kg/min, titrate daily dose <10 mg/kg	D	100%	?	ND	ND	Yes	ND
2.5–15 μg/kg/min, titrate	D	100%	100%	No	No	No	No
0.5–20 μg/kg/min, titrate	D	100%	100%	No	No	No	No
15–75 μg/kg i.v. load, then 2.5–15 mg q6h p.o.	D	100%	50–75%	ND	ND	ND	ND
2–12 μg/min, titrate	D	100%	100%	No	No	No	No
100 mg prn	D	100%	100%	No	ND	No	No
1–3 mg/kg qd Individualize	D	100% Individualize	75–100% Individualize	Yes	Yes	Yes	Yes
Anesthesia induction	D	100%	100%	No	No	ND	ND
Anesthesia induction	D	100%	75%	ND	ND	ND	ND
0.25–5 mg tid	D	100%	100%	ND	ND	ND	ND
0.5–5 mg tid	D	100%	100%	No	ND	N0	No

TABLE 3.6. (*Continued*)

THERAPEUTIC CATEGORY **Drug Class** *Drug*	V_d[b] (liter/kg) Normal	$t_{1/2}\beta$ (hr) CL_{CR} (ml/min) >50	<10	PPB (%) Normal	fe (%)
Diazepam (parenteral)	0.7–3.4	20–90	20–90	94–98	<1
Active metabolites; main metabolite does not appear to accumulate in RF; PPB decreased in ESRD; V_d increased in ESRD.					
Flurazepam	3.4	47–100	47–100	96.6	<1
Active metabolite.					
Lorazepam	0.9–1.3	10–20	32–70	87	<1
Inactive metabolite.					
Midazolam	1–6.6	1.2–12.3	1.2–12.3	93–96	<1
PPB decreased in ESRD; renal clearance of active metabolite decreased in ARF.					
Oxazepam	0.6–1.6	5–10	25–90	97	<1
Inactive metabolite; PPB decreased and V_d increased in ESRD.					
Temazepam	1.3–1.5	4–10	ND	96	<1
PPB decreased in renal disease.					
Triazolam	1.1	2–4	2–4	85–95	2
PPB correlates with α-1 acid glycoprotein concentration.					
Miscellaneous agents					
Buspirone	5	2–4	5.8	95	<1
Active metabolite accumulates in ESRD, metabolite PPB 35–41%.					
Chloral hydrate	0.6	7–14	ND	70–80	<1
Active metabolite.					
Haloperidol (parenteral)	14–21	10–36	ND	90–92	1
Lithium carbonate	0.5–0.9	14–28	40	None	95
Dosage should be individualized using patient-specific parameters calculated from plasma concentrations. Plasma levels rebound after hemodialysis.					
Phenothiazines					
Chlorpromazine (parenteral)	21	11–42	11–42	91–99	<1
Promethazine (parenteral)	Large	9–12	ND	76–93	ND
Excessive sedation					
Tricyclic antidepressants					
Dosage reductions indicated for elderly and dehabilitated patients; daily doses should be divided initially and then consolidated in a single hs dose.					
Amitriptyline	6–36	24–40	24–40	96	<2
Reduce dose in elderly.					
Desipramine	28–60	12–54	ND	90	2
Active metabolites.					
Doxepin	9–33	8–25	10–30	95	0
PPB decreased in ESRD.					
Imipramine	9–15	6–20	ND	96	<2
Active metabolites.					

Dose for patients with CL_{CR} = >50 ml/min	Adjustment for Renal Failure			Removed Significantly by			
	Method	CL_{CR} = 10–50 ml/min	CL_{CR} = <10 ml/min	HD	PD	CAVH/CVVH	CAVHD/CVVHD
5–20 mg prn	D	100%	100%	No	ND	No	No
15–30 mg hs	D	100%	100%	No	ND	ND	ND
1–2 mg bid-tid	D	100%	100%	No	ND	No	No
titrate	D	100%	50–100%	No	ND	No	No
10–30 mg tid, qid	D	100%	100%	No	ND	No	No
15–30 mg hs	D	100%	100%	No	ND	No	No
0.125–0.25 mg hs	D	100%	100%	No	ND	No	No
5–10 mg tid	D	100%	50%	?	ND	ND	ND
250 mg tid 500–1000 mg hs	D	ND	Avoid	?	ND	ND	ND
1–5 mg prn	D	100%	100%	No	No	No	No
0.9–2.1 g qd in divided doses	D	Individualize 50–75%	Individualize 25–50%	Yes	No	Yes	Yes
25–50 mg q3–4h	D	100%	100%	No	No	No	No
12.5–50 mg q4h	D	100%	100%	ND	ND	ND	ND
100–300 mg/d	D	100%	100%	No	No	No	No
100–300 mg/d	D	100%	100%	No	No	No	No
100–300 mg/d	D	100%	100%	No	No	No	No
100–300 mg/d	D	100%	100%	No	No	No	No

TABLE 3.6. *(Continued)*

THERAPEUTIC CATEGORY / ***Drug Class*** / *Drug*	V_d[b] *(liter/kg) Normal*	$t_{1/2}\beta$ *(hr)* CL_{CR} *(ml/min)* >50	<10	*PPB (%) Normal*	*fe (%)*
Nortriptyline	15–23	25–38	15–66	95	2
Protriptyline	15–31	54–98	ND	92	0
Other antidepressants					
Fluoxetine	35	2–3 d	2–3 d	95	<2.5
Active metabolite, which is hepatically metabolized with $t_{1/2}$ 7–9 d.					
Paroxetine	ND	17.3	29.7 min CL_{CR} <30	95	2
Dose-dependent pharmacokinetics.					
Sertraline	ND	26	NC	98	<1
Mildly active metabolite.					
Narcotics and narcotic antagonists					
Alfentanil	0.3–1	1–3	1–3	88–95	<1
Dosage ranges widely; PPB decreased in ESRD.					
Butorphanol	9–11	2–4	ND	80	<5
Codeine	3–4	4.4	13.0	7	0
Active metabolites that accumulate in ESRD; narcosis reported in RF on standard doses.					
Fentanyl	2–4	2–7 min	NC	80–84	8
Transdermal patch available for chronic pain control					
Meperidine	4–5	2–7	2–7	70	1–25
Normeperidine, an active metabolite, accumulates in ESRD ($t_{1/2}$–34h) and may cause seizures. CNS excitatory effects not reversed by naloxone. PPB reduced in ESRD. One-time doses OK in ESRD, but avoid chronic use.					
Methadone	3–6	13–58	ND	60–90	24
Fecal elimination is increased in ESRD. Acidic urine increases renal elimination.					
Morphine (parenteral)	3.5	1–4	1–4	20–30	6–10
Active metabolite which accumulates in ESRD					
Naloxone	3	1–1.5	ND	54	0
Propoxyphene	16	9–15	12–20	78	25
Active metabolite norpropoxyphene accumulates in ESRD and may cause cardiac toxicity. Cardiac toxicity not reversed by naloxone.					
Sufentanil	2–3	2–5 min	2–5 min	92	6
Nonnarcotic analgesics					
Dosage ranges widely.					
Acetaminophen	1–2	2	2	20–30	3
Metabolites may accumulate in ESRD.					

Dose for patients with CL_{CR} = >50 ml/min	*Adjustment for Renal Failure*			*Removed Significantly by*			
	Method	*CL_{CR} = 10–50 ml/min*	*CL_{CR} = <10 ml/min*	*HD*	*PD*	*CAVH/CVVH*	*CAVHD/CVVHD*
100–300 mg/d	D	100%	100%	No	No	No	No
15–60 mg/d	D	100%	100%	No	No	No	No
20–80 mg q AM	D	100%	100%	No	No	No	No
20–50 mg q AM	D	50–100%	50%	ND	ND	ND	ND
50–200 mg q AM	D	100%	100%	ND	ND	ND	ND
Anesthetic induction	D	100%	100%	ND	ND	ND	ND
2 mg q3–4h	D	ND	ND	ND	ND	ND	ND
30–60 mg q4–6h	D	75–100%	25–50%	ND	ND	No	No
Anesthetic induction	D	100%	100%	NA	NA	NA	NA
50–100 mg q3–4h	D	50–100%	Avoid	No	No	ND	ND
2.5–10 mg q6–8h	D	100%	100%	No	No	ND	ND
2–10 mg q4h	D	75%	50%	No	ND	No	No
0.4–2 mg	D	100%	100%	ND	ND	ND	ND
65 mg tid-qid	D	100%	Avoid	No	No	ND	ND
Anesthetic induction	D	100%	100%	No	No	No	No
650 mg q4h	I	q6h	q6h	No	No	No	No

TABLE 3.6. *(Continued)*

THERAPEUTIC CATEGORY / ***Drug Class*** / *Drug*	V_d[b] *(liter/kg)* *Normal*	$t_{1/2}\beta$ *(hr)* CL_{CR} *(ml/min)*		*PPB (%)* *Normal*	*fe (%)*
		>50	*<10*		
Aspirin May decrease GFR when renal blood flow is prostaglandin dependent. Excretion enhanced in alkaline urine. May add to uremic GI and hematologic symptoms. PPB reduced in ESRD. Low-dose once-daily therapy for prophylaxis may be cautiously used in ESRD.	0.1–0.2	2–3	2–3	80–90	1.4
Ketorolac May decrease GRF when renal blood flow is prostaglandin dependent.	0.11–0.33	3.8–6.3	9–10	99	60
MISCELLANEOUS AGENTS					
Antithrombotic agents					
Dipyridamole	2.4	12	ND	99	Small
Heparin Half-life increases with dose, titrate dose to APTT.	0.06–0.1	0.3–2	0.3–2	>90	0
Streptokinase ESRD patients may be predisposed to bleeding complications; other dosage regimens have been used.	0.016	1–1.5	ND	ND	0
Ticlopidine Neutropenia; active metabolite in rats, ? in humans; $t_{1/2}$ increases after multiple doses.	ND	24–36	ND	98	<1
Warfarin Titrate dose to INR or PT.	0.15	35–45	35–45	99	0
Anticonvulsants Monitor serum levels.					
Carbamazepine Dosage should be individualized using patient-specific parameters calculated from plasma concentrations. Active metabolite with anticonvulsant and toxic effects, carbamazepine induces its own metabolism; other anticonvulsants induce metabolism; $t_{1/2}$ decreases with chronic therapy and with other concomitant anticonvulsant therapy.	0.8–1.8	24–40 h single dose; 6–25 h chronic dosing	NC	75	2–3
Ethosuximide	0.7	35–55	35–55	10	12–20
Phenytoin Dosage should be individualized using patient-specific parameters calculated from plasma concentrations. Measure free levels in renal insufficiency or failure.	1	24	24	90	2

Dose for patients with CL_{CR} = >50 ml/min	Adjustment for Renal Failure			Removed Significantly by			
	Method	CL_{CR} = 10–50 ml/min	CL_{CR} = <10 ml/min	HD	PD	CAVH/CVVH	CAVHD/CVVHD
650 mg q4h	I	q4–6h	Avoid	Yes	No	No	Yes
30–60 mg load 15–30 mg q6h	D	100%	15 mg q6h	ND	ND	ND	ND
75 mg tid	D	100%	100%	ND	ND	ND	ND
5000 U load 800–1500 U/h	D	100%	100%	No	No	No	No
1.5 mU over 60 min or 250,000 U load, 100,000 U/h	D	100%	100%	ND	ND	ND	ND
250 mg bid	D	100%	100%	ND	ND	ND	ND
10 mg load × 2–3 d 2–10 mg/d	D	100%	100%	No	No	No	No
200 mg bid to 1200 mg/d in divided doses	D	100% Individualize	100% Individualize	No	No	No	No
500–1500 mg/d	D	100%	100%	Yes	Yes	ND	ND
18 mg/kg load, 200– 500 mg/d	D	100% Individualize	100% Individualize	No	No	No	No

TABLE 3.6. *(Continued)*

THERAPEUTIC CATEGORY / ***Drug Class*** / *Drug*	$V_d{}^b$ *(liter/kg)* *Normal*	$t_{1/2}\beta$ *(hr)* CL_{CR} *(ml/min)*		*PPB (%)* *Normal*	*fe (%)*
		>50	*<10*		
Phenytoin continued PPB decreased and V_d increased in RF. Dose-dependent pharmacokinetics.					
Primidone	0.6	5–15	5–15	20	40
Partially converted to phenobarbital and other metabolites with long half-life, monitor phenobarbital and primidone levels.					
Sodium valproate	0.2	9–18	6–15	90	1–3
Decreased PPB in uremia; $t_{1/2}$ decreases with polytherapy; monitoring total drug concentrations in ESRD may be misleading.					
ANTIHISTAMINES					
H-1 antagonists					
Diphenhydramine	3.3–6.8	3.4–9.3	ND	80	2
Hydroxyzine	19.5	14–20	ND	ND	0
Active metabolite excreted by the kidney.					
Antiulcer agents					
Dosage of H_2 blockers (cimetidine, famotidine, ranitidine) should be guided by gastric pH monitoring in the acute care setting.					
Cimetidine (parenteral)	0.8–1.3	1.5–2	5	20	50–70
Inhibition of tubular secretion of creatinine. Mental confusion in patients with renal or hepatic disease.					
Famotidine (parenteral)	0.8–1.4	2.5–4	12–19	15–22	65–80
Omeprazole	0.4–0.5	0.5–1	0.5–1	95	<1
Ranitidine (parenteral)	1.1–1.9	1.5–3	6–9	15	80
Arthritis and gout agents					
Allopurinol	0.5	2–8	2–8	<5	30
Renal excretion of active metabolite (oxypurinol) with half-life of 25 h.					
Colchicine (oral)	470–700	9–20	40	31	5–17
Enterohepatic recycling of colchicine and metabolites. Acute: doses given until pain relief or GI symptoms appear. Avoid prolonged use in CL_{CR} <50 ml/min.					
Bronchodilators					
Albuterol (oral)	2–2.5	4	Increased	7	51–64
Aerosol available.					
Diphylline	0.8	1.8–2.3	12	<3	85
Ipratropium	4.6	1.6	ND	ND	ND

Dose for patients with CL_{CR} = >50 ml/min	Adjustment for Renal Failure			Removed Significantly by			
	Method	CL_{CR} = 10–50 ml/min	CL_{CR} = <10 ml/min	HD	PD	CAVH/CVVH	CAVHD/CVVHD
250–500 mg qid	D, I	Individualize	Individualize	Yes	ND	ND	ND
15–60 mg/kg qd divided bid-qid	D	100%	100%	No	No	No	No
25–50 mg q6–8h	D	100%	100%	No	No	No	No
25–100 mg q6h	D	?	?	No	No	ND	ND
300 mg q6h or 37.5–50 mg/h	D, I	q8–12h 25–37.5 mg/h	q12h 18–25 mg/h	Yes	No	No	No
20–40 mg q12h	I	q12–24h	q24h	No	No	No	Yes
20–40 mg qd	D	100%	100%	No	No	No	No
50 mg q8h or 6.25 mg/h	I	q12h	q24h	Yes	No	No	No
300 mg/d	D, I	150 mg qd	100 mg q24–72h	Yes	ND	ND	ND
Acute: 0.5–1.3 mg, then 0.5–0.65 mg q1–2h prn Chronic: 0.5–0.65 mg qd or qod	I	?	?	No	ND	ND	ND
2–4 mg tid-qid	D	75%	50%	ND	ND	ND	ND
15 mg/kg/d	D	50%	25%	Yes	ND	ND	ND
2 inhalations qid	D	100%	100%	No	No	No	No

TABLE 3.6. *(Continued)*

THERAPEUTIC CATEGORY / *Drug Class* / *Drug*	V_d[b] *(liter/kg)* *Normal*	$t_{1/2}\beta$ *(hr)* CL_{CR} *(ml/min)* >50	<10	*PPB (%)* *Normal*	*fe (%)*
Terbutaline	0.94	14	ND	25	50
Large first-dose effect. Parenteral doses should be avoided in ESRD. Oral doses unchanged. Aerosol available.					
Theophylline	0.3–0.7	4–12	4–12	55	18
May exacerbate uremic gastrointestinal symptoms. Doses are expressed in terms of aminophylline. Monitor plasma levels of theophylline.					
Corticosteroids					
Betamethasone (parenteral)	1.4	5.5	ND	65	5
Cortisone (oral)	ND	0.5–2	3.5	90	0
Dexamethasone	0.8–1	3–4	ND	70	2.6
Oral and i.v. dose equivalent.					
Hydrocortisone	ND	1.5–2	1.5–2	ND	0
Oral and i.v. dose equivalent.					
Methylprednisolone	1.2–1.5	2.3	2.3	78	4.9
Prednisolone	2.2	2.5–3.5	2.5–3.5	Saturable	26
Oral and i.v. dose equivalent.					
Prednisone	0.97	2.5–3.5	2.5–3.5	Saturable	3
Triamcinolone (oral)	1.4–2.1	1.9–6	1.9–6	ND	ND
Hypoglycemic agents					
Titrate insulin and oral hypoglycemic agents with blood glucose monitoring.					
Acetohexamide	0.21	1–1.3	1–1.3	65–90	<1
May falsely elevate serum creatinine level. Active metabolite with half-life of 5–8 h. Prolonged hypoglycemia in azotemic patients.					
Chlorpropamide	0.09–0.27	24–42	50–200	88–96	20
Prolonged hypoglycemia in azotemic patients.					
Glipizide	0.13–0.16	2–7	ND	97	4–5.7
Inactive metabolites.					
Glyburide	0.16–0.3	7–10	ND	99	50
Active metabolite prolongs hypoglycemic effect in rats.					
Insulin	0.15	2–4	13	5	0
Renal metabolism of insulin decreases with azotemia.					
Tolazamide	ND	4–7	ND	94	7
Weakly active metabolites.					
Tolbutamide	0.1–0.15	4–6	4–6	95–97	0
Some patients may require divided doses.					
Miscellaneous drugs					
Metoclopramide	2–3.4	2.5–4	14–15	40	10–22
Extrapyramidal side effects common in ESRD.					

Dose for patients with CL_{CR} = >50 ml/min	*Adjustment for Renal Failure*			*Removed Significantly by*			
	Method	*CL_{CR} = 10–50 ml/min*	*CL_{CR} = <10 ml/min*	*HD*	*PD*	*CAVH/ CVVH*	*CAVHD/ CVVHD*
2.5–5 mg tid	D	50%	Avoid	ND	ND	ND	ND
6 mg/kg load, 0.5–0.7 mg/kg/h	D	100%	100%	Yes	ND	No	No
0.5–9 mg/d	D	100%	100%	ND	ND	ND	ND
25–500 mg/d	D	100%	100%	No	ND	ND	ND
0.75–9 mg/d	D	100%	100%	ND	ND	ND	ND
20–500 mg/d	D	100%	100%	ND	ND	ND	ND
10–150 mg qd	D	100%	100%	Yes	ND	ND	ND
5–60 mg/d	D	100%	100%	Yes	ND	No	No
5–60 mg/d	D	100%	100%	No	ND	ND	ND
4–48 mg/d	D	100%	100%	ND	ND	ND	ND
250–1500 mg/d	I	Avoid	Avoid	ND	No	ND	ND
100–500 mg/d	I	Avoid	Avoid	ND	No	ND	ND
2.5–15 mg/d	D	100%	100%	ND	ND	ND	ND
2.5–20 mg/d	D	Avoid	Avoid	No	No	No	No
Variable	D	75%	50%	No	No	No	No
100–500 mg/d	D	100%	100%	ND	ND	ND	ND
1–2 g/d	D	100%	100%	No	No	No	No
10–15 mg qid	D	75%	50%	No	ND	No	No

TABLE 3.6. *(Continued)*

THERAPEUTIC CATEGORY / *Drug Class* / *Drug*	V_d[b] *(liter/kg) Normal*	$t_{1/2}\beta$ *(hr)* CL_{CR} *(ml/min)* >50	<10	*PPB (%) Normal*	*fe (%)*
Cyclosporine	3.5–7.4	3–16	3–16	96–99	<1
N-Acetylcysteine	0.34	2.3	ND	ND	30
Dosage indicated is for treatment of acetaminophen overdose.					
Pentoxifylline	2.4	0.8	0.8	0	0
Neuromuscular agents					
Alfentanil	0.3–1	1.4–2	1.4–2	88–95	<1
Atracurium	0.15–0.18	0.3–0.4	0.3–0.4	82	0
Etomidate	2–4.5	4–5	4–5	75	0
Gallamine	0.21–0.24	2.3–2.7	6–20	30–70	85–100
If blockade not responsive to neostigmine, dialysis may be useful.					
Ketamine	1.8–3.1	2–3.5	2–3.5	ND	2–3
Metocurine	0.42–0.57	3.5–5.8	11.4	35	45–60
Neostigmine	0.5–1	1.3–3	3	0	67
Pancuronium	0.15–0.38	2.3	4.3–8.2	70–85	30–40
Active metabolite, which can accumulate in renal insufficiency.					
Pyridostigmine	0.8–1.4	1.5–2	6	ND	80–90
Renal excretion decreased by basic drugs.					
Succinylcholine	ND	3	ND	ND	0
Hyperkalemia in ESRD.					
Sufentanil	1.7–5.2	2	2	92	1–2
Tubocurarine	0.22–0.39	2–4	5.5	30–50	40–60
Prolonged neuromuscular blockade reported in ESRD.					
Vecuronium	0.18–0.27	0.5–1.3	0.5–1.3	30	25
Active metabolite, which can accumulate in renal insufficiency.					

[a]Data compiled from Refs. 11–68.

[b]V_d, volume of distribution; APTT, activated partial thromboplastin time; CAVH/CAVHD, continuous arteriovenous hemofiltration or hemodialysis; CL, clearance CVVH/CVVHD, continuous venovenous hemofiltration or hemodialysis; D, dose ESRD, end-stage renal disease; Fe(%), fraction of systemically available drug excreted unchanged in the urine; GFR, glomerular filtration rate; HD, hemodialysis; I

Dose for patients with CL_{CR} = >50 ml/min	Adjustment for Renal Failure			Removed Significantly by			
	Method	CL_{CR} = 10–50 ml/min	CL_{CR} = <10 ml/min	HD	PD	CAVH/CVVH	CAVHD/CVVHD
3–10 mg/kg/d	D	100%	100%	No	No	ND	ND
140 mg/kg load, 70 mg/kg q4h for 17 doses	D	100%	100%	ND	ND	ND	ND
400 mg tid	D	100%	100%	ND	ND	ND	ND
8–245 µg/kg load, 0.5–3 µg/kg*min	D	100%	100%	ND	ND	ND	ND
0.4–0.5 mg/kg load, 0.08–0.1 mg/kg q15–25 min	D	100%	100%	ND	ND	ND	ND
0.2–0.6 mg/kg	D	100%	100%	ND	ND	ND	ND
0.5–1.5 mg/kg	D	Avoid	Avoid	NA	NA	NA	NA
1–4.5 mg/kg	D	100%	100%	ND	ND	ND	ND
0.2–0.4 mg/kg	D	Avoid	Avoid	ND	ND	ND	ND
15–375 mg/d	D	50%	25%	ND	ND	ND	ND
0.04–0.1 mg/kg	D	50%	Avoid	ND	ND	ND	ND
60–1500 mg/d	D	35%	20%	ND	ND	ND	ND
0.3–1.1 mg/kg load, 0.04–0.07 mg/kg prn	D	100%	100%	ND	ND	ND	ND
1–30 µg/kg	D	100%	100%	ND	ND	ND	ND
0.1–0.2 mg/kg	D	50%	Avoid	ND	ND	ND	ND
0.08–0.1 mg/kg load, 0.01–0.05 mg/kg	D	100%	Avoid	ND	ND	ND	ND

interval; INR, international normalized ratio; LOAD, loading dose; MTT, methylthiotetrazole; NA, not applicable; NC, no change; ND, no data; PPB(%), plasma protein binding percent; PD, peritoneal dialysis; PT, prothrombin time; RF, renal failure; t½β, terminal elimination half-life; ?, data equivocal or insufficient to make recommendations.

TABLE 3.7. Diuretic Classes

Agents	*Site of Action*	*Usual Dose (24 h)*	$t_{1/2}$	*Metabolism*
Carbonic anhydrase inhibitors (acetazolamide)	Proximal tubule	250–500 mg	5 h	Excreted unchanged in urine
Osmotic diuretics (mannitol)	Proximal tubule; loop of Henle	0.25 g/kg	Dependent on GFR; usually 30–60 min	Excreted unchanged in urine
Loop diuretics	Loop of Henle			Both hepatic and renal metabolism
Furosemide		20–80 mg	1 to 2 h	
Bumetanide		1–2 mg	1 to 2 h	
Ethacrynic acid		50–200 mg	1 to 2 h	
Thiazides	Distal tubule	See Table 3.8		
Potassium-sparing diuretics	Collecting duct			Hepatic and renal metabolism
Spironolactone		25–200 mg	20 h	
Triamterene		50–200 mg	3–5 h	
Amiloride		5–10 mg	6–9 h	

TABLE 3.8. Thiazide Diuretics

Thiazides	*Dose*	*Frequency*	*Route*	*Comments*
Bendroflumethizide	25–200 mg	qd–bid	p.o.	
Benzthiazide	25–200 mg	qd	p.o.	
Chlorothiazide	500 mg–2 g	qd–bid	p.o. i.v.	Only i.v. thiazide
Chlorthalidone	12.5–150 mg	qd	p.o.	
Cyclothiazide	1–2 mg	qd	p.o.	
Hydrochlorothiazide	12.5–150 mg	qd	p.o.	
Hydroflumethiazide	25–200 mg	qd–bid	p.o.	
Indapamide	2.5–5 mg	qd	p.o.	? Less effect on lipids
Methyclothiazide	2.5–10 mg	qd	p.o.	
Metolazone	0.5–10 mg	qd	p.o.	Marked differences between formulations
Polythiazide	1–4 mg	qd	p.o.	
Quinethazone	25–200 mg	qd–bid	p.o.	
Trichloromethiazide	1–4 mg	qd–bid	p.o.	

TABLE 3.9. Agents Used in the Treatment of Hyperkalemia[a]

Agent	*Mechanism*	*Dosage*
Calcium gluconate (10%)	Direct antagonism	10–20 ml i.v. over 2–5 min
Sodium bicarbonate (8.4%)	Redistribution	50 ml i.v. over 1–5 min; can be repeated
Glucose/insulin	Redistribution	2–3 g glucose/1 unit regular insulin; bolus: 50 ml D50W with 10 U regular insulin.
Sodium polystyrene sulfonate (SPS, Kayexalate)	Increased elimination	15–60 g p.o. or rectally as retention enema up to 3–4 times/day; Sorbitol to be given concomitantly with SPS p.o.
β_2 agonists	Redistribution	Nebulized treatment of 20 mg albuterol in 4 ml normal saline inhaled over 10 min
Dialysis	Increased elimination	—

[a]Compiled from Refs. 69 and 70.

REFERENCES

1. Cockcroft DW, Gault MH: Prediction of creatinine clearance from serum creatinine. *Nephron* 16:31–41, 1976.
2. Mawer CE, Knowles BR, Lucas SB, Stirland RA, Tooth JA: Computer-assisted prescribing of kanamycin for patients with renal insufficiency. *Lancet* i:12–15, 1972.
3. Keller E, Reetze P, Schollmeyer P: Drug therapy in patients undergoing continuous ambulatory peritoneal dialysis: clinical pharmacokinetic considerations. *Clin Pharmacokinet* 18:104–117, 1990.
4. O'Brien MA, Mason NA: Systemic absorption of intraperitoneal antimicrobials in continuous ambulatory peritoneal dialysis. *Clin Pharm* 11:246–254, 1992.
5. Paap CM, Nahata MC, Mentser MA, Mahan JD, Puri SK, Hubbard JA: Cefotaxime and metabolite disposition in two pediatric continuous ambulatory peritoneal dialysis patients. *Ann Pharmacother* 26:341–343, 1992.
6. Rubin J: Vancomycin absorption from the peritoneal cavity during dialysis-related peritonitis. *Perit Dial Int* 10:283–285, 1990.
7. Sennesael JJ, Maes VA, Pierard D, Debeukelaer SH, Verbeelen DL: Streptomycin pharmacokinetics in relapsing mycobacterium xenopi peritonitis. *Am J Nephrol* 10:422–425, 1990.
8. Debruyne D, Ryckelynck J-P, Moulin M, Hurault de Ligny B, Levaltier B, Bigot M-C: Pharmacokinetics of fluconazole in patients undergoing continuous ambulatory peritoneal dialysis. *Clin Pharmacokinet* 18:491–498, 1990.
9. Dahl K, Walstad RA, Widerøe T-E: The effect of peritonitis on the transperitoneal transport of cefuroxime in patients of CAPD treatment. *Nephrol Dial Transplant* 5:275–281, 1990.
10. Burgess ED, Gill MJ: Intraperitoneal administration of acyclovir in patients receiving continuous ambulatory peritoneal dialysis. *J Clin Pharmacol* 30:997–1000, 1990.

Onset of Action	Special Considerations
Immediate	Monitor with continuous ECG; calcium and sodium bicarbonate are incompatible.
Minutes	Alkaline load.
Minutes	Monitor blood sugar to prevent hypoglycemia.
2–12 h	Approximately 1 mEq K^+ adsorbed per gram of Kayexalate administered. Monitor for fluid, electrolyte, and GI disturbances; concomitant sorbitol to be administered for prevention of fecal impaction. Rectal route less effective.
30 min	Potassium-lowering effect extremely variable among patients. Combined therapy with insulin and glucose may be more effective than either therapy alone.
2–4 h	Feasibility includes appropriate access and availability.

11. Chan GLC, Matzke GR: Effects of renal insufficiency on the pharmacokinetics and pharmacodynamics of opioid analgesics. *Drug Intell Clin Pharm* 21:773–783, 1987.
12. Glare PA, Walsh TD: Clinical pharmacokinetics of morphine. *Ther Drug Monit* 13:1–23, 1991.
13. St. Peter WL, Redic-Kill KA, Halstenson CE: Clinical pharmacokinetics of antibiotics in patients with impaired renal functions. *Clin Pharmacokinet* 22:169–210, 1992.
14. Bunke CM, Aronoff GR, Luft FC: Pharmacokinetics of common antibiotics used in continuous ambulatory peritoneal dialysis. *Am J Kidney Dis* 3:114–117, 1983.
15. AHFS Drug Information 93—American Hospital Formulary Service, Bethesda, MD, American Society of Hospital Pharmacists, 1993.
16. Evans WE, Schentag JJ, Jusko WJ (eds): *Applied Pharmacokinetics—Principles of Therapeutic Drug Monitoring,* ed 3. Applied Therapeutics, Vancouver, 1992.
17. *Facts and Comparisons.* Facts and Comparisons, Inc., St. Louis, 1993.
18. Goodman GA, Rall TW, Nies AS, Taylor P (eds): *The Pharmacological Basis of Therapeutics,* ed 8. Pergamon Press, Elmsford, NY, 1990.
19. Achtert G, Scherrmann JM, Christen MO: Pharmacokinetics/bioavailability of colchicine in healthy male volunteers. *Eur J Drug Metab Pharmacokinet* 14:317–322, 1989.
20. Agoston S, Vandenbrom RHG, Wierda JMKH: Clinical pharmacokinetics of neuromuscular blocking drugs. *Clin Pharmacokinet* 22:94–115, 1992.
21. Barrie JR, Mousdale S: Ciprofloxacin levels in a patient undergoing veno-venous haemodiafiltration. *Intensive Care Med* 18:437–438, 1992.
22. Blackwell BG, Leggett JE, Johnson CA, Zimmerman SW, Craig WA: Ampicillin and sulbactam pharmacokinetics and pharmacodynamics in continuous ambulatory peritoneal dialysis (CAPD). *Perit Dial Int* 10:221–226, 1990.

23. Boelaert J, Daneels R, Van Landuyt HW, Schurgers M: Multiple dose pharmacokinetics of acyclovir in patients on continuous ambulatory peritoneal dialysis (abstract). *Antimicrob Agents Chemother* 142, 1985.
24. Boulieu R, Bastien O, Bleyzac N: Pharmacokinetics of ganciclovir in heart transplant patients undergoing continuous venovenous hemodialysis. *Ther Drug Monit* 15:105–107, 1993.
25. Brass C, Galgiani JN, Blaschke TF, Defelice R, O'Reilly RA, Stevens DA: Disposition of ketoconazole, an oral antifungal, in humans. *Antimicrob Agents Chemother* 21:151–158, 1982.
26. Burgess ED, Blair AD: Pharmacokinetics of ceftizoxime in patients undergoing continuous ambulatory peritoneal dialysis. *Antimicrob Agents Chemother* 24:237–239, 1983.
27. Davenport A, Goel S, Mackenzie JC: Neurotoxicity of acyclovir in patients with end-stage renal failure treated with continuous ambulatory peritoneal dialysis. *Am J Kidney Dis* 20:647–649, 1992.
28. Debruyne D, Ryckelynck J-P: Clinical pharmacokinetics of fluconazole. *Clin Pharmacokinet* 24:10–27, 1993.
29. Debruyne D, Ryckelynck J-P, Hurault de Ligny B, Moulin M: Pharmacokinetics of piperacillin in patients on peritoneal dialysis with and without peritonitis. *J Pharm Sci* 79:99–102, 1990.
30. Doyle GD, Laher M, Kelly JG, Byrne MM, Clarkson A, Zussman BD: The pharmacokinetics of paroxetine in renal impairment. *Acta Psychiatr Scand* 80(suppl 350):89–90, 1989.
31. Driessen JJ, Vree TB, Guelen PJM: The effects of acute changes in renal function on the pharmacokinetics of midazolam during long-term infusion in ICU patients. *Acta Anaesthesiol Belg* 42:149–155, 1991.
32. Fitzgerald J: Narcotic analgesics in renal failure. *Conn Med* 55:701–704, 1991.
33. Fletcher CV, Beatty C, Balfour Jr HH: Ganciclovir disposition in patients with renal insufficiency: implications for dose adjustment (abstract). *Pharmacotherapy* 11:277, 1991.
34. Gross ML, Somani P, Ribner BS, Raeader R, Freimer EH, Higgins Jr JT: Ceftizoxime elimination kinetics in continuous ambulatory peritoneal dialysis. *Clin Pharmacol Ther* 34:673–680, 1983.
35. Guay DRP, Awni WM, Findlay JWA, et al: Pharmacokinetics and pharmacodynamics of codeine in end-stage renal disease. *Clin Pharmacol Ther* 43:63–71, 1988.
36. Halvorsen MB, Whitmer JT, Halstenson CE: Hemodialysis clearance of encainide and metabolites. *Ther Drug Monit* 13:375–378, 1991.
37. Harford AM, Sica DA, Tartaglione T, Polk RE, Dalton HP, Poyner W: Vancomycin pharmacokinetics in continuous ambulatory peritoneal dialysis patients with peritonitis. *Nephron* 43:217–222, 1986.
38. Hoyer J, Schulte K-L, Lenz T: Clinical pharmacokinetics of angiotensin converting enzyme (ACE) inhibitors in renal failure. *Clin Pharmacokinet* 24:230–254, 1993.
39. Hui KK, Duchin KL, Kripalani KJ, Chan D, Kramer PK, Yanagawa N: Pharmacokinetics of fosinopril in patients with various degrees of renal function. *Clin Pharmacol Ther* 49:457–467, 1991.
40. Ito MK, Smith AR, Lee ML: Ticlopidine: a new platelet aggregation inhibitor. *Clin Pharm* 11:603–617, 1992.
41. Johnson C, Zimmerman S, Leggett J, et al: Pharmacokinetics and pharmacodynamics of ampicillin/sulbactam in CAPD patients (abstract). *Perit Dial Int* 7(suppl):S40, 1987.
42. Johnson RJ, Blair AD, Ahmad S: Ketoconazole kinetics in chronic peritoneal dialysis. *Clin Pharmacol Ther* 37:325–329, 1985.
43. Josselson J, Narang PK, Adir J, Yacobi A, Sadler JH: Bretylium kinetics in renal insufficiency. *Clin Pharmacol Ther* 33:144–150, 1983.

44. Kaiser G, Ackermann R, Sioufi A: Pharmacokinetics of a new angiotensin-converting enzyme inhibitor, benazepril hydrochloride, in special populations. *Am Heart J* 117:746–751, 1989.
45. Keller E, Fecht H, Böhler J, Schollmeyer P: Single-dose kinetics of imipenem/cilastatin during continuous arteriovenous haemofiltration in intensive care patients. *Nephrol Dial Transplant* 4:640–645, 1989.
46. Kelly JG, O'Malley K: Clinical pharmacokinetics of the newer ACE inhibitors. *Clin Pharmacokinet* 19:177–196, 1990.
47. Kirch W, Ramsch KD, Duhrsen U, Ohnhaus EE: Clinical pharmacokinetics of nimodipine in normal and impaired renal function. *Int J Clin Pharmacol Res* 4:381–384, 1984.
48. Kowalsky SF, Echols M, Schwartz MT, Bailie GR, McCormick E: Pharmacokinetics of ciprofloxacin in subjects with varying degrees of renal function and undergoing hemodialysis or CAPD. *Clin Nephrol* 39:53–58, 1993.
49. Lawless ST, Restaino I, Azin S, Corddry D: Effect of continuous arteriovenous haemofiltration on pharmacokinetics of amrinone. *Clin Pharmacokinet* 25:80–82, 1993.
50. Lowenthal DT, Saris SD, Paran E, Cristal N: The use of transdermal clonidine in the hypertensive patient with chronic renal failure. *Clin Nephrol* 39:37–42, 1993.
51. Marquardt ED, Ishisaka DY, Batra KK, Chin B: Removal of ethosuximide and phenobarbital by peritoneal dialysis in a child. *Clin Pharm* 11:1030–1031, 1992.
52. Murdoch D, McTavish D: Sertraline. A review of its pharmacodynamic and pharmacokinetic properties, and therapeutic potential in depression and obsessive-compulsive disorder. *Drugs* 44:604–624, 1992.
53. Ochs HR, Rauh HW, Greenblatt DJ, Kaschell HJ: Clorzepate dipotassium and diazepam in renal insufficiency: serum concentrations and protein binding of diazepam and desmethyldiazepam. *Nephron* 37:100–104, 1984.
54. Parker CJR, Jones JE, Hunter JM: Disposition of infusions of atracurium and its metabolite, laudanosine, in patients in renal and respiratory failure in an ITU. *Br J Anaesth* 61:531–540, 1988.
55. Prendergast BD: Glyburide and glipisize, second-generation oral sulfonylurea hypoglycemic agents. *Clin Pharm* 3:473–485, 1984.
56. Przechera M, Bengel D, Risler T: Pharmacokinetics of imipenem/cilastatin during continuous arteriovenous hemofiltration. *Contrib Nephrol* 93:131–134, 1991.
57. Rello J, Roglan A, García-Cases C, Jané F, Net A: Effect of continuous arteriovenous hemodialysis on ganciclovir pharmacokinetics. *Drug Intell Clin Pharm* 24:544–545, 1990.
58. Rivey MP, Taylor JW, Mullenix TA: DIAS rounds—drug information analysis service. *Drug Intell Clin Pharm* 23:687–689, 1989.
59. Rosansky SJ, Johnson KL, McConnell J: Use of transdermal clonidine in chronic hemodialysis patients. *Clin Nephrol* 39:32–36, 1993.
60. Ruedy J: The effects of peritoneal dialysis on the physiological disposition of oxacillin, ampicillin and tetracycline in patients with renal disease. *Can Med Assoc J* 94:257–261, 1966.
61. Sabouraud A, Rochdi M, Urtizberea M, Christen MO, Achtert G, Scherrmann JM: Pharmacokinetics of colchicine: a review of experimental and clinical data. *Gastroenterology* 30(suppl 1):35–39, 1992.
62. Schentag JJ: Cefmetazole sodium: pharmacology, pharmacokinetics, and clinical trials. *Pharmacotherapy* 11:2–19, 1991.
63. Schmith VD, Piraino B, Smith RB, Kroboth PD: Alprazolam in end-stage renal disease. I. Pharmacokinetics. *J Clin Pharmacol* 31:571–579, 1991.
64. Segredo V, Caldwell JE, Matthay MA, Sharma ML, Gruenke LD, Miller RD: Persistent paralysis in critically ill patients after long-term administration of vecuronium. *N Engl J Med* 327:524–528, 1992.

65. Sica DA: Kinetics of angiotensin-converting enzyme inhibitors in renal failure. *J Cardiovasc Pharmacol* 20(Suppl 10):S13–S20, 1992.
66. SmithKline Beecham Pharmaceuticals: *Package insert for Paxil™ brand of paroxetine hydrochloride tablets,* (unpublished data), 1993.
67. Somani P, Freimer EH, Gross ML, Higgins Jr JT: Pharmacokinetics of imipenem-cilastatin in patients with renal insufficiency undergoing continuous ambulatory peritoneal dialysis. *Antimicrob Agents Chemother* 32:530–534, 1988.
68. Wallace SL, Singer JZ, Duncan GJ, Wigley FM, Kuncl RW: Renal function predicts colchicine toxicity: guidelines for the prophylactic use of colchicine in gout. *J Rheumatol* 18:264–269, 1991.
69. Heim-Duthoy KL, Kalil RSN, Kasiske BL: Acute renal failure. In DiPiro JT, Talbert RL, Hayes PE, Yee GC, Matzke GR, Posey LM (eds): *Pharmacotherapy: a Pathophysiologic Approach.* Appleton & Lange, Norwalk, CT, pp 660–672, 1993.
70. Allon M, Copkney C: Albuterol and insulin for treatment of hyperkalemia in hemodialysis patients. *Kidney Int* 38:869–872, 1990.

CHAPTER

4

Pharmacotherapy in Liver Failure[a]

Patients with liver disease are commonly treated with one or more different drugs in an effort to alleviate the numerous pathologic changes often associated with this and/or other concurrent disease processes. Commonly used drugs include diuretics, antibiotics, sedatives, and antiinflammatory, cardiovascular, and cancer chemotherapeutic agents. Of importance are the effects of liver disease on the absorption, distribution, elimination, and pharmacologic response to these drugs. Such changes may require reductions in drug dosage in order to avoid drug toxicity. The understanding of how liver disease can influence drug disposition and dosage requirements entails an appreciation for

1. The various types of functions that the liver performs;
2. The pathologic changes produced by liver disease and how these changes alter hepatic function; and
3. The parameters that influence drug disposition and how they are affected by liver disease.

[a] This chapter was contributed by Cheryl A. Kubisty, M.D., Patricia A. Arns, M.D., Peter J. Wedlund, Ph.D., and Robert A. Branch, M.D.

LIVER FUNCTION IN HEALTH AND DISEASE: IMPLICATIONS FOR DRUG DISPOSITION

HEPATIC FUNCTION

The liver plays an important role in the metabolism and elimination of drugs that may be too lipophilic to be removed efficiently by the kidneys. This function is carried out by a number of different enzymes located in liver cells. For example, one group of isoenzymes, referred to collectively as the cytochromes P-450, is important for carrying out many of the mixed function oxidative reactions that convert lipophilic compounds into more water-soluble products. Other enzymes in the liver may further transform these metabolites (or other drugs) by conjugating them with sugars, amino acids, sulfates, or acetate to form products that can be more readily eliminated in the bile or removed by the kidney. Still other liver enzymes (i.e., esterases, deaminases, hydrolases, and reductases) are important for the metabolic transformation and elimination of certain drugs and endogenous chemicals.

Many of these homeostatic and metabolic functions are compromised when the liver is damaged by different etiologic agents such as chemicals (including drugs) and diseases. The actual degree of damage to liver hemoperfusion, biliary excretion, and synthetic and metabolic functions in the liver can vary widely and therefore lead to variable changes in drug disposition within each disease entity (62, 102). Such changes in drug disposition reflect, to some extent, the degree to which the liver is impaired. For example, alcoholic liver disease can range from fatty liver, with little or no change in the disposition of most drugs, to severe cirrhosis, with major changes in the disposition of certain classes of drugs. Hepatic neoplasms also show great variability in the effect on drug disposition, depending on type (primary versus secondary), size, invasiveness, and vascularity of tumor mass. Moreover, certain acute injuries to the liver, as seen in viral hepatitis, may affect the disposition of some drugs, but this effect may be reversible as the injury subsides.

Hepatic reserves may help to maintain liver functions, and changes in drug metabolism may be slight since few, if any, liver functions are performed at 100% of their capacity (44). For example, under normal conditions, urea formation from ammonia and amino acids occurs at 60% of capacity. Glucose maintenance requires only 20% of liver function. Bilirubin elimination must fall below 10% of normal before jaundice develops, and albumin and clotting factors are synthesized by only a small percentage of the total liver cells at any one time. Furthermore, these and other liver processes may be increased when demand is increased. As a result, it is often difficult to determine the extent of liver damage caused by an agent because reserve and repair mechanisms tend to maintain hepatic function.

Such reserve and recuperative properties are obviously advantageous for the liver. This regenerative capability allows the liver to recover completely following acute liver insult. Even when the damage is extensive, if the causative agent is removed, the liver is capable of full recovery. However, if the etiologic agent is not removed so that the liver becomes exposed to chronic damage, then hepatic reserves may become seriously depleted. A limited repertoire of liver responses to such chronic damage will result in a characteristic pathophysiologic state of cirrhosis. Under such circumstances, significant changes in drug disposition may occur. The level of cytochrome P-450 enzymes in the liver, for example, may decline (37, 65, 143, 147, 159), and this change can seriously impair the liver's ability to metabolize endogenous products and drugs (32, 56, 112, 159, 160). Deterioration in other liver functions (i.e., the removal of bilirubin and fatty acids and the synthesis of plasma proteins) may lead to further alterations in drug disposition by influencing drug binding and distribution in the body (15, 167, 176).

ARCHITECTURE AND BLOOD FLOW IN CIRRHOSIS

The development of cirrhosis begins with initial hepatocellular damage-producing inflammation, followed by phagocytic removal of dead or necrotic cells. This damage stimulates the secretion of collagen by fibroblasts, while the damaged and dead cells are repaired or replaced. As the damage continues, further collagen secretion is coupled with retraction of collagen fibrils. This leads to the formation of bands of connective scar tissue, inducing a deformation of normal architecture characteristic of cirrhosis. In compensation for hepatocellular damage, hepatocyte regeneration may lead to the clustered formation of new hepatocytes, which later form liver nodules. These nodules may increase in size and further distort the normal liver architecture.

As the liver architecture becomes distorted, the resistance to the flow of blood through the liver is increased. This increase, in turn, causes the portal venous pressure to increase. To alleviate an increased pressure, portal venous blood is shunted around the liver through collateral channels directly into the systemic circulation (43). The development of these collateral channels for shunting the portal venous blood occurs primarily where tributaries of the portal venous system lie in close proximity to those of the systemic circulation (i.e., submucosa of the esophagus, stomach, rectum, left renal vein, and abdomen).

The development of collateral channels for the shunting of portal venous blood around the liver can alter the effective hepatic blood flow and the amount of drug reaching the systemic circulation after oral administration (53, 127, 132, 155). These and other changes in drug disposition may require the dosage of some drugs to be reduced.

In addition, recent studies have shown that hepatic disease may also alter the microcirculation of the liver. Sinusoidal plasma in the healthy liver has direct access to the hepatocyte. Although the sinusoid is lined by endothelial cells, this is not a continuous layer; there is an incomplete basal lamina, and endothelial cells contain multiple fenestrations. Between the sinusoidal endothelium and the hepatocyte is the space of Disse, which contains the microvilli of hepatic cells, reticular fibers, and fat storage cells. Alcoholic liver disease is associated with an increase in type III collagen in the space of Disse, formation of a basal lamina, and a decrease in the number of fenestrations and porosity of the endothelial cell as seen with scanning electron microscopy (55, 87, 121, 158). This endothelialization transforms sinusoids into capillary-like channels and limits the access of the contents of sinusoidal blood to the hepatocyte. Studies using multiple indicator dilution techniques support the concept that conversion of loose interendothelial cell junctions to tight endothelial cell junctions may provide a barrier to the movement of molecules into the proximity of the hepatocyte (59–61). This intrahepatic shunting could be of importance in the diffusion of albumin and other large molecules, including protein-bound substances such as drugs, which may result in decreased ability for drug metabolism by the liver.

RENAL FUNCTION

Hemodynamic changes may also be present in the kidneys of patients with liver disease. Renal blood flow has been shown to be decreased in many patients with cirrhosis (137–139). Glomerular filtration rate is variable in cirrhosis, but may be decreased in patients with ascites (76). Moreover, the handling of electrolytes by the kidneys is disturbed in patients with cirrhosis. Renal sodium retention is a well-known phenomenon associated with this disease and contributes to the development of ascites. With progression of liver disease, a number of these factors will further depress kidney function to the point of renal failure (149). It follows that drugs having a major renal route of elimination may have an altered disposition in patients with liver disease, because of the secondary development of functional renal failure.

CHARACTERISTICS OF DRUG DISPOSITION

Whether pathologic changes associated with liver disease require an alteration in a normal drug regimen is determined by the dispositional characteristics of the drug and the biologic determinants of the system (12, 41, 180). Drug disposition, which includes both the distribution and elimination of drug, is determined in part by the physical properties of the drug. Important characteristics include molecular size, charge, pK_a, and lipid solubility. These factors will determine distribution as well as the route of elimination. In general, water-soluble drugs have a small volume of distribution and can be eliminated unchanged in urine, and lipid-soluble drugs have a large volume of distribution and require metabolism to more water-soluble moieties. Depending on the physical characteristics of any given drug, the balance of physiologic factors influencing that drug's disposition will vary. These physiologic factors have the potential to be altered by disease states. Thus, the influence of any one disease process can be complex; it can be mediated by a variety of factors and can influence the disposition of different drugs to a variable extent.

DISTRIBUTION

The major aspects of distribution affected by liver disease are volume of distribution (V_d) and plasma protein binding. Conceptually, the apparent volume of distribution is the volume into which a drug distributes in the body when it is at equilibrium and is related to the pool from which the drug concentration is measured. It is a theoretical concept and reflects the partitioning of drug between the fluid compartments in the body (e.g., plasma, interstitial fluid, and intracellular fluid). It is calculated by the equation:

$$V_d = D/Cp \qquad (1)$$

where D represents the fraction of the dose absorbed and Cp is drug concentration at equilibrium. One way that liver disease can affect the V_d is by the production of ascites, which may produce an increase in the body's total fluid compartment. For example, propranolol has been shown to exhibit a 2-fold increase in V_d in patients with ascites, regardless of the extent of protein binding (18).

Most drugs in plasma are reversibly bound to proteins, such as albumin, globulin, α-1-acid glycoprotein, lipoproteins, ceruloplasmin, and transferrin. Acidic drugs commonly bind to albumin, whereas basic drugs more commonly bind to α-1-acid glycoprotein. Only unbound drug is available for distribution into tissues and capable of evoking a pharmacologic response (68, 82, 84, 126, 150). The extent of protein binding is therefore important in determining both pharmacologic response and drug disposition.

Cirrhosis causes a number of alterations that can also influence the binding of drugs within the blood, including (*a*) a decrease in serum albumin levels, (*b*) the appearance of altered or defective plasma proteins, and (*c*) the accumulation of endogenous and exogenous compounds that can displace drugs from protein binding sites. For example, acute viral hepatitis or primary biliary cirrhosis can lead to elevated serum bilirubin levels. The strong affinity of bilirubin for protein binding sites on albumin and the elevated levels are in part responsible for the displacement of some acidic drugs from the protein (15, 167, 182). Taken together, these factors can produce alterations in drug binding to proteins and in the unbound serum drug concentrations. As a result, changes may occur in drug distribution and elimination and pharmacologic response.

With a decrease in drug binding to plasma or blood proteins, more drug may become available for distribution into tissues, increasing the drug's apparent volume of distribution. This change can alter the drug's elimination half-life independently of any change in drug metabolism. The reason for this change is apparent from the dependence of the half-life ($t_{1/2}$) on both its total clearance from the blood (Cl) and its apparent volume of distribution (V_d), according to the equation:

$$t_{1/2} = 0.693\ V_d / Cl \qquad (2)$$

As a result of this dependence, the half-life of a drug can be a misleading parameter when one is attempting to determine the effect(s) of liver disease on drug elimination. For example, an increase in the apparent volume of distribution of a drug may lead to a prolongation in its elimination half-life in the absence of any real change in metabolic drug elimination. An example of this phenomenon is the increase in the half-life of lorazepam (79) in patients with liver disease. This prolongation has been explained entirely by an increase in drug distribution secondary to decreased plasma binding, rather than by a reduction in clearance.

In addition to influencing drug distribution, changes in protein binding can influence drug elimination. A change in the free fraction of a drug in the blood can lead to an increase in the

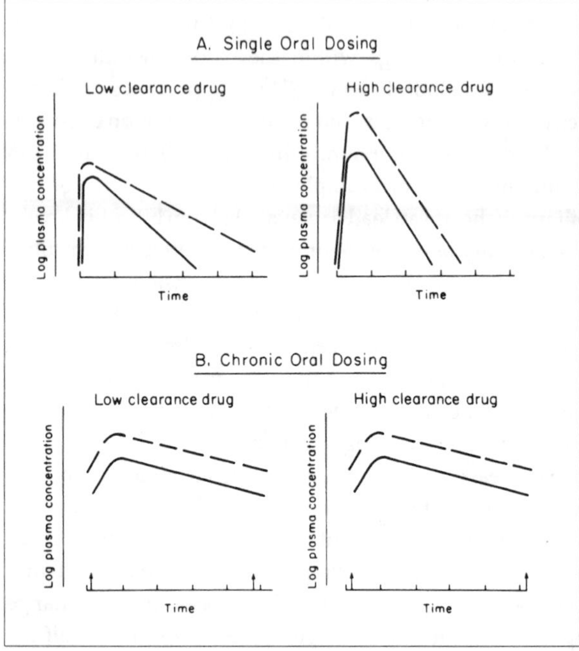

FIGURE 4.1. The effects of single (**A**) and chronic (**B**) oral dosing on low-clearance (enzyme-limited) and high-clearance (flow-limited) drugs in patients with cirrhosis (*dashed lines*) and in normal subjects (*solid lines*). *Arrows* indicate dosage interval for chronic dosing graphs.

amount of drug available to the drug-metabolizing enzymes and therefore to an increase in the total clearance of some drugs. This increase can shorten the half-life of a drug in the absence of any change in the activity of drug-metabolizing enzymes. Indeed, the decrease in the half-life of tolbutamide (182) in acute viral hepatitis has been attributed solely to a decrease in its binding to plasma proteins, since it has been shown that even though total (free + bound) clearance of tolbutamide increases, protein binding decreases and free clearance remains unchanged.

The effect of protein binding on drug disposition is difficult to predict. At present, there are no guidelines for predicting the effect of liver disease on drug binding. However, two general rules may provide some insight into the more important factors influencing the extent of change: (*a*) If protein binding is altered by a particular liver disease, the degree of liver damage will influence the extent of change in drug binding to plasma proteins. (*b*) Changes in the extent of binding to plasma proteins will tend to be greater for extensively bound drugs (i.e., >60% bound) than for poorly bound drugs (i.e., <60% bound). Although these are general rules that have their exceptions, they should provide some appreciation for the effects of liver disease on plasma protein binding.

ELIMINATION

Elimination of drug is defined as the irreversible loss of drug from the site of measurement and includes both metabolism and excretion. Clearance is an important parameter that relates drug concentration to the rate of elimination, thereby providing a measure of efficiency of the elimination process. By definition, total or systemic clearance is a measure of the amount of plasma cleared of drug per unit time. This measure can be obtained from measurements of drug concentration in plasma after single doses (Equation 2) or at steady state:

$$Cl = rate\ of\ drug\ administration/Cp_{ss} \qquad (3)$$

where Cp_{ss} is the steady-state plasma concentration. Clearance is independent of the mechanism of elimination involved, and if multiple routes of elimination occur concurrently, it provides an estimate of the sum of these processes.

When the rate of elimination is proportional to the amount of drug present, this is known as a first-order process. Clearance of drug is constant (linear) over a range of concentrations. Not all drugs undergo first-order kinetics; however, in some instances dose-dependent elimination occurs. Clearance in these cases is nonlinear and will vary depending on the achieved concentration of drug.

Clearance can also be described as the efficiency of removal of drug across an organ of elimination, the two major organs being liver and kidney. Hepatic clearance, (Cl_H), reflects the efficiency with which the liver irreversibly removes drug from the blood. It is determined by both the fraction of drug removed or extracted *(E)* from the blood during passage through the liver and the liver blood flow (Q_H). The relationship between these parameters is given by the equation:

$$Cl_H = Q_H E \quad (4)$$

Drugs that are given orally must first pass through the liver before reaching the systemic circulation. If hepatic enzymes extract drug from the blood as it passes through, then the fraction *(F)* of the total dose entering the general circulation is reduced. For drugs that are completely absorbed from the gastrointestinal tract, this fraction *F* (or bioavailability) is determined from the drug's extraction *(E)* by the liver according to the equation:

$$F = 1 - E \quad (5)$$

The ability of the liver to extract a drug is, in turn, dependent on three separate factors: (*a*) the intrinsic activity of metabolic enzymes and transport processes within the liver that irreversibly remove drug from the blood, (*b*) the fraction of total drug in blood that is free to interact with enzymes responsible for its elimination, and (*c*) the rate at which drug passes or flows through the liver (129, 144, 179).

The irreversible removal of drug from the blood may be carried out by a number of separate enzymes in the liver. For simplicity, however, the elimination process is often considered as if it results only from a single enzyme system. Thus, metabolic and transport processes responsible for drug removal by the liver, defined as the free intrinsic drug clearance (Cl^u_{int}) can be described by a simple Michaelis-Menten equation as:

$$Cl^u_{int} = V_{max} / (K_m + C^u_L) \quad (6)$$

where V_{max} represents the maximal rate of irreversible drug elimination by all liver enzymes, K_m is the Michaelis-Menten constant for the overall enzymatic removal process, and C^u_L is the concentration of unbound or free drug in liver.

The second factor that can contribute to the extraction of a drug by the liver is the free fraction of drug in blood (f_B). If the unbound fraction of total drug in the blood changes, then the free drug concentration at the site of elimination will also change. For some drugs, changes in binding can alter hepatic extraction by metabolic and transport enzymes in the liver.

Finally, the total amount of drug extracted by the liver is dependent on the rate at which the drug is delivered to the enzymes responsible for its elimination. This rate of delivery is determined by the liver blood flow (Q_H) perfusing functional hepatocytes. If intrinsic clearance is high, flow becomes the rate-limiting factor, and reductions in flow will not change hepatic extraction but rather will reduce hepatic clearance. If, on the other hand, intrinsic clearance is low, then as flow is decreased, hepatic extraction will increase and hepatic clearance will not be influenced by blood flow.

The relationship of the extraction (E) of a drug by the liver with its free intrinsic clearance (Cl^u_{int}), free fraction in the blood (f_B), and the total effective liver blood flow (Q_H) is given by the equation:

$$E = f_B Cl^u_{int} / (Q_H + f_B Cl^u_{int}) \quad (7)$$

If Equation 7 is now substituted into Equation 4, which defines hepatic clearance, the expression obtained relates hepatic clearance with three variables: f_B, Q_H, and Cl^u_{int}. Thus, hepatic clearance may be written as:

$$Cl_H = Q_H E = Q_H f_B Cl^u_{int} / (Q_H + f_B Cl^u_{int}) \quad (8)$$

Although these relationships may appear complex, it is important to recognize that hepatic clearance is determined by only these three physiologic variables, each of which can be changed independently by liver disease. The effect on drug disposition of any one of these variables can be anticipated by knowing the relative importance of each of these variables to that drug's disposition. This concept has been used to provide a framework for the classification of drugs into a system in which those drugs sharing a rate-limiting characteristic are grouped together.

DRUGS CLASSIFIED BY DISPOSITIONAL CHARACTERISTICS

Flow-limited Drugs. When the total intrinsic clearance ($f_B Cl^u_{int}$) of a drug is large relative to liver blood flow (Q_H), such that $E > 0.6$, hepatic clearance of the drug becomes dependent on liver blood flow (Equation 8). The rate at which the liver is able to remove these drugs from the blood is limited by their rate of presentation to the liver. Theoretically, metabolism and protein binding should not affect hepatic clearance of these drugs. Accordingly, this class of drugs is referred to as blood flow-limited and is sensitive to factors that can alter the effective liver blood flow. It should be noted that if the disease process reduces the intrinsic clearance so that it is less than the liver blood flow, the drug will lose its flow-sensitive characteristics.

Enzyme-limited Drugs. When the total intrinsic clearance of a drug is small relative to liver blood flow, such that $E < 0.2$, hepatic clearance becomes essentially dependent on the intrinsic activity of liver enzymes (Equation 8). Factors that influence the ability of the liver enzymes to remove drug become more important in altering drug elimination than changes in liver blood flow. Drugs with this characteristic belong to the class referred to as enzyme limited. This class is further subdivided according to the extent of protein binding.

Enzyme-limited, Binding-insensitive Drugs. For enzyme-limited drugs with low binding to plasma or blood proteins (i.e., <50% bound), a change in plasma protein binding is not an important factor in altering hepatic drug elimination (Equation 8). This drug class is most affected by factors that change the level or activity of liver enzymes (Cl^{u}_{int}) responsible for their elimination. Drugs with these characteristics are referred to as enzyme-limited and binding-insensitive.

Enzyme-limited, Binding-sensitive Drugs. For enzyme-limited drugs that are extensively bound to plasma or blood proteins (i.e., >85% bound), hepatic clearance is sensitive to changes in protein binding in the blood (f_B) and/or liver enzyme activity (Cl^{u}_{int}). Drugs with these characteristics are referred to as enzyme-limited and binding-sensitive. Factors that may alter binding to proteins in the blood or the activity of liver enzymes responsible for drug elimination influence the hepatic clearance of these drugs.

Flow/Enzyme-sensitive Drugs. A drug may not be extensively bound or poorly extracted by the liver, but fall somewhere between the flow-limited and enzyme-limited classes. The clearance of these drugs from the blood may be sensitive to changes in liver blood flow, intrinsic clearance by the liver, and, in some cases, binding to plasma proteins (Equation 8). Drugs with these characteristics are referred to as flow and enzyme sensitive.

Drugs are classified according to this scheme to help provide a better appreciation of the importance of pathophysiologic changes produced by liver disease in altering drug disposition. Certain biologic determinants of metabolism (i.e., disease or genetic predisposition) may change the classification of a given drug for an individual.

It is now known that some people have genetic defects in the metabolism of certain drugs. Fast and slow acetylators of isoniazid have been recognized since the 1950s. More recently, independent genetic polymorphisms have been found for a number of other drugs metabolized by different oxidative enzymes. Poor and extensive metabolizers of debrisoquine, an antihypertensive agent (154), and mephenytoin, an anticonvulsant, are representative examples of two independent routes of oxidative metabolism mediated by cytochrome P-450 $2D_6$ and cytochrome P-450 $2C_{MP}$, respectively. Not only will the effect of liver disease have a greater effect on the clearance of this drug in extensive metabolizers than in poor metabolizers, but the effect of factors such as development of portal-systemic shunts will have a marked influence on systemic availability in extensive but not in poor metabolizer subjects.

INFLUENCE OF LIVER DISEASE ON DRUG DISPOSITION

As mentioned previously, both dispositional characteristics of a drug and biologic determinants of the system involved are important in determining the effects of liver disease on ultimate drug disposition. In the following sections, the effects of liver disease on each of these factors are discussed.

ROUTE OF ELIMINATION

Since there are multiple routes of elimination, only some of which involve the liver, it is important to determine which route is utilized for a given drug. For a drug that is excreted unchanged by the kidney, liver disease should have no effect on disposition, provided that there is no secondary or concomitant renal disease.

There is a strong relationship between the proportion of the drug that is eliminated following oxidative metabolism by the liver and the percentage of decrease in its free clearance caused by cirrhosis. Thus, liver disease has the greatest effect on those drugs that undergo extensive oxidative metabolism.

ROUTE OF METABOLISM

For drugs that are metabolized by the liver, the route of metabolism is also important in determining the effects of liver disease on drug disposition. All metabolic pathways are not affected equally by liver disease. For example, the elimination of lorazepam, morphine, and oxazepam, which are metabolized primarily by conjugation with glucuronic acid, is generally unaltered by liver disease, except in decompensated liver disease (57, 79, 124, 152, 156). The reason for this is unknown. It may reflect the sparing of conjugative pathways of drug metabolism in the liver during liver disease and/or the importance of other organs to the elimination of drugs by this route. This preservation contrasts with reductions in clearance of drugs that are eliminated by oxidative metabolism.

ROUTES AND DURATION OF DRUG ADMINISTRATION

The effect of liver disease on drug disposition is determined by (*a*) the route of drug administration, (*b*) the class to which the drug belongs (i.e., flow-limited, flow/enzyme-sensitive, or enzyme-limited), and (*c*) duration of drug administration.

As noted previously, drugs that are taken orally, unlike those administered intravenously or intramuscularly, pass through the liver before reaching the systemic circulation and target tissues. This provides an opportunity for presystemic elimination, particularly for flow-limited drugs, with their high hepatic extractions, which normally have a low bioavailability. For flow-limited drugs, liver disease may increase their bioavailability. This increased bioavailability is partially explained by a decrease in the efficiency of drug extraction by liver enzymes.

Another important factor contributing to this increase is the rerouting of blood from the portal vein through intrahepatic and extrahepatic portal-systemic shunts in response to portal hypertension caused by liver disease. In severely cirrhotic patients, this shunting may involve 60% or more of portal venous blood flow (46, 163, 164). This shunting allows a large amount of an orally administered drug to bypass the liver altogether and enter the systemic circulation directly. As a result of the changes in bioavailability of flow-limited drugs, peak blood concentrations following single oral dose administration are substantially higher in patients with cirrhosis than in normal subjects (Fig. 4.1). In contrast, the bioavailability of enzyme-limited drugs is high in normal subjects and remains unaffected in liver disease. Thus, peak concentrations following single oral dose administration are the same in cirrhotic and normal subjects (Fig. 4.1).

The case is somewhat different for chronic oral therapy: drug blood levels accumulate to an approximately steady-state situation that is dependent on drug clearance, the fraction of the dose that reaches the systemic circulation, and the dosage interval (Equation 3). Reductions in clearance resulting from liver disease create the potential for excessive drug accumulation during chronic therapy for both flow-limited and enzyme-limited drugs (Fig. 4.1). This may require dosage reduction in order to obtain the desired therapeutic objective.

In summary, the influence of liver disease on drug disposition is a function of how a drug is handled in healthy subjects. For flow-limited drugs, initial blood concentrations following intravenous or intramuscular administration can be expected to be similar in cirrhotic and normal subjects, whereas peak blood concentrations are higher in cirrhotic patients after single oral dose administration or at steady state during chronic therapy. In contrast, enzyme-limited drugs can be expected to have similar initial blood concentrations after both intravenous and single oral dose administration in cirrhotic and normal subjects, but increased blood concentrations at steady state during chronic therapy in cirrhotic subjects.

SEVERITY OF LIVER DISEASE

The type and severity of liver disease are variables that influence drug disposition. Not all drugs that undergo extensive oxidative metabolism are affected to an equal extent by all liver diseases. Acute viral hepatitis, for example, has no effect on the metabolic elimination (Cl^{u}_{int}) of tolbutamide, warfarin, diphenylhydantoin, or antipyrine (15, 36, 80, 182, 183), whereas it does produce changes in metabolic elimination of hexobarbital, meperidine, and chlordiazepoxide (178). These observations might reflect differences in the degree to which different oxidative pathways of drug elimination are affected by liver disease, but more likely reflect the differences in the severity of the disease process in patients used for the separate studies. Thus, it may not be possible to find any change in the metabolic elimination of drugs in patients with mild or moderate forms of hepatitis. Certainly, the levels of cytochrome P-450 drug-metabolizing enzymes are not altered in liver biopsies from such patients (37). With more extensive liver damage from viral hepatitis or other causes, the level of these enzymes declines (37, 147). This decline should cause a decrease in the free intrinsic clearance of those drugs that are oxidatively metabolized in the liver by this enzyme system (95).

DRUG INTERACTIONS IN LIVER DISEASE

Patients with liver disease are often on a multidrug regimen. Certain drugs are well-known to affect drug metabolism either by induction or inhibition of metabolic enzymes.

Phenobarbital, pentobarbital, tolbutamide, and phenytoin act as metabolic inducers, increasing the synthesis of metabolic enzymes. The administration of enzyme-inducing drugs to patients with moderate liver disease may offset the disease-induced decrease in cytochrome P-450 enzymes. This effect, however, is limited. With an increase in the severity of liver damage, liver reserves may become too depressed for drug administration to exert much of an effect on either the level or activity of these enzymes (37, 159).

Cimetidine, on the other hand, a drug commonly used in the treatment of patients with alcoholic liver disease, has been shown to decrease total plasma clearance of theophylline (161), chlordiazepoxide (106), as well as numerous other drugs, in both control and cirrhotic subjects. It is believed that cimetidine interferes with oxidative metabolism but does not alter hepatic blood flow (106). Consequently, patients with liver disease may have an additional risk of impaired drug metabolism. The study by Nelson and colleagues (106) showed the decrease in plasma clearance of chlordiazepoxide to be greater in the control group than in the cirrhotic group, suggesting that the greater the initial microsomal function, the greater the effect of an inhibitor. However, it should be emphasized that this further decrease in drug metabolism may still be of importance in a patient with liver disease who may already have decreased metabolic function.

RECOMMENDATIONS FOR DOSAGE ADJUSTMENTS

As seen from the discussion of pharmacokinetic considerations in liver disease, it is not easy to predict the effect of disease on drug disposition in individual patients. Although severity of disease seems to play a major role in distribution and elimination of a drug, there is no good predictor of hepatic function. Despite a considerable effort by a number of investigators (8, 14, 30, 130, 151), there is no useful noninvasive test of liver function to guide dosage adjustments (12, 180). The best that can be said for most of the so-called liver function tests (i.e., serum albumin, prothrombin time, bilirubin, serum glutamic-oxaloacetic and glutamic-pyruvic transaminases (SGOT and SGPT), alkaline phosphatase, etc.) is that they reflect but do not predict the extent of liver damage (44).

Measuring cytochrome P-450 enzyme levels from liver biopsies might be expected to provide a better measure of the degree to which oxidative drug metabolism in the liver has been damaged. The level of these enzymes, however, has not been found to be a useful predictor of the metabolic elimination of drugs by this organ (95, 159). One explanation for the poor predictive value is that this measure fails to account for total hepatic size (130).

Some measures do exist that correlate with drug clearance, such as tests of antipyrine (160), aminopyrine, and indocyanine green clearance; however, these studies are not usually conducted as part of a patient's routine clinical evaluation. Moreover, the correlation coefficients usually approximate only 0.6 in most studies, accounting for only 40% or less of variance. Therefore, a good predictor of hepatic function or drug clearance has not been found; and at the present time, there is not a good hepatic counterpart for glomerular filtration rate, which is a reliable indicator of renal function.

Before considering the influence of liver disease on drug dosage requirements, some mention must be made of the use of drugs in general. There are always risks associated with the use of any drugs, and these risks may become particularly pronounced in patients with liver disease. In a prospective drug-monitoring study of more than 2000 patients, Naranjo and colleagues (103, 104) found the frequency of adverse drug reactions (ADRs) to be higher in patients with cirrhosis than in those with renal disease, other liver diseases, or neither liver nor renal disease. In the group of cirrhotic patients, the frequency of ADRs was significantly correlated with the severity of liver dysfunction as measured by a composite clinical and laboratory index. Thus, consideration should be given to whether the drug is really needed and whether its benefits outweigh the risks. For example, the use of some drugs in patients with liver disease is associated with a particularly high risk, and they should be used with great caution or not at all in these patients (Table 4.1). In general, the drugs listed in Table 4.1 fall into three categories: (*a*) drugs capable of causing liver damage even in normal patients, (*b*) drugs that can further compromise depressed liver functions often found in liver disease patients, and (*c*) drugs that can make the complications of liver disease worse. In the above-cited study, diuretics were found to be the most common cause of ADRs and to cause the most severe reactions.

If drug treatment is required and alternatives are available, it is preferable to use a drug whose disposition is least affected by the liver disease (e.g., a drug that is excreted renally or metabolized by glucuronidation). If a drug must be prescribed that may be affected by the disease process, then a number of factors must be considered, including (*a*) the extent of liver damage, (*b*) the degree of hepatic elimination of the drug, (*c*) the degree of protein binding, (*d*) the class to which the drug belongs (i.e., enzyme-limited, flow/enzyme-sensitive, or flow-limited), (*e*) the route of administration, and (*f*) the duration of administration.

A considerable amount of information has been gathered over the years regarding disposition of specific drugs in liver disease. Most of this work has been done in cirrhosis, a lesser amount in acute viral hepatitis, and very little in other types of liver disease. To help the clinician, Table 4.2 presents a compilation of the dispositional characteristics of a number of drugs in normal subjects, the route of elimination of these drugs, the effect of liver disease on their disposition, and recommendations for adjustment of dose.

For drugs not listed in Table 4.2, general guidelines for dosage adjustment are given in Table 4.3. Although these considerations may not be all-inclusive, they should provide some guidance as to the extent of dosage change required with liver disease.

TABLE 4.1. Drugs That Should Be Used with Caution or Not at All in Liver Disease Patients

Group I: Drugs capable of causing hepatic damage
Acetaminophen
Acetylsalicylic acid
Chlorpromazine
Erythromycin estolate
Methotrexate
Methyldopa
Group II: Drugs that can compromise liver functions
Anabolic and contraceptive steroids
Prednisone (in acute viral hepatitis)
Tetracycline
Group III: Drugs that may make complications of liver disease worse
Cyclooxygenase inhibitors (indomethacin)
Diuretics
Meperidine and other CNS depressants
Morphine
Pentazocine
Phenylbutazone

TABLE 4.2. The Dispositional Characteristics in Normal Subjects and in Patients with Liver Disease, Routes of Elimination, and Recommendations for Dose Adjustment for a Variety of Drugs[a]

Drug	*Protein Binding (%)*	*Volume of Distribution (V_d) (liter/kg)*	*Half-life ($t_{1/2}$) (h)*	*Clearance (Cl) (ml/min)*	*Class*	*Hepatic/Renal Elimination*	*Effect of Liver Disease on Drug Disposition*	*Adjustment of Dose*	*References*
Antibiotic/Antiviral/Antifungal									
Amantadine	—	4.75	20.0	190	—	<10% Hepatic >90% Renal	Negligible unless renal function decreased	None	
Amikacin	5	0.26	2.5	85	—	<5% Hepatic >95% Renal	Negligible unless renal function decreased	None	
Ampicillin	30	0.28	1.0	340	—	<10% Hepatic >90% Renal	$t_{1/2}$ ↑; V_d ↑; Cl →; f_p ? →	None	83
Aztreonam	56	0.15	1.9	70	—	33% Hepatobiliary 66% Renal	$t_{1/2}$ ↑; V_d →; Cl →	Decrease if chronic, high-dosing	86
Carbenicillin	48	0.16	1.0	130	—	<10% Hepatic >90% Renal	Negligible unless renal function decreased	None	52
Cefaclor	24	0.35	1.0	280	—	<10% Hepatic >90% Renal	Negligible unless renal function decreased	None	
Cefamandole	74	0.16	1.0	130	—	<5% Hepatic >95% Renal	Negligible unless renal function decreased	None	
Cefazolin	84	0.15	1.8	68	—	<5% Hepatic >95% Renal	$t_{1/2}$ ↓ ; f_p ↑	None	113

Cefoperazone	90 non-linear	0.20	1.7	80	Enzyme-limited, binding-sensitive	75% Hepatic 25% Renal	$t_{1/2}$ ↑; V_d →; Cl ↓ 60%; f_p ?	Decrease dose	16, 17
Cefotaxime	36	0.24	1.2	94	—	40% Hepatic 60% Renal	$t_{1/2}$ ↑; V_d ?; Cl ?	Unknown	98
Cefotetan	83	0.15	3.7	39.5	—	80% Renal 20% Biliary (unchanged)	Negligible unless renal function decreased	None	
Cefoxitin	73	0.12	1.0	98	—	15% Hepatic 85% Renal	Negligible unless renal function decreased	None	
Ceftazidime	17	0.2	1.7	75	—	10% Hepatic 90% Renal	$t_{1/2}$ ↑; V_d ?; Cl slight ↓	Negligible unless renal function decreased	123
Ceftriaxone	90	0.14	8.4	16	Enzyme-limited, binding-sensitive	60% Hepatobiliary 40% Renal	$t_{1/2}$ →; V_d ↑ if ascites present; Cl →; fp ↑	None	162
Cefuroxime	30	0.33	1.2	210	—	<1% Hepatic >99% Renal	Negligible unless renal function decreased	None	117
Cephalothin	75	0.30	0.60	470	—	30–50% Hepatic 50–70% Renal	$t_{1/2}$ slight ↑; V_d→; Cl ↓	None	113
Chloramphenicol	70	1.0	3.0	170	Enzyme-limited, binding-sensitive	>90% Hepatic <10% Renal Glucuronidation of drug	$t_{1/2}$ ↑; V_d slight ↓; Cl ↓ 65%; f_p ? →; unknown if f_p changes	Decrease dose	101
Ciprofloxacin	30	2.3	4.0	350	—	40% Renal (unchanged) 15% Hepatic	Negligible unless renal function decreased	None	145, 97

TABLE 4.2. *(Continued)*

Drug	*Protein Binding (%)*	*Volume of Distribution (V_d) (liter/kg)*	*Half-life ($t_{1/2}$) (h)*	*Clearance (Cl) (ml/min)*	*Class*	*Hepatic/Renal Elimination*	*Effect of Liver Disease on Drug Disposition*	*Adjustment of Dose*	*References*
Clindamycin	79	0.58	2.0	160	Enzyme-limited, binding-sensitive	90% Hepatic 10% Renal	$t_{1/2}$ slight ↑; V_d →; Cl ↓ 23%; f_p →	Decrease dose in severe cases	10, 51
Doxycycline	82	—	12.0	195	—	<10% Hepatic >90% Renal	Negligible unless renal function decreased	None	
Erythromycin	80	0.77	1.6	600	Enzyme-limited, binding-sensitive	>90% Hepatic <10% Renal	$t_{1/2}$ ↑; no other information	Decrease dose in moderate or severe disease	48, 81
Fluconazole	12	0.8	35	20	—	70% Renal (unchanged) 10% Hepatic	Negligible unless renal function decreased	None	63
Ganciclovir	2	0.5	3.0	185/ 1.73m^2	—	>90% Renal (unchanged)	Negligible unless renal function decreased	None	
Gentamicin	<5	0.25	2.0	100	—	<5% Hepatic >95% Renal	Negligible unless renal function decreased	None	
Imipenem	25	0.33	1.1	186	—	70% Renal (unchanged) 25% Nonspecific hydrolysis	Negligible unless renal function decreased	None	

Isoniazid	<10	0.6	2.0 fast 6.0 slow	480 fast 170 slow	Enzyme-limited, binding-insensitive	85% Hepatic 15% Renal Drug acetylated	$t_{1/2}$ ↑; some assume Cl ↓; genetic differences more important than disease	Decrease dose in severe cases	3
Kanamycin	<10	0.20	3.0	55	—	<5% Hepatic >95% Renal	Negligible unless renal function decreased	None	
Metronidazole	10	0.75	8.0	85	—	>90% Hepatic <10% Renal	$t_{1/2}$ ↑; V_d ↓; Cl ↓	Decrease dose	29, 35
Nafcillin	90	0.4	1.0	580	Enzyme-limited, binding-sensitive	70% Hepatic 30% Renal	$t_{1/2}$ ↑ but little change; V_d ↓; Cl ↓ 50–60%; fp ?→	Decrease dose in moderate or severe disease	90
Neomycin	40	—	2.0	—	—	<5% Hepatic >95% Renal	Negligible unless renal function decreased	None	
Rifampin	85	0.4	2.5	180	Enzyme-limited, binding-sensitive	90% Hepatic 10% Renal	$t_{1/2}$ ↑; V_d ?; Cl ↓; f_p ?	Decrease in severe disease	72, 134
Streptomycin	35	0.26	2.5	85	—	<5% Hepatic >95% Renal	Negligible unless renal function decreased	None	
Sulfamethoxazole	66	0.17	9.0	15	Enzyme-limited, binding-sensitive	70% Hepatic 30% Renal Drug acetylated	Unknown, but probably little change unless there is severe liver disease	Slight decrease	
Tobramycin	<5	0.24	2.5	80	—	<5% Hepatic >95% Renal	Negligible unless renal function decreased	None	

TABLE 4.2. *(Continued)*

Drug	*Protein Binding (%)*	*Volume of Distribution (V_d) (liter/kg)*	*Half-life ($t_{1/2}$) (h)*	*Clearance (Cl) (ml/min)*	*Class*	*Hepatic/Renal Elimination*	*Effect of Liver Disease on Drug Disposition*	*Adjustment of Dose*	*References*
Trimethoprim	45	1.5	12.0	96	—	30% Hepatic 70% Renal	Slight unless renal function decreased	None	
Vancomycin	55	0.4	5.0	80	—	<10% Hepatic >90% Renal	$t_{1/2}$ ↑; V_d →; Cl ↓	Decrease dose	21
Zidovudine	36	1.6	1.1	1900	Flow-limited	14% Renal (unchanged) 74% Hepatic	$t_{1/2}$, Cl, V_d	Decrease dose	165
Analgesic									
Acetaminophen	20	0.9	2.2	350	Flow/enzyme-sensitive	>95% Hepatic <5% Renal Mostly conjugated	$t_{1/2}$ ↑; V_d ?; Cl ↓ 54%; assume f_p →; little change in Cl if albumin >3.5 g/100 ml	Avoid chronic use; single dose—no change	9, 39, 153
Meperidine	65	4.5	4.5	900	Flow/enzyme-sensitive	>95% Hepatic <5% Renal	$t_{1/2}$ ↑; V_d →; Cl ↓ 50%; f_p →	Decrease oral dose by 50% in cirrhosis or acute viral hepatitis	105, 133
Methadone	80	4.0	28	150	Enzyme-limited, binding-sensitive	80% Hepatic 20% Renal	$t_{1/2}$ ↑ with severe liver disease; Cl →; V_d ↑ slightly	None or decrease	107, 108

Morphine	35	3.7	2.0	1200	Flow-limited	90% GI tract and liver, 10% renal Extensive glucuronidation	$t_{1/2}$ →; V_d →; Cl →; f_p →, by some reports f_p ↑	None, but avoid in severe liver disease	119, 124, 125
Pentazocine	65	5.4	4.5	1000	Flow-limited	>95% Hepatic <5% Renal	$t_{1/2}$ ↑; V_d →; Cl ↓ 50%	Decrease oral dose by ⅔	105, 132
Propoxyphene	75	16	12	1200	Flow-limited	>95% GI tract and liver; <2% renal	$t_{1/2}$ ↑ slightly; V_d ?; Cl ↓ 25%; f_p →	Decrease oral dose by 50%	42
Anticancer									
Adriamycin	50	2.5	20	100	Enzyme-limited, binding-insensitive	>95% Hepatic <5% Renal Most biliary Active metabolite	$t_{1/2}$ ↑; V_d ?; Cl ?; f_p ?, assume f_p →	Unknown	13
Bleomycin	0	0.3	2.0	120	—	40% Hepatic 60% Renal	Unknown; probably not altered greatly	None ? Perhaps decrease	
Cyclophosphamide	14	0.6	5.0	120	Enzyme-limited, binding-insensitive	90% Hepatic 10% Renal Active metabolite	$t_{1/2}$ ↑; V_d ?→; Cl ↓ 43%; f_p ?→	Unknown	70, 175
Cytosine arabinoside	13	2.5	2.5	800	—	Extensive extrahepatic elimination; 40% renal	No data; probably little effect	None	
Etoposide	—	.28	5.6	39	—	65% Hepatic 35% Renal	$t_{1/2}$ →; V_d →; Cl →	None	31, 49
5-Fluorouracil	—	0.5	0.1	—	Flow-limited	Hepatic and extrahepatic; <5% Renal	Some decrease in clearance expected	Probable slight decrease	

TABLE 4.2. *(Continued)*

Drug	*Protein Binding (%)*	*Volume of Distribution (V_d) (liter/kg)*	*Half-life ($t_{1/2}$) (h)*	*Clearance (Cl) (ml/min)*	*Class*	*Hepatic/Renal Elimination*	*Effect of Liver Disease on Drug Disposition*	*Adjustment of Dose*	*References*
Methotrexate	50	0.5	9.0	80	—	15% Hepatic; mostly biliary; 85% Renal	No data; probably little effect. Drug is hepatotoxic and should be avoided if possible.	None	
Antiepileptic									
Carbamazepine	75	1.1	18.0 induced	—	Enzyme-limited, binding-sensitive	>98% Hepatic <2% Renal	No data; expect a decrease in clearance and increase in $t_{1/2}$	Probably decrease dose	
Diphenylhydantoin	92	0.65	15.0 nonlinear	40	Enzyme-limited, binding-sensitive	>95% Hepatic <5% Renal	AVH $t_{1/2}$ →; Cl →; f_p ↑. Cirrhosis f_p ↑	Decrease dose in moderate to severe liver disease	15, 119
Phenobarbital	50	0.8	100	8	Enzyme-limited, binding-insensitive	75% Hepatic 25% Renal	$t_{1/2}$ ↑; presumed Cl ↓	Decrease with severe liver disease	7
Valproic acid	89 nonlinear	12	0.14	30	Enzyme-limited, binding-sensitive	>98% Hepatic <25% Renal	$t_{1/2}$ ↑; V_d slightly ↑; Cl ↓ 40%; f_p ↑	Decrease dose	88

Antipyretic/ Antiinflammatory									
Antipyrine	<10	0.58	12	50	Enzyme-limited, binding-insensitive	92% Hepatic 8% Renal	$t_{1/2}$ ↑; V_d ↑ or →; *Cl* ↓ 60% or more, but actual decrease in *Cl* depends on disease	Not used clinically	23, 34, 54, 64, 80, 93, 96, 100, 130, 157, 159, 166
Dexameth-asone	68	0.75	3.25	260	Flow/enzyme-sensitive	>97% Hepatic <3% Renal	f_p→; V_d →; $t_{1/2}$ ↑; *Cl* ↓	Decrease dose	71
Fenprofen	>99	0.10	1.5	200	Enzyme-limited, binding-sensitive	>98% Hepatic <2% Renal	No data; would expect *fp* ↑; $t_{1/2}$ ↑; *Cl* ↑ or →	Decrease dose	
Ibuprofen	>99	0.15 *V* area *F*	2.0	52	Enzyme-limited, binding-sensitive	>99% Hepatic <1% Renal	$t_{1/2}$ slightly ↑ in severe LD; V_d ?; *Cl* ?	Decrease in severe liver disease if high doses	69
Indomethacin	90	0.17	8.0	125	Enzyme-limited, binding-sensitive	>98% Hepatic <2% Renal	$t_{1/2}$ ↑; no other information. Assume *Cl* ↓, f_p ↑	Decrease dose as required	50
Naproxen	99.6	0.10	14.0	5	Enzyme-limited, binding-sensitive	>90% Hepatic <10% Renal	$t_{1/2}$ ↑; V_d →; *Cl* ↓ 28%; f_p ?	Decrease dose in moderate to severe disease	24, 184
Phenylbu-tazone	98.5	0.17	70	2	Enzyme-limited, binding-sensitive	>99% Hepatic <1% Renal	$t_{1/2}$ ↑ or →; f_p ↑ ; V_d ?; *Cl* ? Assume *Cl* ↓ with liver disease	Decrease dose	20

TABLE 4.2. *(Continued)*

Drug	Protein Binding (%)	Volume of Distribution (V_d) (liter/kg)	Half-life ($t_{1/2}$) (h)	Clearance (Cl) (ml/min)	Class	Hepatic/Renal Elimination	Effect of Liver Disease on Drug Disposition	Adjustment of Dose	References
Prednisolone	80	0.6	3.0	180	Enzyme-limited, binding-sensitive	>85% Hepatic <15% Renal	$t_{1/2}$ →; V_d →; Cl →; f_p → or ↑. Drug little affected by liver disease.	None	71, 171
Salicylic acid	80–95 dose dependent	0.17 dose dependent	2.4–19	13 in therapeutic range	—	2–30% Renal; dose dependent	$t_{1/2}$ →; V_d →; Cl ?; f_p ↑	None	141
Sulfinpyrazone	99	0.06	6.0	23	Enzyme-limited, binding-sensitive	65% Hepatic 35% Renal	No data; would expect some decrease in *Cl* with liver disease	Slight decrease in dose	
Cardiovascular									
Atenolol	<5	0.55	6.5	55–130	—	10% Hepatic 90% Renal	$t_{1/2}$ →; V_d →; Cl →	None	74
Captopril	27	0.7	1.9	13.3/kg	—	40% Renal 50% Hepatic	Negligible unless renal function decreased	None	
Digitoxin	95	0.60	180	2.5	Enzyme-limited, binding-sensitive	70% Hepatic 30% Renal	$t_{1/2}$ → or ↓; Cl ↑ or →; f_p ↑	None	73, 109
Digoxin	30	6.0	35	150	—	30% Hepatic 70% Renal	Appears negligible	None	88

Disopyramide	80	non-linear	1.0	8	100	—	45% Hepatic 55% Renal	No data; would not expect a tremendous change in liver disease	Probably slight decrease	
Enalapril	50		1.0	4.0	125	Flow/enzyme-sensitive	Rapidly hydrolyzed to active enalaprilat in the liver, 60% excreted in the urine	$t_{1/2}$ enalaprilat C_{max} enalaprilat	None	11, 115
Esmolol	55		1.2	0.15	310/kg	—	80% Renal (rapidly hydrolyzed to inactive product in blood)	Negligible	None	22
Isradipine	95		3.0	8.0	1400	Flow-limited	<90% Hepatic	Cl, C_{max}, AUC, $t_{1/2}$, V_d	Decrease dose	1, 28
Labetalol	50		11.5	3.0	1600	Flow-limited	>95% Hepatic <5% Renal	$t_{1/2}$ →; V_d ↓; Cl → or ↓; f_p ?, assume ↑	Decrease oral dose; decrease i.v. dose to much smaller extent	53
Lidocaine	65	non-linear	1.1	2.0	1000	Flow-limited	97% Hepatic 3% Renal	$t_{1/2}$ ↑; V_d ↑ or →; Cl ↓ ~ 50%; f_p ? Low therapeutic ratio. Decrease in Cl depends on severity of disease	Decrease dose by 50% in severe liver disease	4, 39, 58, 168–170, 181

TABLE 4.2. *(Continued)*

Drug	*Protein Binding (%)*	*Volume of Distribution (V_d) (liter/kg)*	*Half-life ($t_{1/2}$) (h)*	*Clearance (Cl) (ml/min)*	*Class*	*Hepatic/Renal Elimination*	*Effect of Liver Disease on Drug Disposition*	*Adjustment of Dose*	*References*
Lisinopril	<10	1.8	12	106	—	3% Hepatic 97% Unchanged 70% Fecal 30% Renal	Negligible unless renal function decreased	None	
Lorcainide	70	12.9	8.0	1700	Flow-limited	98% Hepatic 2% Renal	$t_{1/2}$ ↑; V_d →; Cl ↓ 29%; f_p ↑ slightly. Cl_{int} exhibits a very large decrease	Decrease dose	78
Metoprolol	10	3.2	4.0	800	Flow-limited	95% Hepatic 5% Renal	$t_{1/2}$ ↑; V_d ↑ slightly; Cl ↓ 23%; f_p ? assumed unaffected	Decrease dose slightly	135
N-Acetyl-procainamide	10	1.4	8.0	210	—	20% Hepatic 80% Renal	No data; expect little change unless renal function altered	None	
Nifedipine	98	1.0	3.0	600	Flow-limited, binding-sensitive	100% Hepatic	$t_{1/2}$ ↑; V_d →; Cl ↓; f_p ↑	Decrease dose	75
Pindolol	57	6.2	3.5	300	Enzyme-limited, binding-insensitive	70% Hepatic 30% Renal	Not affected by AVH. Cirrhosis Cl ↓ slightly and renal excretion of drug is increased	Some decrease in severe liver disease	114

Prazosin	97	1.3	3.0	450	Flow-limited	95% Hepatic 5% Renal	No data—would expect $t_{1/2}$ ↑; Cl ↓; f_p ↑	Decrease dose	
Procainamide	15	2.2	3.0	600	—	45% Hepatic 55% Renal Drug acetylated	$t_{1/2}$ ↑; V_d ?; Cl ? probably decreased slightly	Some minor decrease in dose	33
Propranolol	95	4.0	4.0	850	Flow-limited	>95% Hepatic <5% Renal	$t_{1/2}$ ↑; V_d ↑; Cl ↓ ~ 60%; f_p ↑. Tremendous decrease in Cl_{int}. Flow/enzyme-limited in cirrhosis	Decrease dose depending on extent of damage	19, 129, 185
Quinidine	85	3.0	6.0	330	Flow/enzyme-sensitive	80% Hepatic 20% Renal	$t_{1/2}$ ↑; V_d ↑; Cl →; f_p ↑; Cl_{int} decreased significantly	Decrease dose	5, 128
Tocainide	10	3.0	13	150	Enzyme-limited	60% Hepatic 40% Renal	$t_{1/2}$ ↑; V_d ?; Cl ↓	Decrease dose	120
Verapamil	92	6.7	3.5	1570	Flow-limited	95% Hepatic 5% Renal	$t_{1/2}$ ↑; V_d ↑; Cl ↓ 60%; f_p →; Cl_{int} decreases even more than 60%	Decrease dose by 50% in severe liver disease	155, 186
Diuretic									
Bumetanide	?	9.45	1.0	129	—	36% Hepatic 64% Renal	$t_{1/2}$ ↑; V_d ↓; Cl ↓	Minor decrease in dose	89
Furosemide	95	0.15	1.0	170	—	35% Hepatic 65% Renal	$t_{1/2}$ ↑ or →; V_d ↑ or →; Cl →; f_p ↑; the change in f_p compensates for decrease in Cl_{int} of liver	None or slight decrease in severe cases	40, 172, 174

TABLE 4.2. *(Continued)*

Drug	Protein Binding (%)	Volume of Distribution (V_d) (liter/kg)	Half-life ($t_{1/2}$) (h)	Clearance (Cl) (ml/min)	Class	Hepatic/Renal Elimination	Effect of Liver Disease on Drug Disposition	Adjustment of Dose	References
Hydrochlorothiazide	95	1.5	2.5	480	—	<10% Hepatic >90% Renal	No data; probably little affected unless renal function altered	None	
Spironolactone	98	—	20	—	Enzyme-limited, binding-sensitive, and extrahepatic metabolism	>85% Hepatic <15% Renal	No apparent change in drug disposition with liver disease; $t_{1/2} \rightarrow$	None	2, 146
Triamterene	50	2.5	2.0	1000	Flow-limited	95% Hepatic 5% Renal	$Cl \downarrow$; $f_p \rightarrow$; expect $t_{1/2} \uparrow$	Decrease dose	173
Sedative/Hypnotic									
Amylobarbital	60	1.2	21	35	Enzyme-limited, binding-insensitive	>95% Hepatic <5% Renal	$t_{1/2} \uparrow$; $V_d \rightarrow$; $Cl \downarrow$ 55%; $f_p \uparrow$. Little change if albumin >3.5 g/100 ml	Decrease dose	91
Chlordiazepoxide	96	0.3	12 age-dependent	20	Enzyme-limited, binding-sensitive	>99% Hepatic <1% Renal	$t_{1/2} \uparrow$; $V_d \uparrow$; $Cl \downarrow$ 60%; $f_p \uparrow$. Both AVH and cirrhosis affect drug	Decrease dose	141, 142

Diazepam	99	1.2	45	28	Enzyme-limited, binding-sensitive	>97% Hepatic <3% Renal	$t_{1/2}$ ↑; V_d ↑; *Cl* ↓ 50%; f_p ↑. AVH and cirrhosis increase $t_{1/2}$. Large therapeutic index—safe	Single dose, no change; chronic, decrease dose	77, 92, 110
Flumazenil	40	0.85	0.8	1201	Flow-limited	>90% Hepatic	$t_{1/2}$, *Cl*, V_d	? Decrease dose	66
Hexobarbital	47	1.2	6.0	232	Enzyme-limited, binding-insensitive	>99% Hepatic <1% Renal	$t_{1/2}$ ↑; V_d →; *Cl* ↓ 62% (*Cl* decreased in AVH and cirrhosis, *Cl* → in cholestasis); f_p →	Decrease during chronic dosing	136
Lorazepam	90	1.3	12.0	53	Enzyme-limited, binding-sensitive	>98% Hepatic <2% Renal Extensive glucuronidation	$t_{1/2}$ ↑; V_d ↑; *Cl* →; f_p ↑. Neither AVH nor cirrhosis affects drug dosing	None	79
Methohexital	—	61	2.0	829	Flow/enzyme-sensitive	>90% Hepatic <10% Renal	No data; assume *Cl* ↓, $t_{1/2}$ ↑	Probably decrease dose	
Midazolam	—	1.3	1.6	624	Flow-limited	>95% Hepatic <5% Renal	$t_{1/2}$ ↑; V_d slightly ↑; *Cl* ↓	Decrease dose	6, 85
Nitrazepam	87	1.9	26	63	Enzyme-limited	>99% Hepatic <1% Renal Mainly nitro-reduction	$t_{1/2}$ →; V_d →; *Cl* →; f_p ↑	None	67

TABLE 4.2. *(Continued)*

Drug	Protein Binding (%)	Volume of Distribution (V_d) (liter/kg)	Half-life ($t_{1/2}$) (h)	Clearance (Cl) (ml/min)	Class	Hepatic/Renal Elimination	Effect of Liver Disease on Drug Disposition	Adjustment of Dose	References
Oxazepam	90	1.6	6.0	140	Enzyme-limited, binding-sensitive	>99% Hepatic <1% Renal Extensive glucoronidation	$t_{1/2}$ →; V_d →; Cl →; f_p →. Neither AVH nor cirrhosis alters disposition significantly	None	152
Pentobarbital	65	1.0	30	30	Enzyme-limited, binding-sensitive	99% Hepatic <1% Renal	No data; expect Cl ↓, $t_{1/2}$ ↑	Single dose, no change; chronic, lower dose	148
Primidone	19	0.86	17	41	—	60% Hepatic 40% Renal (in children)	$t_{1/2}$ →; V_d slight ↑; Cl slight ↑ in hepatitis	None	131
Temazepam	98	1.2	14	80	—	>98% Hepatic <2% Renal Mainly glucuronidation	$t_{1/2}$ →; V_d →; Cl →; f_p →	None	111
Others									
Alfentanil	90	0.28	1.5	200	Flow/enzyme-sensitive	99% Hepatic 1% Renal	$t_{1/2}$ ↑; V_d →; Cl ↓; f_p ↑ (dose-dependent)	Decrease dose	38
Atracurium	—	0.16	0.33	385		Hofmann elimination; autometabolism	$t_{1/2}$ →; V_d ↑; Cl →; long $t_{1/2}$ of metabolite	Decrease dose if long-term use	177

Caffeine	31	0.54	6.0	63	Enzyme-limited, binding-insensitive	95% Hepatic 5% Renal	$t_{1/2}$ ↑ slightly; V_d →; Cl ↓ 40%; f_p ↑; large therapeutic ratio	None	30
Chlormethiazole	64	0.12	7.0	1100	Flow-limited; vitamin B substitute	>99% Hepatic <1% Renal	$t_{1/2}$ ↑; V_d →; Cl ↓ 28%; f_p ↑	Probably not necessary	127
Cimetidine	20	1.1	2.3	550	—	40% Hepatic 60% Renal	$t_{1/2}$ →; V_d ↑ or ↓ or →; Cl → or ↓; f_p changes assumed unimportant. Drug associated with increased incidence of mental confusion in cirrhotics	Decrease dose in severe liver disease	26, 45, 106
Clofibrate (CPIB)	95	0.15	18.0	8	Enzyme-limited, binding-sensitive	90% Hepatic <10% Renal Glucuronidation of metabolite	$t_{1/2}$ →; V_d ↑ slightly; Cl →; f_p ↑. AVH does not alter Cl; cirrhosis does have an effect on Cl_{int} ↓ 50%	Decrease dose in cirrhosis by 50%	46
Diphenhydramine	78	6.5	9.5	696	Flow-limited	>98% Hepatic <2% Renal	$t_{1/2}$ ↑; V_d →; free Cl ↓; total Cl →; f_p ↑	Decrease dose	94
Doxacurium	30	0.22	1.5	190	—	>90% Renal	Negligible unless renal function decreased	None	27
Famotidine	17	1.1	3.3	430	—	70% Renal (unchanged) 30% Hepatic	Negligible unless renal function decreased	None	116
Fentanyl	80	3.5	4.0	750	—	92% Hepatic 8% Renal	$t_{1/2}$ →; V_d →; Cl →	None	47

TABLE 4.2. *(Continued)*

Drug	*Protein Binding (%)*	*Volume of Distribution (V_d) (liter/kg)*	*Half-life ($t_{1/2}$) (h)*	*Clearance (Cl) (ml/min)*	*Class*	*Hepatic/Renal Elimination*	*Effect of Liver Disease on Drug Disposition*	*Adjustment of Dose*	*References*
Omeprazole	95	0.35	0.75	550	Flow-limited	>90% Hepatic	$t_{1/2}$, Cl,	None	140
Ranitidine	15	1.5	2.3	600	—	30% Hepatic 70% Renal	$t_{1/2}$ →; V_d →; Cl → or ↓	None	99, 118
Sulfisoxazole	92	0.15	6.6	20	Enzyme-limited, binding-sensitive	50% Hepatic 50% Renal Acetylation	$t_{1/2}$ →; V_d ↑; Cl ↑; f_p ↑	None	25
Theophylline	52	0.5	8.0	45	Enzyme-limited, binding-sensitive	91% Hepatic 9% Renal	$t_{1/2}$ ↑; V_d → cirrhosis, ↑ hepatitis and cholestasis; Cl ↓ 55%; f_p ↑. Low therapeutic index caution	Decrease dose by 50%	161
Thiopental	85	2.3	9.0	275	Enzyme-limited	>99% Hepatic <1% Renal	$t_{1/2}$ →; V_d →; Cl →; f_p ↑	Uncertain; may need to decrease dose	122
Tolbutamide	98	0.15	5.0	20.0	Enzyme-limited, binding-sensitive	95% Hepatic 5% Renal	$t_{1/2}$ slightly ↑ or →; V_d →; Cl ↑; f_p ↑. AVH has been reported to increase rate of elimination	None; probably not used in liver disease	167, 182

Warfarin	99	0.20	23	8.0	Enzyme-limited, binding-sensitive	99% Hepatic 1% Renal	$t_{1/2}$ →; V_d →; Cl →; f_p →. AVH no effect, but may be related to extent of liver damage	None; probably not used in liver disease	181

[a] GI, gastrointestinal; AVH, acute viral hepatitis; LD, liver disease.

TABLE 4.3. Considerations for Drug Dosage Adjustments in Liver Disease Patients

Extent of Change in Drug Dose	*Conditions or Requirements to Be Satisfied*
No change or minor change in dose	1. Mild liver disease 2. Extensive elimination of drug by kidneys and no renal dysfunction 3. Elimination by pathways of metabolism spared by liver disease 4. Drug is enzyme-limited and given acutely 5. Drug is flow/enzyme-sensitive and given acutely only by i.v. route 6. No alteration in drug sensitivity
Decrease in dose of up to 25%	1. Elimination by the liver does not exceed 40% of the dose; no renal dysfunction 2. Drug is flow-limited and given by i.v. route, with no large change in protein binding 3. Drug is flow/enzyme-limited and given acutely by oral route 4. Drug has a large therapeutic ratio
Decrease in dose of >25%	1. Drug metabolism is affected by liver disease; drug administered chronically 2. Drug has a narrow therapeutic range; protein binding altered significantly 3. Drug is flow-limited and given orally 4. Drug is eliminated by kidneys and renal function severely affected 5. Altered sensitivity to drug due to liver disease

ACKNOWLEDGMENT

This work was supported in part by U.S. Public Health Service Grant GM 31304.

REFERENCES

1. Abernethy D, Schwartz JB: Pharmacokinetics of calcium antagonists under development. *Clin Pharmacokinet* 15:1–14, 1988.
2. Abshagen U, Rennekamp H, Luszpinski G: Disposition kinetics of spironolactone in hepatic failure after single doses and prolonged treatment. *Eur J Clin Pharmacol* 11:169–176, 1977.
3. Acocella G, Bonollo L, Garimoldi M, Mainardi M, Tenconi LT, Hicolis FB: Kinetics of rifampin and isoniazid administered alone and in combination to normal subjects and patients with liver disease. *Gut* 13:47–53, 1972.
4. Adjepon-Yamoah KK, Himmo J, Prescott LF: Gross impairment of hepatic drug metabolism in a patient with chronic liver disease. *Br Med J* 4:387–388, 1974.
5. Affrime A, Reidenberg MM: The protein binding of some drugs in plasma from patients with alcoholic liver disease. *Eur J Clin Pharmacol* 8:267–269, 1975.
6. Allonen H, Zieglar G, Koltz U: Midazolam kinetics. *Clin Pharmacol Ther* 30:653–660, 1981.
7. Alvin J, Meltorse T, Hoyumpa A, Bush MT, Schenker S: The effect of liver disease in man on the disposition of phenobarbital. *J Pharmacol Exp Ther* 192:224–235, 1975.
8. Andreasen PB, Greisen G: Phenazone metabolism in patients with liver disease. *Eur J Clin Invest* 6:21–26, 1976.
9. Andreasen PB, Hutters L: Paracetamol (acetaminophen) clearance in patients with cirrhosis of the liver. *Acta Med Scand Suppl* 624:99–105, 1979.
10. Avant GR, Schenker S, Alford RH: The effect of cirrhosis on the disposition and elimination of clindamycin. *Am J Dig Dis* 20:223–230, 1975.
11. Baba T, Murabayashi S, Tomiyama T, Takebe K: The pharmacokinetics of enalapril in patients with compensated liver cirrhosis. *Br J Clin Pharmacol* 29:766–769, 1990.
12. Bass N, Williams R: Guide to drug dosage in hepatic disease. *Clin Pharmacokinet* 15:396–420, 1988.
13. Benjamin RS: Clinical pharmacology of adriamycin (NSC-123127). *Cancer Chemother Rep* 6:183–185, 1975.
14. Bircher J, Blankart R, Halpern A, Hacki W, Laissue J, Preisig R: Criteria for assessment of functional impairment in patients with cirrhosis of the liver. *Eur J Clin Invest* 3:72–85, 1973.
15. Blaschke TF, Meffin PJ, Melmon KL, Rowland M: Influence of acute viral hepatitis on phenytoin kinetics and protein binding. *Clin Pharmacol Ther* 17:685–691, 1975.
16. Boscia JA, Korzeniowski OM, Kobasa WD, Rocha H, Levison ME, Kaye D: Pharmacokinetics of cefoperazone in normal subjects and patients with hepatosplenic schistosomiasis. *J Antimicrob Chemother* 12:407–410, 1983.
17. Boscia JA, Korzeniowski OM, Snepar R, Kobasa WD, Levison ME, Kaye D: Cefoperazone pharmacokinetics in normal subjects and patients with cirrhosis. *Antimicrob Agents Chemother* 23:385–389, 1983.
18. Branch RA, James J, Read AE: A study of factors influencing drug disposition in chronic liver disease, using the model drug (+)-propranolol. *Br J Clin Pharmacol* 3:243–249, 1976.
19. Branch RA, Shand DG: Propranolol disposition in chronic liver disease: a physiological approach. *Clin Pharmacokinet* 1:264–279, 1976.

20. Brodie MJ, Boobis S: The effect of chronic alcoholic ingestion and alcoholic liver disease on binding of drugs to serum proteins. *Eur J Clin Pharmacol* 13:435–438, 1978.
21. Brown N, Ho DHW, Fong KL, Bogerd L, Maksymiuk A, Bolivar R, Fainstein V, Bodey GP: Effects of hepatic function on vancomycin clinical pharmacology. *Antimicrob Agents Chemother* 23:603–609, 1983.
22. Buchi KN, Rollins DE, Tolman KG, Achari R, Drissel D, Hulse JD: Pharmacokinetics of esmolol in hepatic disease. *J Clin Pharmacol* 27:880–884, 1987.
23. Burnett DA, Barak AJ, Tuma DJ, Sorrell MF: Altered elimination of antipyrine in patients with acute viral hepatitis. *Gut* 17:341–344, 1976.
24. Calvo MV, Dominguez-Gil A, Macias JG, Dietz JL: Naproxen disposition in hepatic and biliary disorders. *Int J Clin Pharmacol Ther Toxicol* 18:242–246, 1980.
25. Cello JP, Oie S: Binding and disposition of sulfisoxazole in alcoholic cirrhosis. *J Pharmacokinet Biopharm* 13:1–12, 1985.
26. Cello JP, Oie J: Cimetidine disposition in patients with Laennec's cirrhosis during multiple dosing therapy. *Eur J Clin Pharmacol* 25:223–229, 1983.
27. Cook DR, Freeman J, Lai A, Robertson K, Kang Y, Stiller R, Aggarwal S, Abou-Donia M, Welch R: Pharmacokinetics and pharmacodynamics of doxacurium in normal patients and in those with hepatic or renal failure. *Anesth Analg* 72:145–150, 1991.
28. Cotting J, Reichen J, Kutz K, Laplanche R, Nuesch E: Pharmacokinetics of isradipine in patients with chronic liver disease. *Eur J Clin Pharmacol* 38:599–603, 1990.
29. Daneshmend TK, Homeida M, Kaye CM, Elamin AA, Roberts CJC: Disposition of oral metronidazole in hepatic cirrhosis and in hepatosplenic schistosomiasis. *Gut* 23:807–813, 1982.
30. Desmond PV, Patwardhan RV, Johnson RF, Schenker S: Impaired elimination of caffeine in cirrhosis. *Dig Dis Sci* 25:193–197, 1980.
31. D'Incalci M, Rossi C, Zucchetti M, Urso R, Cavalli F, Mangioni C, Williams Y, Sessa C: Pharmacokinetics of etoposide in patients with abnormal renal and hepatic function. *Cancer Res* 46:2566–2571, 1986.
32. Doshi J, Luisada-Oppe A, Leevy CM: Microsomal pentobarbital hydroxylase activity in acute viral hepatitis. *Proc Soc Exp Biol Med* 140:492–495, 1975.
33. duSouich P, Erill S: Metabolism of procainamide and *p*-aminobenzoic acid in patients with chronic liver disease. *Clin Pharmacol Ther* 22:588–595, 1977.
34. El-Raghy I, Back DJ, Osman F, Nafeh MA, Orme M L'E: The pharmacokinetics of antipyrine in patients with graded severity of schistosomiasis. *Br J Clin Pharmacol* 20:313–316, 1985.
35. Farrell G, Baird-Lambert J, Cvejic J, Buchanan N: Disposition and metabolism of metronidazole in patients with liver failure. *Hepatology* 4:722–726, 1984.
36. Farrell GC, Cooksley WGE, Hart P, Powell LW: Drug metabolism in liver disease. Identification of patients with impaired hepatic drug metabolism. *Gastroenterology* 75:580–588, 1978.
37. Farrell GC, Cooksley WGE, Powell LW: Drug metabolism in liver disease: activity of hepatic microsomal metabolizing enzymes. *Clin Pharmacol Ther* 26:483–492, 1979.
38. Ferrier C, Marty J, Bouffard Y, Haberer JP, Levron JC, Duvaldestin P: Alfentanil pharmacokinetics in patients with cirrhosis. *Anesthesiology* 62:480–484, 1985.
39. Forrest JAH, Finlayson NDC, Adjepon-Yamoah KK, Prescott LF: Antipyrine, paracetamol, and lidocaine elimination in chronic liver disease. *Br Med J* 1:1384–1387, 1977.
40. Fuller R, Hoppel C, Ingalls ST: Furosemide kinetics in patients with hepatic cirrhosis with ascites. *Clin Pharmacol Ther* 30:461–467, 1981.

41. Gelman CR, Rumack BH: DRUGDEX® Information System. Micromedix, Inc., Denver, CO.
42. Giacomini KM, Giacomini JC, Gibson TP, Levy G: Propoxyphene and norpropoxyphene plasma concentrations after oral propoxyphene in cirrhotic patients with and without surgically constructed portacaval shunt. *Clin Pharmacol Ther* 28:417–424, 1980.
43. Giargcau AJ, Chalmers TC: The natural history of cirrhosis. I. Survival with esophageal varices. *N Engl J Med* 268:469–473, 1963.
44. Goldberg D, Brown D: Advances in the application of biochemical tests to diseases of the liver and biliary tract: their role in diagnosis, prognosis, and the elucidation of pathogenetic mechanisms. *Clin Biochem* 20:127–148, 1987.
45. Grahnen A, Jameson S, Lööf L, Tyllström J, Lindström B: Pharmacokinetics of cimetidine in advanced cirrhosis. *Eur J Clin Pharmacol* 26:347–355, 1984.
46. Groszman R, Kotelanski B, Khatri IM, Cohn JN: Quantitation of portasystemic shunting from the splenic and mesenteric beds in alcoholic liver disease. *Am J Med* 53:715–722, 1972.
47. Haberer JP, Schoeffler P, Couderc E, Duvaldestin P: Fentanyl pharmacokinetics in anaesthetized patients with cirrhosis. *Br J Anaesth* 54:1267–1270, 1982.
48. Hall KW, Nightingale CH, Gibaldi M, Nelson E, Bates TR, Disanto AR: Pharmacokinetics of erythromycin in normal and alcoholic liver disease subjects. *J Clin Pharmacol* 22:321–325, 1982.
49. Hande KR, Wedlund PJ, Noone RM, Wilkinson GR, Greco FA, Wolff SN: Pharmacokinetics of high-dose etoposide (VP-16-213) administered to cancer patients. *Cancer Res* 44:379–382, 1984.
50. Helleberg L: Clinical pharmacokinetics of indomethacin. *Clin Pharmacokinet* 6:245–258, 1981.
51. Hinthorn DR, Baker LH, Romig DR, Hassanien K, Liu C: Use of clindamycin in patients with liver disease. *Antimicrob Agents Chemother* 9:498–501, 1976.
52. Hoffman TA, Cestero R, Bullock WE: Pharmacodynamics of carbenicillin in hepatic and renal failure. *Ann Intern Med* 73:173–178, 1970.
53. Homeida M, Jackson L, Roberts CJC: Decreased first-pass metabolism of labetalol in chronic liver disease. *Br Med J* 2:1048–1050, 1978.
54. Homeida M, Roberts CJC, Halliwell M, Read AE, Branch RA: Antipyrine clearance per unit volume liver: an assessment of hepatic function in chronic liver disease. *Gut* 20:596–601, 1979.
55. Horn T, Christofferson P, Henriksen JH: Alcoholic liver injury: defenestration in noncirrhotic livers—a scanning electron microscopic study. *Hepatology* 7:77–82, 1987.
56. Howden C, Birnie G, Brodie M: Drug metabolism in liver disease. *Pharmacol Ther* 40:439–474, 1989.
57. Hoyumpa A, Schenker S: Is glucuronidation truly preserved in patients with liver disease? *Hepatology* 13(4):786–795, 1991.
58. Huet P, Lelorier J: Effects of smoking and chronic hepatitis B on lidocaine and indocyanine green kinetics. *Clin Pharmacol Ther* 28:208–215, 1980.
59. Huet P-M, Goresky CA, Villeneuve J-P, Marleau D, Lough JO: Assessment of liver microcirculation in human cirrhosis. *J Clin Invest* 70:1234–1244, 1982.
60. Huet P-M, Pomier-Layrargues G, Villeneuve J-P, Varin F, Viallet A: Intrahepatic circulation in liver disease. *Semin Liver Dis* 6:277–286, 1986.
61. Huet P-M, Villeneuve J-P, Pomier-Layrargues G, Marleau D: Hepatic circulation in cirrhosis. *Clin Gastroenterol* 14:155–168, 1985.
62. Huet P-M, Villeneuve J-P: Determinants of drug disposition in patients with cirrhosis. *Hepatology* 3(6):913–918, 1983.

63. Humphrey MJ, Jevons S, Tarbit MH: Pharmacokinetic evaluation of UK-49,858, a metabolically stable triazole antifungal drug, in animals and humans. *Antimicrob Agents Chemother* 28:648–653, 1985.
64. Ishizaki T, Chiba K, Sasaki T: Antipyrine clearance in patients with Gilbert's syndrome. *Eur J Clin Pharmacol* 27:297–302, 1984.
65. Iqbal S, Vickers C, Elias E: Drug metabolism in end-stage liver disease: in vitro activities of some phase I amd phase II enzymes. *J Hepatol* 11:37–42, 1990.
66. Janssen U, Walker S, Maier K, von Gaisberg U, Klotz U: Flumazenil disposition and elimination in cirrhosis. *Clin Pharmacol Ther* 46:317–323, 1989.
67. Jochemsen R, Van Beusekom BR, Spoelstra P, Janssens AR, Breimer DD: Effect of age and liver cirrhosis on the pharmacokinetics of nitrazepam. *Br J Clin Pharmacol* 15:295–302, 1983.
68. Johannessen SI, Gerna M, Bakke J, Strandjord RE, Morselli PL: CSF concentrations and serum protein binding of carbamazepine and carbamazepine-10gll-epoxide in epileptic patients. *Br J Clin Pharmacol* 3:575–582, 1976.
69. Juhl RP, VanThiel DH, Dittert LW, Albert KS, Smith RB: Ibuprofen and sulindac kinetics in alcoholic liver disease. *Clin Pharmacol Ther* 34:104–109, 1983.
70. Juma FD: Effect of liver failure on the pharmacokinetics of cyclophosphamide. *Eur J Clin Pharmacol* 26:591–593, 1984.
71. Kawai S, Ichikawa Y, Homma M: Differences in metabolic properties among cortisol, prednisolone, and dexamethasone in liver and renal diseases. Accelerated metabolism of dexamethasone in renal failure. *J Clin Endocrinol Metab* 60:848–854, 1985.
72. Kenny MT, Strates B: Metabolism and pharmacokinetics of the antibiotic rifampin. *Drug Metab Rev* 12:159–218, 1981.
73. Kirch W, Ohnhaus EE, Dylewicz P, Pabst J, Storstein L: Bioavailability and elimination of digitoxin in patients with hepatorenal insufficiency. *Am Heart J* 111:325–329, 1986.
74. Kirch W, Schafer-Korting M, Mutschler E, Ohnhaus EE, Braun W: Clinical experience with atenolol in patients with chronic liver disease. *J Clin Pharmacol* 23:171–177, 1983.
75. Kleinbloesem CH, van Harten J, Wilson JPH, Danhof M, van Brummelen P, Breimer DD: Nifedipine: kinetics and hemodynamic effects in patients with liver cirrhosis after intravenous and oral administration. *Clin Pharmacol Ther* 40:21–28, 1986.
76. Klinger EL, Vaamonde CA, Vaamonde LS, Lancestremere RG, Morosi HJ, Frisch E, Papper S: Renal function changes in cirrhosis of the liver. *Arch Intern Med* 125:1010–1015, 1970.
77. Klotz U, Antonin KH, Brugel H, Bieck PR: Disposition of diazepam and its major metabolite desmethyldiazepam in patients with liver disease. *Clin Pharmacol Ther* 21:430–436, 1977.
78. Klotz U, Fischer C, Muller-Seydlitz P, Schulz J, Mueller WA: Alterations in the disposition of differently cleared drugs in patients with cirrhosis. *Clin Pharmacol Ther* 26:221–227, 1979.
79. Kraus JW, Desmond PV, Marshall JP, Johnson RF, Schenker S, Wilkinson GR: Effects of aging and liver disease on disposition of lorazepam. *Clin Pharmacol Ther* 24:411–419, 1978.
80. Krausz Y, Zylber-Katz E, Levy M: Antipyrine clearance and its correlation to routine liver function tests in patients with liver disease. *Int J Clin Pharmacol Ther Toxicol* 18:253–257, 1980.
81. Kroboth PD, Brown A, Lyon JA, Kroboth FJ, Juhl RP: Pharmacokinetics of single-dose erythromycin in normal and alcohol liver disease subjects. *Antimicrob Agents Chemother* 21:135–140, 1982.

82. Levy G: Effect of plasma protein binding of drugs on duration and intensity of pharmacological activity. *J Pharm Sci* 65:1264–1265, 1976.
83. Lewis GP, Jusko WJ: Pharmacokinetics of ampicillin in cirrhosis. *Clin Pharmacol Ther* 18:475–484, 1975.
84. Lima JJ, Boudoulas H, Blanford M: Concentration-dependence of disopyramide binding to plasma protein and its influence on kinetics and dynamics. *J Pharmacol Exp Ther* 219:741–747, 1981.
85. MacGilchrist AJ, Birnie GG, Cook A, Scobie G, Murray T, Watkinson G, Brodie MJ: Pharmacokinetics and pharmacodynamics of intravenous midazolam in patients with severe alcoholic cirrhosis. *Gut* 27:190–195, 1986.
86. MacLeod CM, Bartley EA, Payne JA, Hudes E, Vernam K, Devlin RG: Effects of cirrhosis on kinetics of aztreonam. *Antimicrob Agents Chemother* 26:493–497, 1984.
87. Mak KM, Lieber CS: Alterations in endothelial fenestrations in liver sinusoids of baboons fed alcohol: a scanning electron microscopic study. *Hepatology* 4:386–391, 1984.
88. Malini PL, Sarti F, Dal Monte PR, Grepioni A, Boschi S, Ambrosioni E: Effect of chronic liver disease on plasma levels and metabolism of digoxin and betamethyl digoxin. *Int J Clin Pharmacol Res* 1:21–27, 1982.
89. Marcantonio LA, Auld WHR, Murdock WR, Purohit R, Skellern GG, Howes CA: The pharmacokinetics and pharmacodynamics of the diuretic bumetanide in hepatic and renal disease. *Br J Clin Pharmacol* 15:245–252, 1983.
90. Marshall JP, Salt WB, Elam RO, Wilkinson GR, Schenker S: Disposition of nafcillin inpatients with cirrhosis and extrahepatic biliary obstruction. *Gastroenterology* 73:1388–1392, 1977.
91. Mawer GE, Miller NE, Turnberg LA: Metabolism of amylobarbitone in patients with chronic liver disease. *Br J Pharmacol* 44:549–560, 1972.
92. McConnell JB, Curry SH, Davis M, Williams R: Clinical effects and metabolism of diazepam in patients with chronic liver disease. *Clin Sci* 63:75–80, 1982.
93. Mehta MU, Venkataramanan R, Burckart GJ, Ptachcinski RJ, Yang SL, Gray JA, Van Thiel DH, Starzl TE: Antipyrine kinetics in liver disease and liver transplantation. *Clin Pharmacol Ther* 39:372–377, 1986.
94. Meredith CG, Christian CD Jr, Johnson RF, Madhavan SV, Schenker S: Diphenhydramine disposition in chronic liver disease. *Clin Pharmacol Ther* 35:474–479, 1984.
95. Meyer B, Luo H, Bargetzi M, Renner E, Stalder G: Quantitation of intrinsic drug-metabolizing capacity in human liver biopsy specimens: support for the intact-hepatocyte theory. *Hepatology* 13(3):475–481, 1991.
96. Miguet J-P, Vuitton D, Deschamps J-P, Allemand H, Joanne C, Bechtel P, Carayon P: Cholestasis and hepatic drug metabolism: comparison of metabolic clearance rate of antipyrine in patients with intrahepatic or extrahepatic cholestasis. *Dig Dis Sci* 26:718–722, 1981.
97. Montay G, Gaillot J: Pharmacokinetics of fluoroquinolones in hepatic failure. *J Antimicrob Chemother* 26(suppl B):61–67, 1990.
98. Moreau L, Durand H, Biclet P: Cefotaxime concentrations in ascites. *J Antimicrob Chemother* 6(suppl A):121–122, 1980.
99. Morichau-Beauchant M, Houin G, Mavier P, Alexandre C, Dhumeaux D: Pharmacokinetics and bioavailability of ranitidine in normal subjects and cirrhotic patients. *Dig Dis Sci* 31:113–118, 1986.
100. Narang APS, Datta DV, Nath N, Mathur VS: Impairment of hepatic drug metabolism in patients with acute viral hepatitis. *Eur J Drug Metab Pharmacokinet* 7:255–258, 1982.
101. Narang APS, Datta DV, Nath N, Mathur VS: Pharmacokinetic study of chloramphenicol in patients with liver disease. *Eur J Clin Pharmacol* 20:479–483, 1981.

102. Narang APS, Kaur U, Bambery P: Drug metabolism and liver disease in India. *Drug Metab Rev* 23:65–81, 1991.
103. Naranjo CA, Busto U, Janecek E, Ruiz I, Roach CA, Kaplan K: An intensive drug monitoring study suggesting possible clinical irrelevance of impaired drug disposition in liver disease. *Br J Clin Pharmacol* 15:451–458, 1983.
104. Naranjo CA, Busto U, Mardones R: Adverse drug reactions in liver cirrhosis. *Eur J Clin Pharmacol* 13:429–434, 1978.
105. Neal EA, Meffin PJ, Gregory PB, Blaschke TF: Enhanced bioavailability and decreased clearance of analgesics in patients with cirrhosis. *Gastroenterology* 77:96–102, 1979.
106. Nelson DC, Avant GR, Speeg Jr KV, Hoyumpa Jr AM, Schenker S: The effect of cimetidine on hepatic drug elimination in cirrhosis. *Hepatology* 5:305–309, 1985.
107. Novick DM, Kreek MJ, Arns PA, Lau LL, Yancovitz SR, Gelb AM: Effect of severe alcoholic liver disease on the disposition of methadone in maintenance patients. *Alcoholism* 9:349–354, 1985.
108. Novick DM, Kreek MJ, Fanizza AM, Yancovitz SR, Gelb AM, Stenger RJ: Methadone disposition in patients with chronic liver disease. *Clin Pharmacol Ther* 30:353–362, 1981.
109. Ochs HR, Greenblatt DJ, Bodem G, Dengler HJ: Disease-related alterations in cardiac glycoside disposition. *Clin Pharmacokinet* 7:434–451, 1982.
110. Ochs HR, Greenblatt DJ, Eckardt B, Harmatz JS, Shader RI: Repeated diazepam dosing in cirrhotic patients: accumulation and sedation. *Clin Pharmacol Ther* 33:471–476, 1983.
111. Ochs HR, Greenblatt DJ, Verburg-Ochs B, Matlis R: Temazepam clearance is unaltered in cirrhosis. *Am J Gastroenterol* 81:80–84, 1986.
112. Oellerich M, Burdelski M, Lautz HU, Schulz M, Schmidt FW, Herrmann H: Lidocaine metabolite formation as a measure of liver function in patients with cirrhosis. *Ther Drug Monit* 12:219–226, 1990.
113. Ohashi K, Tsunoo M, Tsuneoka K: Pharmacokinetics and protein binding of cefazolin and cephalothin in patients with cirrhosis. *J Antimicrob Chemother* 17:347–351, 1986.
114. Ohnhaus EE, Münch U, Meier J: Elimination of pindolol in liver disease. *Eur J Clin Pharmacol* 22:247–251, 1982.
115. Ohnishi A, Tsuboi Y, Ishizaki T, Kubota K, Ohno T, Yoshida H, Kanezaki A, Tanaka T: Kinetics and dynamics of enalapril in patients with liver cirrhosis. *Clin Pharmacol Ther* 45:657–665, 1989.
116. Ohnishi K: Effects of hepatic disease on the pharmacokinetics of famotidine and effects of famotidine on hepatic hemodynamics and peptic ulcer. *Hepatogastroenterology* 37:6–10, 1990.
117. Okolicsanyi L, Venuti M, Orlando R, Xerri L, Pugina M: Pharmacokinetic studies of cefuroxime in patients with liver cirrhosis. *Arzneimittelforschung* 7:777–782, 1982.
118. Okolicsanyi L, Venuti M, Strazzabosco M, Orlando R, Nassuato G, Iemmolo RM, Lirussi R, Muraca M, Pastorino AM, Castelli G: Oral and intravenous pharmacokinetics of ranitidine in patients with liver cirrhosis. *Int J Clin Pharmacol Ther Toxicol* 22:329–332, 1984.
119. Olsen GD, Bennett WM, Potter GA: Morphine and phenytoin binding to plasma proteins in renal and hepatic failure. *Clin Pharmacol Ther* 17:677–684, 1976.
120. Oltmanns D, Pottage A, Endell W: Pharmacokinetics of tocainide in patients with combined hepatic and renal dysfunction. *Eur J Clin Pharmacol* 25:787–790, 1983.
121. Orrego H, Medline A, Blendis LM, Rankin JG, Kreaden DA: Collagenisation of the Disse space in alcoholic liver disease. *Gut* 20:673–679, 1979.
122. Pandele G, Chaux F, Salvadori C, Farinotti M, Duvaldestin P: Thiopental pharmacokinetics in patients with cirrhosis. *Anesthesiology* 59:123–126, 1983.

123. Pasko MT, Beam TR, Spooner JA, Camara DS: Safety and pharmacokinetics of ceftazidime in patients with chronic hepatic dysfunction. *J Antimicrob Chemother* 15:365–374, 1985.
124. Patwardhan R, Johnson R, Sheehan J, Desmond P, Wilkinson G, Hoyumpa A, Branch R, Schenker S: Morphine metabolism in cirrhosis. *Gastroenterology* 80:1344, 1981.
125. Patwardhan RV, Johnson RF, Hoyumpa A, Sheehan JJ, Desmond PV, Wilkinson GR, Branch RA, Schenker S: Normal metabolism of morphine in cirrhosis. *Gastroenterology* 81:1006–1011, 1981.
126. Pearson RM, Breckenridge AM: Renal function, protein binding and pharmacological response to diazoxide. *Br J Clin Pharmacol* 3:169–175, 1976.
127. Pentikainen PJ, Neuvonen PJ, Jostell K-G: Pharmacokinetics of chlormethiazole in healthy volunteers and patients with cirrhosis of the liver. *Eur J Clin Pharmacol* 17:275–284, 1980.
128. Perez-Mateo M, Erill S: Protein binding of salicylates and quinidine in plasma from patients with renal failure, chronic liver disease and chronic respiratory insufficiency. *Eur J Clin Pharmacol* 11:225–231, 1977.
129. Pessayre D, Lebrec D, Descatorie V, Peignoux M, Benhamou J-P: Mechanism for reduced drug clearance in patients with cirrhosis. *Gastroenterology* 74:566–571, 1978.
130. Pirttiaho HI, Sotaniemi EA, Ahlqvist J, Pitkanen U, Pelkonen RO: Liver size and indices of drug metabolism in alcoholics. *Eur J Clin Pharmacol* 13:61–67, 1978.
131. Pisani F, Perruca E, Primerano G, D'Agostino AA, Petrelli RM, Fazio A, Oteri G, Di Perri R: Single-dose kinetics of primidone in acute viral hepatitis. *Eur J Clin Pharmacol* 27:465–469, 1984.
132. Pond SM, Tong T, Benowitz NL, Jacob P: Enhanced bioavailability of pethidine and pentazocine in patients with cirrhosis of the liver. *Aust N Z J Med* 10:515–519, 1980.
133. Pond SM, Tong T, Benowitz NL, Jacob P, Rigod J: Presystemic metabolism of meperidine to normeperidine in normal and cirrhotic subjects. *Clin Pharmacol Ther* 30:183–188, 1981.
134. Pozzi E, Menghini P: Blood levels of rifampicin in liver diseases. *Int J Clin Pharmacol* 10:44–49, 1974.
135. Regardh G-G, Jordo L, Ervik M, Lundborg P, Olsson R, Ronn O: Pharmacokinetics of metoprolol in patients with hepatic cirrhosis. *Clin Pharmacokinet* 6:375–388, 1981.
136. Richter E, Breimer DD, Zilly W: Disposition of hexobarbital in intra- and extrahepatic cholestasis in man and the influence of drug metabolism-inducing agents. *Eur J Clin Pharmacol* 17:197–202, 1980.
137. Ring-Larsen H: Renal blood flow in cirrhosis: relation to systemic and portal haemodynamics and liver function. *Scand J Clin Lab Invest* 37:635–642, 1977.
138. Ring-Larsen H, Birger H, Henriksen JH, Christensen NJ: Sympathetic nervous activity and renal and systemic hemodynamics in cirrhosis: plasma norepinephrine concentration, hepatic extraction, and renal release. *Hepatology* 2:304–310, 1982.
139. Ring-Larsen H, Henriksen JH: Pathogenesis of ascites formation and hepatorenal syndrome: humoral and hemodynamic factors. *Semin Liver Dis* 6:341–352, 1986.
140. Rinetti M, Regazzi MB, Villani P, Tizzoni M, Sivelli R: Pharmacokinetics of omeprazole in cirrhotic patients. *Arzneimittelforschung* 41(I):420–422, 1991.
141. Roberts MS, Rumble RH, Wanwimolruk S, Thomas D, Brooks PM: Pharmacokinetics of aspirin and salicylate in elderly subjects and in patients with alcoholic liver disease. *Eur J Clin Pharmacol* 25:253–261, 1983.
142. Robinson JD, Whitney HAK Jr, Guisti DL, Morgan DD, Mendenhall CL: The absorption of intramuscular chlordiazepoxide (Librium) in patients with severe alcoholic liver disease. *Int J Clin Pharmacol Ther Toxicol* 21:433–438, 1983.

143. Roos F, Zysset T, Reichen J: Differential effect of biliary and micronodular cirrhosis on oxidative drug metabolism. *Biochem Pharmacol* 41(10):1513–1519, 1991.
144. Rowland M, Benet LZ, Graham GG: Clearance concepts in pharmacokinetics. *J Pharmacol Biopharm* 1:123–136, 1973.
145. Ruhnke M, Trautmann M, Borner K, Hopfenmuller W: Pharmacokinetics of ciprofloxacin in liver cirrhosis. *Chemotherapy* 36:385–391, 1990.
146. Sadee W, Schroder R, Leitner E, Dagcioglu M: Multiple dose kinetics of spironolactone and canrenoate-potassium in cardiac and hepatic failure. *Eur J Clin Pharmacol* 7:195–200, 1974.
147. Schoene B, Fleischmann RA, Remmer H: Determination of drug metabolizing enzymes in needle biopsies of human liver. *Eur J Clin Pharmacol* 4:65–73, 1972.
148. Sessions JT, Minkel HP, Bullard JC, Ingelfinger FJ: The effect of barbiturates in patients with liver disease. *J Clin Invest* 33:1116–1127, 1954.
149. Shear L, Kleinerman J, Gabuzda GJ: Renal failure in patients with cirrhosis of the liver. *Am J Med* 39:184–198, 1965.
150. Shoeman DW, Azarnoff DL: Diphenylhydantoin potency and plasma protein binding. *J Pharmacol Exp Ther* 195:84–86, 1975.
151. Shreeve WW, Shoop JD, Ott DG, McInteer BB: Test for alcoholic cirrhosis by conversion of ^{14}C- or ^{13}C-galactose to expired CO_2. *Gastroenterology* 71:98–101, 1976.
152. Shull HJ, Wilkinson GR, Johnson R, Schenker S: Normal disposition of oxazepam in acute viral hepatitis and cirrhosis. *Ann Intern Med* 84:420–425, 1976.
153. Siegers C-P, Oltmanns D, Younes M: Effect of alcohol and chronic liver disease on the metabolic disposal of paracetamol in man. *Hepatogastroenterology* 28:304, 1981.
154. Sloan TP, Lancaster R, Shah RR, Idle JR, Smith RL: Genetically determined oxidation capacity and the disposition of debrisoquine. *Br J Clin Pharmacol* 15:443–450, 1983.
155. Somogyi A, Albrecht M, Kliens G, Schafer K, Eichelbaum M: Pharmacokinetics, bioavailability and ECG response of verapamil in patients with liver disease. *Br J Clin Pharmacol* 12:51–60, 1981.
156. Sonne J, Andreasen PB, Loft S, Dossing M, Andreasen F: Glucuronidation of oxazepam is not spared in patients with hepatic encephalopathy. *Hepatology* 11(6):951–956, 1990.
157. Sotaniemi EA, Luoma PV, Jarvensiva PM, Sotaniemi KA: Impairment of drug metabolism in polycystic non-parasitic liver disease. *Br J Clin Pharmacol* 8:331–335, 1979.
158. Sotaniemi EA, Niemaïa O, Risteli L, Stenb̈ack F, Pelkonen RO, Lahtela JT, Risteli J: Fibrotic process and drug metabolism in alcoholic liver disease. *Clin Pharmacol Ther* 40:46–55, 1986.
159. Sotaniemi EA, Pelkonen RO, Puukka M: Measurement of hepatic drug-metabolizing enzyme activity in man. *Eur J Clin Pharmacol* 17:267–274, 1980.
160. St. Peter J, Awni W: Quantifying hepatic function in the presence of liver disease with phenazone (antipyrine) and its metabolites. *Clin Pharmacokinet* 20(1):50–65, 1991.
161. Staib AH, Schuppan D, Lissner R, Zilly W, Bomhard GV, Richter E: Pharmacokinetics and metabolism of theophylline in patients with liver diseases. *Int J Clin Pharmacol Ther Toxicol* 18:500–502, 1980.
162. Stoeckel K, Tuerk H, Trueb V, McNamara PJ: Single-dose ceftriaxone kinetics in liver insufficiency. *Clin Pharmacol Ther* 36:500–509, 1984.
163. Syrota A, Paraf A, Gaudebout C, Desgrez A: Significance of intra- and extrahepatic portasystemic shunting in survival of cirrhotic patients. *Dig Dis Sci* 26:878–885, 1981.

164. Syrota A, Vinot J-M, Paraf A, Roucayrol JC: Scintillation splenoportography: hemodynamic and morphological study of the portal circulation. *Gastroenterology* 71:652–659, 1976.

165. Taburet A-M, Naveau S, Zorza G, Colin J-N, Delfraissy J-F, Chaput J-C, Singlas E: Pharmacokinetics of zidovudine in patients with liver cirrhosis. *Clin Pharmacol Ther* 47:731–739, 1990.

166. Teunissen MWE, Spoelstra P, Koch CW, Weeds B, Van Duyn W, Janssens AR, Breimer DD: Antipyrine clearance and metabolite formation in patients with alcoholic cirrhosis. *Br J Clin Pharmacol* 18:707–715, 1984.

167. Thiessen JJ, Sellers EM, Denbeigh P, Dolman L: Plasma protein binding of diazepam and tolbutamide in chronic alcoholics. *J Clin Pharmacol* 16:345–351, 1976.

168. Thomson PD, Melmon KL, Richardson JA, Cohn K, Steinbrunn W, Cudihee R, Rowland M: Lidocaine pharmacokinetics in advanced heart failure, liver disease, and renal failure in humans. *Ann Intern Med* 78:499–508, 1973.

169. Thomson PD, Rowland M, Melmon KL: The influence of heart failure, liver disease, and renal failure on the disposition of lidocaine in man. *Am Heart J* 82:417–421, 1971.

170. Tschang C, Steiner JA, Hignite CE, Huffman DH, Azarnoff DL: Systemic availability of lidocaine in patients with liver disease (abstract). *Clin Res* 25:609A, 1977.

171. Uribe M, Summerskill WHJ, Go VLW: Comparative serum prednisone and prednisolone concentrations following administration to patients with chronic active liver disease. *Clin Pharmacokinet* 7:452–459, 1982.

172. Verbeeck RK, Patwardhan RV, Villeneuve J-P, Wilkinson GR, Branch RA: Furosemide disposition in cirrhosis. *Clin Pharmacol Ther* 31:719–725, 1982.

173. Villeneuve J-P, Rocheleau F, Raymond G: Triamterene kinetics and dynamics in cirrhosis. *Clin Pharmacol Ther* 35:831–837, 1984.

174. Villeneuve J-P, Verbeeck RK, Wilkinson GR, Branch RA: Furosemide kinetics and dynamics in patients with cirrhosis. *Clin Pharmacol Ther* 40:14–20, 1986.

175. Wagner VT, Heydrich D, Bartels H, Hohorst HJ: The influence of damaged liver parenchyma, renal insufficiency and hemodialysis on the pharmacokinetics of cyclophosphamide and its activated metabolites. *Arzneimittelforschung* 30:1588–1592, 1980.

176. Wallace S, Brodie MJ: Decreased drug binding in serum from patients with chronic hepatic disease. *Eur J Clin Pharmacol* 9:429–432, 1976.

177. Ward S, Weatherley BC: Pharmacokinetics of atracurium and its metabolites. *Br J Anaesth* 58:6S–10S, 1986.

178. Wilkinson GR: The effects of liver disease and aging on the disposition of diazepam, chlordiazepoxide, oxazepam and lorazepam in man. *Acta Psychiatr Scand* 274:561–573, 1978.

179. Wilkinson GR, Shand DG: A physiological approach to hepatic drug clearance. *Clin Pharmacol Ther* 18:377–390, 1975.

180. Williams RL: Drug administration in hepatic disease. *N Engl J Med* 309(26):1616–1622, 1983.

181. Williams RL, Blaschke TF, Meffin PJ, Melman KL, Rowland M: Influence of viral hepatitis on the disposition of two compounds with high clearance: lidocaine and indocyanine green. *Clin Pharmacol Ther* 20:290–299, 1976.

182. Williams RL, Blaschke TF, Meffin PJ, Melmon KL, Rowland M: Influence of acute viral hepatitis on disposition and plasma binding of tolbutamide. *Clin Pharmacol Ther* 21:301–309, 1977.

183. Williams RL, Schary WL, Blaschke TF, Meffin PJ, Melmon KL, Rowland M: Influence of acute viral hepatitis on disposition and pharmacological effect of warfarin. *Clin Pharmacol Ther* 20:90–97, 1976.

184. Williams RL, Upton RA, Cello JP, Jones RM, Blitstein M, Kelly J, Nierenburg D: Naproxen disposition in patients with alcoholic cirrhosis. *Eur J Clin Pharmacol* 27:291–296, 1984.
185. Wood AJJ, Kornhauser DM, Wilkinson GR, Shand DG, Branch RA: The influence of cirrhosis on steady-state blood concentrations of unbound propranolol after oral administration. *Clin Pharmacokinet* 3:478–487, 1978.
186. Woodcock BG, Rietbrock I, Vohringer HF, Rietbrock N: Verapamil disposition in liver disease and intensive care patients: kinetics, clearance and apparent blood flow relationships. *Clin Pharmacol Ther* 29:27–34, 1981.

CHAPTER

5

Pharmacotherapy in Pulmonary Disease[a]

PHARMACOLOGIC APPROACH TO THE PATIENT WITH PULMONARY DISEASE

ASTHMA

Aerosolized β_2 agonists are the initial drugs of choice for management of acute bronchospasm. The high margin of safety for inhaled β_2 agonists allows these agents to be given as frequently as q20 minutes × the first 3 doses, then repeated q hour in severe cases (1). Sequential inhalation may maximize the therapeutic effects of β-adrenergic agonists by allowing better penetration of the bronchodilator aerosol after some bronchodilation has been achieved (2). Continuous nebulization has also been used (3), but the efficacy of this mode of delivery has yet to be shown.

In most patients with an attack of bronchospasm, especially if airway narrowing is predominantly due to spasm and not to mucosal edema, control can be achieved with aerosolized β_2

[a]The material in this chapter was contributed by the following: The opening text and Tables 5.2, 5.5, and 5.7 were contributed by Henry J. Silverman, M.D.; Tables 5.1, 5.3, 5.4, 5.6, and 5.9 were contributed by Marissa Seligman, Pharm.D.; Table 5.8 was contributed by Bertil K. J. Wagner, Pharm.D., David M. Angaran, M.S., F.C.C.P., F.A.S.H.P., and David W. Fuhs, M.S., Pharm.D.; Tables 5.10 and 5.11 were contributed by Robert Chin Jr., M.D., F.C.C.P., Donald Charles Eagerton, M.D., and Michael Salem, M.D.; Table 5.12 was contributed by Daniel J. Lebovitz, M.D., and Michael D. Reed, Pharm.D., F.C.C.P., F.C.P.

agonists within the first hour (4). Intravenous aminophylline should not be part of the initial management of acute severe bronchospasm, because this agent in combination with a sympathomimetic is neither additive nor synergistic and may increase the toxicity of inhaled β-adrenergic agonists (5, 6). Intravenous steroids may be administered as part of initial treatment in patients who present with severe bronchospasm (peak expiratory flow rate (PEFR) < 100 liters/min).

Status asthmaticus is present when there is no improvement or further deterioration occurs after initial treatment. At this time, concern with the inability of an aerosol dose to penetrate the lower airways due to mucus plugs and/or airway edema may warrant the use of s.c. or i.v. preparations. Corticosteroids should also be administered, if not already given, and intravenous aminophylline should be started at this time. Magnesium sulfate may also be administered as a 1.2-g bolus in 50 ml of saline over 20 minutes.

Although anticholinergic agonists should not be used as primary therapy because of their slow time course of action and medium potency, their administration may help prolong the duration of bronchodilation. Aerosolized corticosteroids have no role during the acute exacerbation of asthma, because they can cause bronchial irritation and potentially worsen the attack. Antibiotics should not be administered unless there is a strong suspicion of pneumonia based on clinical and radiographic findings and the Gram stain (7).

Oxygen therapy should be given to all patients with bronchospasm to mitigate paradoxical bronchodilator-induced hypoxemia and reverse hypoxic pulmonary vasoconstriction. If mechanical ventilation is instituted, sedatives may be useful to minimize peak airway pressure due to agitation; paralyzing agents (vecuronium bromide or pancuronium bromide) may also be beneficial in reducing airway pressures by decreasing chest wall compliance. The anesthetic gases halothane and ether may also cause further bronchodilation. The mucolytic agent *N*-acetylcysteine may be useful when combined with therapeutic bronchoscopy for bronchial lavage to remove tenacious mucus (8).

CHRONIC OBSTRUCTIVE PULMONARY DISEASE

The administration of supplemental, low-flow oxygen is probably the single most useful treatment in most cases of acute exacerbations of chronic obstructive pulmonary disease (COPD) (9). Although COPD is characterized by irreversible airflow obstruction, there may be a reversible component in the setting of an acute exacerbation (10–12) and, therefore, aerosolized β_2 agonists should initially be administered in conjunction with oxygen. If no response occurs, then an aerosolized anticholinergic agent may be helpful. Intravenous aminophylline has not been shown to be helpful in acute exacerbations of COPD (13). The benefit of corticosteroids in the treatment of an acute exacerbation is controversial, but a short-term administration may be warranted in those refractory to initial treatment. Mucolytic agents may be beneficial in the presence of tenacious sputum. *N*-acetylcysteine (1–4 ml of a 10% solution) can be aerosolized with a bronchodilator.

Diuretics are helpful when increased extravascular lung water is present. Antibiotics are useful only when there is evidence for bronchitis or pneumonia (14). Respiratory stimulants may prevent intubation and mechanical ventilation by allowing time for the beneficial actions of bronchodilators, corticosteroids, and oxygen to take effect, but the high incidence of side effects associated with these agents causes their administration to be controversial (15).

ADULT RESPIRATORY DISTRESS SYNDROME

The overall mortality rate of 50–70% associated with adult respiratory distress syndrome (ARDS) has remained unchanged during the past 10–20 years, not only due to the increased prevalence of sicker patients presenting with this syndrome but also to the lack of therapy aimed at treating the underlying pathogenesis.

Recent advances, however, made in elucidating the pathophysiology of this syndrome have started to influence the pharmacologic approach to patients with this syndrome. Briefly, investigators have emphasized the importance of sepsis as a cause of ARDS and have focused on the relationships between endotoxin, macrophages, and circulating cytokines in mediating the manifestations of this syndrome (16–21). Consequently, ARDS is considered as simply the pulmonary component of a generalized panendothelial inflammation affecting multiple organs and caused by circulating mediators released in response to systemic sepsis, trauma, or another major insult.

The appreciation that nosocomial infections, especially pneumonia, enhance the mortality rate in patients with ARDS (22–25) has led to strategies aimed at preventing these infections. One strategy involves selective decontamination of the digestive tract (SDD) with the use of oral and systemic antibiotics. The rationale for this therapy is to suppress the growth of potentially pathogenic aerobic Gram-negative gut bacteria that may aspirate directly into the lungs or invade the systemic circulation via bacterial translocation (15, 26–28). Although several studies have reported a decrease in the incidence of nosocomial pneumonias in patients treated with a SDD protocol, compared to that of control patients, only two studies have shown a significant decrease in mortality (29).

Gastric acid neutralization with H_2-receptor antagonists or antacids with subsequent gastric microbial growth may increase the incidence of aspiration pneumonia. Studies comparing sucralfate, a cytoprotective agent that has in vitro antibacterial properties, with pH-altering agents have suggested a decreased incidence of nosocomial pneumonias with this agent (30–32) and, therefore, its use should be considered in patients tolerating enteral feedings.

The demonstration of pathological oxygen supply dependency in ARDS leading to tissue hypoxia and subsequent multiple organ failure has led several investigators to suggest therapy aimed at maximizing oxygen delivery (33–35). Methods to minimize oxygen demand may also be beneficial in restoring the balance between oxygen demand and uptake. Fever, increased work of breathing, anxiety, and the metabolic stresses of sepsis, trauma, and the associated tissue repair processes all increase the metabolic demand for oxygen. Hence, antipyretics to correct hyperthermia, as well as agents to induce sedation and muscular paralysis, may be beneficial. No study, however, has yet demonstrated that optimizing DO_2 and VO_2 enhances survival.

The central role that endotoxin may play in initiating the immunoinflammatory cascade has led to investigations on the efficacy of antibodies to endotoxin in sepsis. Initial studies with antiendotoxin antibodies were optimistic (36, 37), but recent studies employing monoclonal antibodies have been less impressive (38, 39).

Tumor necrosis factor (TNF), a mediator released by macrophages in response to endotoxin, may play a role in promoting lung injury (40–42). Recent animal studies have demonstrated the efficacy of antibodies to TNF in endotoxin shock (43, 44) and, currently, phase I as well as phase III clinical trials are underway to determine the safety and efficacy of such antibodies in humans with the sepsis syndrome.

Therapeutic strategies have also focused on modulating the inflammatory response in ARDS. Nonsteroidal antiinflammatory drugs that inhibit cyclooxygenase products have reduced the extent of pulmonary injury in animal models of sepsis and ARDS (45–47). Promising results have been observed in initial clinical trials, using ibuprofen (48–59). Corticosteroids and prostaglandin E_1 (PGE_1) have not been shown to benefit patients with ARDS (60–64).

Survival statistics demonstrating that approximately only 10% of patients die from respiratory failure (23) suggest that therapeutic strategies focused on alleviating pulmonary injury may not be rewarding. Indeed, newer ventilatory strategies, including extracorporeal techniques, have not enhanced survival in patients with ARDS (51). However, hyperoxia lung damage is a concern, because elevated concentrations of oxygen must be given to patients due to increased pulmonary shunting. Some pulmonary oxygen toxicity could be avoided if intracellular PO_2 monitoring indicated adequate cellular oxygenation at lower FIO_2 levels. Unfortunately, current therapeutic prescription of oxygen is based empirically on arterial PO_2, which does not reflect the adequacy of cellular oxygen utilization. Hence, the lowest possible concentration of oxygen that maintains tissue oxygenation should be administered in order to avoid further pulmonary injury from hyperoxia. At the present time, it is recommended that PEEP be employed to maintain the PAO_2 > 60 mm Hg at an FIO_2 at or below 0.6. Surfactant may help with limiting the use of high concentrations of oxygen, but it awaits further clinical trials before its safety and efficacy can be assessed.

PULMONARY EMBOLISM

Treatment of pulmonary embolism begins with a high level of suspicion, followed by appropriate diagnostic studies, which has been the focus of several reviews (52–55). When pulmonary embolism is initially suspected and there are no contraindications to its use, heparin therapy should begin with a loading dose of 5000–10,000 units, followed by a maintenance infusion of 1000–2000 units/h, which is continued for 7–10 days if a pulmonary embolism is confirmed. Therapy is monitored by the partial thromboplastin time (PTT) and a therapeutic effect is achieved when the baseline PTT is 1.5–2.0 times that of the control. The PTT is checked q12h for 2 days, then daily if the patient remains stable. Oral anticoagulation with warfarin is begun 1 or 2 days after heparin therapy has been initiated and is monitored by the prothrombin time (PT), with the dose titrated to maintain the PT 1½–2 times above the control value.

Thrombolytic therapy should probably be reserved for those patients with hemodynamic compromise; although studies have shown more rapid resolution of pulmonary emboli with thrombolytic agents (56, 57), the 8% overall mortality rate of treated pulmonary embolism has not been improved with thrombolytic therapy (58). Streptokinase is given intravenously as a 250,000-unit bolus over 30 minutes, followed by a maintenance infusion of 100,000 units/h for 24 hours. If after 2–3 hours the thrombin time cannot be prolonged despite an infusion rate in excess of 200,000 units/h, the patient is probably resistant to streptokinase due to circulating antistreptococcal antibodies in high titer. Consequently, urokinase should be administered. After 24 hours, thrombolytic therapy is discontinued, and the patient is started on heparin in a full anticoagulant dose as soon as the thrombin time, followed serially every few hours after discontinuation of streptokinase, falls to within 2½ times the control value.

Tissue plasminogen activator is also effective for thrombolytic therapy in patients with pulmonary emboli and is administered intravenously as an initial bolus of 20 mg over 1 hour, followed by an infusion of 10 mg/h for a total dose of 40–100 mg (59, 65).

In addition to lytic therapy, pulmonary embolism associated with hemodynamic compromise should be supported with fluids to elevate right ventricular preload and to permit more effective right ventricular emptying against the acute increase in afterload and, if necessary, sympathomimetic agents should be given to improve right ventricular function (66).

PULMONARY HYPERTENSION

Pulmonary hypertension is most amenable to pharmacologic therapy in disorders in which active vasoconstriction plays a major pathogenic role and includes patients with COPD or primary pulmonary hypertension.

Chronic Obstructive Pulmonary Disease. In patients with COPD, reversible pulmonary hypertension is due to hypoxic vasoconstriction, which occurs from alterations in pulmonary gas exchange. Several efforts can be used that are directed toward this pathophysiologic mechanism. One, inhaled bronchodilators (β_2 agonists and/or anticholinergic agents), can improve alveolar ventilation and alleviate alveolar hypoxia by producing bronchodilation and enhanced mucociliary clearance. Subcutaneous administration of terbutaline (0.25 mg) can also effect pulmonary vasodilation and provide inotropic support for the right side of the heart (67, 68). Theophylline, in addition to its bronchodilator effects, may also improve right ventricular function and cause pulmonary vasodilation.

Supplemental oxygen should be administered chronically only when the initial hypoxemia has failed to respond to intensive pharmacotherapy, which may take up to 3 months. Presently, oxygen is recommended for patients with either a $PO_2 <$ 55 mm Hg while breathing room air or a PO_2 of 55–65 mm Hg in the presence of secondary erythrocytosis, mental dysfunction responsive to oxygen, or cor pulmonale.

The treatment of right heart failure in cor pulmonale is guided by the presence of the patient's symptoms. Diuretics can treat systemic venous congestion and peripheral edema and relieve dyspnea by reducing pulmonary capillary congestion and extravascular lung water. Diuretics may also enhance left ventricular function by reducing the size of the right ventricle, which can impair left ventricular (LV) filling when dilated (69). Diuretics must be given cautiously, because excessive reduction in right ventricular end-diastolic volume may cause cardiac output to decrease, and excessive use may generate a metabolic alkalosis, which can depress ventilation and thereby elicit alveolar and arterial hypoxemia.

Digitalis has been shown to be useful only in patients with both right and left ventricular function (70–72). Although this agent increases right ventricular contractility, it can also cause pulmonary vasoconstriction (73). This effect, coupled with the enhanced risk of digitalis toxicity in the presence of hypoxemia, acidosis, catecholamine excess, and hypokalemia, has led to the disuse of digitalis in most patients with pulmonary hypertension (74).

Vasodilators should be considered only when conventional therapy and oxygen have failed to ameliorate signs of right ventricular failure in view of the potential adverse consequences of these agents. Hence, careful assessment of their effects on hemodynamics and oxygenation must be undertaken, which usually requires invasive right-sided catheterization.

If vasodilators are used, a beneficial hemodynamic response to a vasodilator is considered when (*a*) pulmonary vascular resistance is reduced by more than 20% and cardiac output is increased or unchanged and (*b*) pulmonary arterial pressure is decreased or unchanged and systemic blood pressure is not significantly reduced (75).

Vasodilator therapy in COPD patients includes the use of hydralazine, nitrates, or calcium channel blockers. Results with hydralazine have been mixed, with some studies showing beneficial hemodynamic effects (76–81), while others indicate limited or detrimental effects, such as excessive ventilation causing increased dyspnea (82–84). Nitrates have produced significant reductions in pulmonary arterial pressure and pulmonary vascular resistance, but due to their vasodilating effects, cardiac output usually falls (76).

Nifedipine often produces an acute decrease in pulmonary vascular resistance, an increase in cardiac output and, in many cases, decreases in pulmonary artery pressure (85–90). A decrease in PAO_2 may occur in some patients as a result of an unfavorable influence on pulmonary ventilation-perfusion relationships caused by reversal of hypoxic vasoconstriction, but this effect is usually mild, and oxygen delivery still may be increased because of the favorable effect of nifedipine on cardiac output. Use of nifedipine should probably be limited to the short-term management of acute decompensations of cor pulmonale, because one study showed lack of long-term hemodynamic effects with this agent, as well as a paradoxical detrimental interaction with concurrent oxygen use (85). Diltiazem and verapamil have not been shown to have an effect on pulmonary hemodynamics in COPD patients (91, 92). PGE_1 has demonstrated favorable hemodynamic effects in acutely decompensated chronic lung disease (93).

MUCOLYTICS

Although the use of physical methods to improve mucus clearance is well-known to the critical care physician, the use and efficacy of pharmacologic methods has been largely ignored due to the lack of well-designed clinical trials, the lack of objective measures of benefit, and uncertainty about the type of patients who are likely to benefit from this therapeutic modality.

Respiratory tract secretions in the tracheobronchial tree originate mainly from the submucosal bronchial glands and goblet cells. The submucosal glands are well-supplied by cholinergic fibers from the vagus nerve and, when stimulated, produce a fluid of relatively low viscosity. These glands are poorly supplied by sympathomimetic nerves. In contrast, the goblet cells are not controlled by the autonomic nervous system but respond to irritants by secreting a relatively viscous product (94).

Reduced mucociliary clearance may be due to an ineffective cough, abnormalities in ciliary function, enhanced epithelial permeability, or alterations in the viscoelasticity properties of the bronchial mucus (94–99). Mucous hypersecretion with retained secretions is seen in patients with asthma, chronic bronchitis, and heavy smokers.

Drugs that decrease mucus clearance include atropine, an anticholinergic agent, which acts by either reducing submucosal gland and epithelial secretions or by inhibiting ciliary activity (100–102). Ironically, atropine could have a beneficial effect on the low-viscosity secretions in the bronchorrhea that sometimes occurs in asthma (103). Results demonstrating the effect of aerosolized ipratropium, a synthetic quaternary anticholinergic, on mucociliary function have been conflicting (104–107), but it is probably safe to administer it with careful monitoring.

Mucociliary clearance may be enhanced by the use of β_2-adrenergic agonists (108–110) and theophyllines (111–113). Some of the improvement in clearance from bronchodilators may be due to enhanced cough based on bronchodilation and a higher peak flow rate. Corticosteroids may improve mucociliary clearance by reducing mediator-induced mucus secretion or by their effects on epithelial inflammation (114–117).

Mucoregulatory drugs have no effect on the mucus already formed but stimulate the activity of the secreting cells. These drugs include bromhexine, carbocysteine, sobrerol, letosteine, and strepronine. Studies with these agents, however, have shown conflicting results (118).

Mucolytics, in contrast, act by breaking up mucoprotein molecules in the mucus already formed in the air passages, promoting expectoration and resorption of the secretions, thus creating the conditions for rapid improvement in mucociliary transport. The best-studied mucolytic agent is *N*-acetylcysteine (119). This agent may be administered topically, orally, or intravenously. It possesses a free sulfhydryl group that can rupture disulfide chemical bonds. The aerosol can induce bronchospasm, which is prevented by concomitant bronchodilator therapy. The aerosol dose is 1–4 ml of a 10% solution of *N*-acetylcysteine, administered every 3–6 hours with a bronchodilator.

Iodide has had long-standing popularity as an oral or intravenous agent with both mucoregulatory and mucolytic effects

(119–122). Iodide can be given as a saturated solution of potassium iodide (SSKI) (10–20 drops in a beverage 3–4 times/day). Side effects include an offensive taste and gastric irritation. A less toxic product is iodinated glycerol (Organidin), which has shown improvement in the clinical status of patients with chronic bronchitis and asthmatics (123). The oral dosage for adults is 60–120 mg 4 times/day.

SURFACTANT

Surfactant, a surface-active physiochemical agent that lines the alveolar surface of the lung (124), reduces surface tension (125) at the air-liquid interface at low end-expiratory volumes, increases lung compliance, and aids in keeping the alveoli dry as an "antiedema" factor (126). The importance of surfactant was recognized more than 50 years ago by Von Neergaard (127), who described how the lungs were more difficult to inflate with air than with fluid and by Avery and Mead (128), who demonstrated that the lungs of infants with hyaline membrane disease had a much higher surface tension than that found in normal lungs.

The components of natural pulmonary surfactant are lipids, proteins, and carbohydrates (129, 130). Phospholipids are the major components of surfactant, making up 80–90% of its weight. The two major classes of phospholipids are phosphatidylcholine and phosphatidylglycerol, with dipalmitoylphosphatidylcholine (DPPC) as the main surface active component. The functions of the other surfactant lipids are less well defined. At least three lung-specific proteins (apoproteins) have been shown to be associated with pulmonary surfactant (131). Although still in dispute, it has become increasingly evident that these proteins aid in spreading surfactant on the alveolar surface, regulate surfactant phospholipid metabolism, and play a role in the immune defense system of the lung. The functional significance of the carbohydrate components remains to be established.

Pulmonary surfactant is secreted from the type II pneumocyte into the alveolar lumen. The surfactant is packaged and stored as lipid bilayers in lamellar bodies, which are exocytosed into the alveolar lumen. Ninety to ninety-five percent of secreted alveolar surfactant is recycled, reprocessed, refined, and repackaged for resecretion via the type II cells. A small fraction of surfactant undergoes macrophage degradation.

Clearance of surfactant material from the alveolar space of normal lungs appears to occur with a half-life of about 20 hours (130). There does not seem to be a large intracellular or extracellular reserve of alveolar surfactant. A number of studies have shown that a variety of agents can stimulate surfactant secretion, including adrenergic agonists, prostaglandins, and cholinergic agonists (132).

Whereas a quantitative surfactant deficiency exists in neonatal respiratory distress syndrome (RDS), animal models of acute lung injury that simulate most of the pathophysiologic and morphologic features of ARDS (133–140), as well as studies in patients with ARDS (141, 142), have demonstrated biochemical and functional deficiencies of surfactant. Mechanisms of surfactant alterations include abnormalities in surfactant production by type II cells and biophysical inhibition of surfactant by constituents of permeability pulmonary edema (136, 137, 143–145). Other postulated mechanisms include attack by proteases present in epithelial lining fluid on surfactant apoproteins (146) and oxygen radical-induced oxidation of lung surfactant apoproteins or peroxidation of lung surfactant lipids (147).

Physiological effects of surfactant include increased pulmonary compliance and decreased shunt, leading to use of lower ventilating pressures and enhanced arterial oxygenation at lower FIO_2. These effects could theoretically reduce the risk of barotrauma and help the patient avoid toxic levels of oxygen, which may decrease the high morbidity and mortality associated with ARDS. Indeed, animal investigations studying the role of surfactant replacement therapy have demonstrated improved pulmonary function, as well as enhanced survival (147–150).

Subsequently, surfactant replacement has shown benefit in newborns at risk of developing or already having established respiratory distress syndrome (151–155). These studies have used natural human surfactant, an animal-based extracted surfactant, or a synthetic surfactant consisting of synthetic DPPC and an alcohol to help with spreading and adsorption (EXOSURF). Specifically, prophylaxis with these types of surfactant has reduced mortality by one-half, whereas surfactant treatment for established RDS has reduced mortality and morbidity due to pneumothorax, pulmonary interstitial emphysema, bronchopulmonary dysplasia, and intraventricular hemorrhage.

The dose of surfactant administered in these studies has varied from 50 to 200 mg of surfactant phospholipid per kilogram in a volume of 2–4 ml. This amount is roughly the size of the alveolar surfactant pool. The surfactant suspension was instilled via a fine-bore feeding tube into the trachea. The response was usually rapid, with an immediate increase in arterial oxygen tension and a decrease in oxygen requirements from around 80%–50% or less within 30 minutes. Reductions in ventilatory settings occurred more slowly. In some babies, these improvements in pulmonary function were sustained after a single dose of surfactant, while in others multiple doses were required to maintain the improvement. Recently, the Food and Drug Administration (FDA) granted approval for use of EXOSURF in newborns at risk of developing or having established RDS.

These encouraging results in RDS have led to investigations assessing the efficacy of surfactant replacement therapy in patients with ARDS. Replacement surfactant treatment in ARDS, compared to that in RDS, is probably more complex due to multiple and ongoing factors causing abnormalities in surfactant. Also to be considered is the delivery of adequate amounts of surface active material to the alveolar air-liquid interface due to the large absolute distances in the adult lung, compared to those in the neonate. Furthermore, injured lung units are closed, thus barring entry to the exogenous material. Techniques used have included selective endobronchial instillation under direct vision with the fiberoptic bronchoscope, as well as continuous nebulization.

Direct instillation of a porcine-derived surfactant have shown transient benefits in oxygenation in case reports (156, 157). Recently, aerosol delivery of EXOSURF in patients with septic-induced ARDS has shown improvement in pulmonary function and a trend toward improved survival (158, 159).

PROSTAGLANDINS

The intimate relationship between the pulmonary system and the prostaglandins is evidenced by the ability of the lungs to synthesize and catabolize many of the prostaglandins and by the potent vasoactive effects of several prostaglandins on the pulmonary system. Although the exact role of alterations in prostaglandin metabolism in acute lung injury remains undefined, recent research has focused on the therapeutic aspects of prostaglandins in lung diseases, especially the two prostaglandins known to vasodilate the pulmonary circulation, prostacyclin (PGI_2, epoprostenol) and PGE_1.

PGI_2 and PGE_1 are naturally occurring prostaglandins and are 20 carbon fatty acid products of the cyclooxygenase pathway of arachidonic acid. They have similar structures and are distinguished by the constituents of the cyclopentane ring and the number of double bonds in the attached 20-carbon unsaturated carboxylic acid side chain. These agents have short half-lives (2–3 minutes), and whereas PGI_2 is mainly metabolized by the liver (160), PGE_1 is rapidly degraded during a single passage through the lungs and, hence, its clearance is decreased with lung injury (161, 162).

In addition to being potent pulmonary vasodilators, properties shared by both agents include systemic vasodilation (163), enhancement of myocardial inotropy (164), inhibition of neutrophil activation (165), stabilization of cell membranes or cytoprotection (166–168), and inhibition of platelet aggregation, although PGI_2 is more powerful (169). One advantage, however, of PGI_2 over PGE_1 appears to be less intense and less prolonged platelet activation after discontinuation (170).

CLINICAL USES

Primary Pulmonary Hypertension. Patients in whom no cause can be found for elevated pulmonary pressures are diagnosed as having primary pulmonary hypertension (PPH) (171). Overall survival at 10 years is less than 10%, due predominantly to right ventricular failure. Several studies have demonstrated the safety and efficacy of PGI_2 in producing pulmonary vasodilation, defined by a greater than 20% drop in pulmonary vascular resistance (171–179). The safety of PGI_2 is attributed to its short half-life, which minimizes the risk of sustained and catastrophic decreases in systemic arterial pressure (180–183). Studies have also shown that the acute response to PGI_2 has predictive value for subsequent oral vasodilator therapy (177, 178, 184, 185). The acutely favorable hemodynamic and symptomatic effects of this agent are maintained during prolonged infusions (175, 179), which makes this drug useful in patients awaiting heart-lung transplantation (175–183). The effect, however, of PGI_2 on long-term survival in PPH remains unknown (186, 187).

PGE_1 has reduced pulmonary vascular resistance in patients with PPH (188–190) and also has predictive value for the response to subsequent oral vasodilator therapy (191, 192). The number of studies evaluating the effects of PGE_1 on PPH are less than those with PGI_2. Furthermore, studies assessing prolonged infusions with PGE_1 have not been performed.

Chronic Obstructive Pulmonary Disease. Pulmonary hypertension complicating COPD is a poor prognostic sign (193) and, hence, an effort to lower pulmonary arterial pressure in order to reduce right ventricular afterload, improve cardiac output, and enhance oxygen delivery may be beneficial to survival. In COPD patients with acutely decompensated chronic lung disease, PGE_1 produced decreases in pulmonary vascular resistance and increases in cardiac output (93). In patients with stable COPD, both PGI_2 and a PGE_1 analog reduced pulmonary vascular resistance and increased oxygen delivery (194, 195). The clinical benefit, however, of pharmacologic reduction in right ventricular afterload in patients with pulmonary hypertension secondary to acute or chronic respiratory failure remains unknown.

Adult Respiratory Distress Syndrome. Therapy with prostaglandins has been suggested for the treatment of ARDS due to their antiinflammatory effect, as well as their vasodilator effect on the pulmonary circulation, because pulmonary hypertension is usually present in ARDS (196). Studies in animal models of ARDS have shown beneficial hemodynamic effects with prostaglandins (197–199). Several reports have documented beneficial effects of PGE_1 on pulmonary vascular resistance, cardiac output, and oxygen delivery in patients with ARDS (200–202). Although one small study demonstrated a trend toward improved survival in predominantly surgical patients with ARDS (203), a large multicenter placebo-controlled trial failed to show a survival benefit with PGE_1 administration (64).

STIMULANTS

Drugs with stimulant actions on the central respiratory system have been used to increase ventilation in patients with chronic COPD, primary alveolar hypoventilation syndrome, and the sleep apnea syndromes. Some respiratory stimulant drugs also appear to have a preferential effect on the activation of upper airway muscles to reverse sleep-related upper airway obstruction.

Doxapram, an analeptic agent, has been used in hastening arousal and reversing ventilatory depression following general anesthesia and to increase ventilation in patients with chronic COPD or with primary alveolar ventilation (204, 205), but its side effects, including hypertension, tachycardia, arrhythmias, and seizures, limit the use of this drug.

Theophylline increases respiratory activity by a direct effect on brainstem respiratory centers (206–208). This agent is effective in the management of idiopathic apnea of prematurity (209, 210) but has not been useful in adults with central sleep apnea (211).

Elevated levels of endogenous progesterone in pregnancy and during the progestational phase of the menstrual cycle lead to an increase in alveolar ventilation. Similarly, the administration of progestational agents has been shown to stimulate breathing in normal individuals and in patients with respiratory disorders (212–215). The oral form of medroxyprogesterone acetate (MPA) has been most widely evaluated for its respiratory stimulatory effects. Following oral administration, the drug is promptly absorbed from the intestinal tract. Metabolism takes place in the liver, but significant quantities are excreted in the urine. This agent has been used to increase alveolar ventilation in patients with COPD or with the obesity hypoventilation syndrome (216, 217). MPA in doses of 60 to

120 mg has had limited success in patients with obstructive sleep apnea (218).

Protriptyline, a tricyclic antidepressant, has been shown to relieve obstructive sleep apnea (219–221), which may be due to a selective activation of motor neurons to upper airway muscles to relieve the upper airway obstruction (222).

Acetazolamide, a reversible inhibitor of carbonic anhydrase, produces a metabolic acidosis and a parallel shift to the left of the ventilatory response to hypercapnia. With a left-shifted hypercapnic response, a smaller degree of hypoventilation is more likely to cause a respiratory stimulus. Acetazolamide has been used successfully to treat central sleep apneas (223), but recent reports have noted that central apneas may be replaced by obstructive apneas (224).

In addition to the discussion above, the following tables are included in this chapter:

1. The classes and receptor actions of beta-adrenergic agents (Table 5.1)
2. Dosages of beta agonists in adults and children (Table 5.2)
3. Beta adrenergic aerosol preparations (Table 5.3)
4. Pharmacokinetics of anticholinergic drugs (Table 5.4)
5. Dosages of anticholinergic drugs (Table 5.5)
6. Two tables on initial iv theophylline rates (Tables 5.6 and 5.7)
7. Adverse effects of theophylline (Table 5.8)
8. Factors affecting theophylline clearance (Table 5.9)
9. Properties of commonly prescribed corticosteroids (Table 5.10)
10. NHLBI Recommended dosage schedules for iv steroids in acute exacerbations of asthma (Table 5.11)
11. Selected compounds used via aerosol to modulate respiratory secretions (Table 5.12)

TABLE 5.1. β-Adrenergic Agents[a]

Drug	Route of Administration			Duration of Action (h)	Receptor		
	Injection	*Inhaled*	*Oral*		β_2	β_1	α
Catecholamines							
Epinephrine	Yes	Yes	No	1–2	+	+	+
Isoproterenol	Yes	Yes	No	2–3	+	+	–
Isoetharine	No	Yes	No	2–3	++	+	–
Bitolterol	No	Yes	No	4–6	++	+	–
Resorcinols							
Metaproterenol	No	Yes	Yes	3–5	++	+	–
Terbutaline	Yes	No	Yes	4–6	++	+	–
Fenoterol	No	Yes	No	4–6	++	+	–
Saligen							
Albuterol	No	Yes	Yes	4–6	++	+	–
Salmeterol	No	Yes	No	1–2	++	±	–
Miscellaneous							
Pirbuterol (Salbutamol)	No	Yes	No	4–6	++	±	–

[a] Adapted from Iafrate RP, Massey ICL, Hendeles L: Current concepts in clinical therapeutics: asthma. *Clin Pharm* 5:206-227, 1986.

TABLE 5.2. β-Adrenergic Agonists

Drug	*Preparation*	*Route of Administration*	*Dosage*
Epinephrine	1 mg/ml	s.c.	Adult: 0.1–0.5 mg, repeated in 20–30 min Pediatric: 0.01 mg/kg
Epinephrine (racemic)	2.25% solution	Aerosol	Adult: 0.3–1.0 ml Pediatric: 0.3–0.6 ml
Isoproterenol	0.5% solution (5 mg/ml)	i.v.	Pediatric: 0.05–1.5 μg/kg/min
Metaproterenol	5% solution	Aerosol	Adult: 0.3 ml (15 mg) q2–4h Pediatric: 0.25–0.5 mg/kg q2–4h
	MDI (0.65 mg/puff)	Aerosol	Adult: 2–3 puffs q2–6h Pediatric: 1–3 puffs q4–6h
Terbutaline	0.1% solution	s.c.	Adult: 0.2–0.4 ml (repeated in 15–30 min) Pediatric: 0.2 mg/kg, max = 6 mg
	MDI (0.2 mg/puff)	Aerosol	Adult: 1–2 puffs q4–6h Pediatric: 1–2 puffs q4–6h
Albuterol	5% solution	Aerosol	Adult: 2.5–5 mg q2–4h Pediatric: 0.05–0.15 mg q4–6h
	MDI (90 mg/puff)	Aerosol	Adult: 1–2 puffs q2–4h Pediatric: 1–2 puffs q4–6h
	5% solution	i.v.	Adult: 100-μg bolus followed by 300 μg in 15 min, 0.05–0.2 μg/kg/min Pediatric: 0.05–0.2 μg/kg/min

TABLE 5.3. β_2-Adrenergic Aerosol Preparations and Dosages[a]

Drug	*Preparations*
Isoproterenol hydrochloride and sulfate	
Various manufacturers	0.25% (1:400) 2.5 mg/ml 0.50% (1:200) 5 mg/ml 1.0% (1:100) 10 mg/ml
Isuprel Mistometer	131 μg/spray
Norisodrine Aerotrol	120 μg/spray
Medihaler-Iso	80 μg/spray
Norisodrine sulfate	110 μg/spray
Isoetharine	
Isoetharine hydrochloride for inhalation	0.1%, 0.125%, 0.2%
Bronkosol	0.25%, 0.5%, 1%
Bronkometer	340 μg/spray
Metaproterenol	
Alupent	5% (50 mg/ml) solution for nebulization
Metaprel	0.6% (15 mg/2.5 ml)
Alupent MDI, Metaprel MDI	0.65 mg/puff, powder suspension
Albuterol	
Ventolin	90 μg/puff, powder suspension
Proventil	0.5% (2.5 mg/ml)
Terbutaline	
Brethaire	0.2 mg/puff, powder suspension
Brethine	0.1% (1 mg/ml) (not FDA approved for this use)
Bitolterol	
Tornalate	0.37 mg/spray
Pirbuterol	
Maxair	0.2 mg/puff, powder suspension
Fenoterol hydrobromide[b]	
Berotec	0.16 mg/puff, powder suspension
Salmeterol[b]	
Serevent	0.25 mg/puff, powder suspension

[a] Originally published in Kelly HW: New beta-2-adrenergic agonist aerosols. *Clin Pharm* 4:393–403, 1985.
[b] Pending FDA approval.

Pediatric Dosages	*Adult Dosages*
0.05–0.1 mg/kg q2–4h	1–2 inhalations of 0.25% solution by hand-bulb nebulizer; via nebulizer q2–4h
1–2 inhalations q4–6h	1–2 sprays q2–4h
0.1–0.2 mg/kg q2–4h	3–5 mg undiluted via nebulizer with oxygen at 4–6 liters/min over 15–20 min q2–4h
	0.5 and 1% solutions diluted 1:3 with 0.9% sodium chloride q2–4h
1–2 sprays q4–6h	1–2 sprays q4–6h
0.25–0.5 mg/kg q2–4h (15 mg maximum single dose)	0.3 ml (15 mg) diluted with 2.5 ml of 0.9% sodium chloride nebulized q2–4h
1–2 puffs q4–6h and before exercise	2–3 puffs q4–6h and before exercise
1–2 puffs q4–6h and before exercise	1–2 puffs q4–6h and before exercise
0.05–0.15 mg diluted with 1–2 ml 0.9% normal saline q4–6h	2.5–5 mg diluted with 0.9% normal saline q4–6h
1–2 puffs q4–6h and before exercise	1–2 puffs q4–6h and before exercise
0.1–0.3 mg/kg q2–6h	5–7 mg undiluted q4–6h
1–3 sprays q4–6h	1–3 sprays q4–6h
1–2 puffs q4–6h	1–2 puffs q4–6h
1–2 puffs q4–6h	1–2 puffs q4–6h
1–2 puffs q12h	1–2 puffs q12h

TABLE 5.4. Bronchodilator Properties of Anticholinergic Drugs[a]

Drug	*Dosages*	*Route of Administration*	*Time of Onset (min)*	*Peak Effect (min)*	*Duration (h)*
Atropine sulfate	0.025–0.075 mg/kg	Inhalation	15–30	30–170	3–5
	0.4–1 mg	Oral	NA	NA	NA
Atropine methonitrate	1–1.5 mg	Inhalation	15–30	40–60	4–6
Glycopyrrolate	0.0044 mg/kg	Inhalation	15–30	30–45	2–8
		Intramuscular	15–30	30–45	2–7
		Subcutaneous			
	0.2 mg	Intravenous	1	NA	NA
Ipratropium	20–40 μg	Inhalation	3–30	90–120	3–8

[a] Adapted from Ziment I, Au JP: Anticholinergic agents. *Clin Chest Med* 7:355–366, 1986.

TABLE 5.5. Anticholinergic Drugs

Drug	*Preparation*	*Route of Administration*	*Dosage*	
Atropine	0.2 (0.5% solution)	Aerosol	Adult:	0.025–0.1 mg/kg q4–6h
			Pediatric:	0.025–0.1 mg/kg q4–6h
Glycopyrrolate	0.02% solution	i.v.	Adult:	0.1–0.2 mg
		Aerosol	Adult:	0.8–1.6 mg q6–8h
Ipratropium	MDI, 20 μg/puff	Aerosol	Adult:	2–4 puffs qid
			Pediatric:	1–2 puffs tid
	0.025% solution (Europe only)	Aerosol	Adult:	100–500 μg q6h

TABLE 5.6. Initial Intravenous Theophylline Maintenance Dosages[a]

Patient Population	*Age*	*Theophylline Infusion Rate[b] (mg/kg/h)*
Neonates	Postnatal age up to 24 days	1 mg/kg q12h[c]
	Postnatal age above 24 days	1.5 mg/kg q12h[c]
Infants	6–52 weeks	0.008 × (age in weeks) + 0.21
Young children	1–9 yr	0.8
Older children	9–12 yr	0.7
Adolescents (smokers)	12–16 yr	0.7
Adolescents (nonsmokers)	12–16 yr	0.5[d]
Adults (healthy, smokers)	16–50 yr	0.7[d]
Adults (healthy, nonsmokers)	Above 16 years (including the elderly)	0.4[d]
Adults with cardiac decompensation, cor pulmonale, or liver dysfunction	Above 16 years	0.2[e]

[a] Originally published in Iafrate RP, Massey KL, Hendeles L: Current concepts in clinical therapeutics: asthma. *Clin Pharm* 5:206–227, 1986. Copyright 1986, American Society of Hospital Pharmacists, Inc. All rights reserved. Used with permission.

[b] Assumes that an appropriate loading dose has been given. To achieve a target concentration of 10 μg/ml. Use lean body weight for obese patients. Although these doses generally are safe, many patients will require higher infusion rates as determined by serial serum measurements. These dosages differ from the current FDA recommendations, which include a higher infusion rate for the first 12 hours. Further dosage reductions may be required for patients who are receiving other drugs that decrease theophylline clearance.

[c] For a target concentration of 7.5 μg/ml (for neonatal apnea).

[d] Not to exceed 900 mg/day unless clinical symptoms and/or serum levels indicate the need for a larger dose.

[e] Not to exceed 400 mg/day unless clinical symptoms and/or serum levels indicate the need for a larger dose.

TABLE 5.7. Initial Intravenous Theophylline Maintenance Dosages

Patient Population	*Theophylline Infusion Rate (mg/kg/h)*
Children 1–9 years old	0.8
Children over 9 years old	0.6
Healthy smokers (adult)	0.8
Healthy nonsmokers (adults)	0.5
Patient age > 60 years	0.3
Congestive heart failure or liver disease	0.2

TABLE 5.8. Adverse Effects of Theophylline[a]

Serum Concentration	*Symptoms*
5–20 µg/ml	Nausea, cramps, insomnia, headache
	Tremor
	Excessive gastric acid secretion
15–35 µg/ml	Nausea, vomiting, diarrhea, stomach ache, headache, irritability, nervousness, insomnia, sinus tachycardia
	Hyperglycemia
>35 µg/ml	Seizures, cerebral hypoxia, arrhythmias, cardio-respiratory arrest, death

[a]Adapted from Hendeles L, Weinberger M: Theophylline: therapeutic use of serum concentration monitoring. In Taylor WJ, Finn AL (eds): *Individual Drug Therapy: Practical*

TABLE 5.9. Factors That Affect Theophylline Clearance[a]

Increase Theophylline Clearance	*Decrease Theophylline Clearance*
Smoking (cigarettes or marijuana)	Hepatic cirrhosis
Phenobarbital	Cor pulmonale
High-protein/low-carbohydrate diet	Congestive heart failure
Charcoal-broiled diet	Propranolol
Phenytoin	Allopurinol (>600 mg/day)
Carbamazepine	Erythromycin
Rifampin	Cimetidine
	Troleandomycin
	Oral contraceptives

[a]Originally published in Iafrate RP, Massey KL, Hendeles L: Current concepts in clinical therapeutics: asthma. *Clin Pharm* 5:206–227, 1986.

Frequency	Duration	Comments
Rare—if dose is slowly titrated over 1–2 weeks	Transient	
Common—if therapeutic serum concentrations are rapidly attained	Transient	Avoided by dose titration
Rare—with concurrent administration of oral β_2-adrenergic agonists	Unknown	Avoided if β_2-agonist is administered by inhalation
Rare		
Common—at serum concentrations >20 μg/ml	Persistent	Decrease dose
Rare—may occur in neonates	Persistent	
Common	Persistent	Minor adverse effects often do not precede life-threatening toxicity

Applications of Drug Monitoring. Gross, Townsend, Frank, Hoffman, New York, 1981, vol 1, pp 32–65. Used with permission.

TABLE 5.10. Properties of Commonly Prescribed Corticosteroids[a]

Agent	*Dose (mg)*	*Mineralocortical Potency*[b]	*Glucocorticoid Potency*[c]	*Duration of Action (h)*
Dexamethasone	0.75	0	25	72
Methylprednisolone	4.0	0.5	5	36
Prednisolone	5.0	0.8	4	24
Prednisone	5.0	0.8	4	24
Cortisol	20.0	1.0	1	8
Hydrocortisone	25.0	1.0	0.8	8
Cortisone	25.0	1.0	0.8	8

[a] From Chernow B: Hormonal and metabolic considerations in critical care medicine. In *Critical Care: State of the Art*. Society of Critical Care Medicine, Fullerton, CA, 1982, vol 3, pp J1.
[b] The higher the number in this column, the more likely the use of the agent will cause metabolic alkalosis.
[c] The higher the number in this column, the more likely the agent will cause suppression of hypothalamic corticotropin-releasing factor (CRF) and pituitary ACTH.

TABLE 5.11. NHLBI Recommended Dosage Schedules for Intravenous Steroids in Acute Exacerbations of Asthma

Methylprednisolone	60–80 mg i.v. bolus	q6–8hr
Hydrocortisone	2.9 mg/kg i.v. bolus	q4h
Hydrocortisone	2.0 mg/kg i.v. bolus	Then 0.5 mg/kg/h continuous i.v. infusion

TABLE 5.12. Selected Compounds Used via Aerosol to Modulate Respiratory Secretions[a]

"Bland" agents
- Water
- Saline
  - Hypotonic (0.45% NaCl)
  - Normal saline (0.9% NaCl)
  - Hypertonic (2–20% NaCl)
- Sodium bicarbonate

Mucolytics
- *N*-acetylcysteine (20%)
- Pancreatic dornase
- rh DNase

Anticholinergics
- Atropine
- Glycopyrrolate
- Ipratropium

[a]See Chapter 35 in *The Pharmacologic Approach to the Critically Ill Patient,* Third Edition, for specific details regarding administration techniques, dose ranges, and associated adverse effects.

REFERENCES

1. Rossing TH, Fanta CH, Goldstein DH, Snapper JR, McFadden Jr ER: Emergency therapy of asthma: comparison of the acute effects of parenteral and inhaled sympathomimetics and infused aminophylline. *Am Rev Respir Dis* 122:365–371, 1980.
2. Heimer D, Shim C, Williams Jr MH: The effects of sequential inhalations of metaproterenol in asthma. *J Allergy Clin Immunol* 66:75–77, 1980.
3. Colacone A, Wolkone N, Stern E, et al: Continuous nebulization of albuterol (salbutamol) in acute asthma. *Chest* 97:693, 1990.
4. Fanta CH, Rossing TH, McFadden Jr ER: Emergency room treatment of asthma: relationships among therapeutic combinations, severity of obstruction and time course of response. *Am J Med* 72:416–422, 1982.
5. Fanta CH, Rossing TH, McFadden Jr ER: Treatment of acute asthma. Is combination therapy with sympathomimetics and methylxanthines indicated? *Am J Med* 80:5–10, 1986.

6. Siegel D, Sheppard D, Gelb A, Weinberg PF: Aminophylline increases the toxicity but not the efficacy of an inhaled beta-adrenergic agonist in the treatment of acute exacerbations of asthma. *Am Rev Respir Dis* 132:283–286, 1985.
7. Graham VAL, Milton AF, Knowles GK, et al: Routine antibiotics in hospital management of acute asthma. *Lancet* ii:418, 1982.
8. Millman M, Good AH, Goldstein IM, et al: Status asthmaticus: use of acetylcysteine during bronchoscopy and lavage to remove mucus plug. *Ann Allergy* 50:85, 1963.
9. Degaute JP, Domenighetti G, Naeije R, et al: Oxygen delivery in acute exacerbation of chronic obstructive lung disease. Effects of controlled oxygen therapy. *Am Rev Respir Dis* 124:26, 1981.
10. Irwin RS, Corraro WM, Erickson AD, et al: A true exacerbation of chronic obstructive bronchitis can be objectively defined. *Am Rev Respir Dis* 123(suppl):57, 1981.
11. Schmidt GA, Hall JB: Acute or chronic respiratory failure: assessment and management of patients with COPD in the emergency setting. *JAMA* 261:3444, 1989.
12. Dull WL, Alexander MR, Sadoul P, et al: The efficacy is isoproterenol inhalation for predicting the response to orally administered theophylline in chronic obstructive pulmonary disease. *Am Rev Respir Dis* 126:656, 1982.
13. Rice KL, Leatherman JW, Duane PG, Snyder LS, Harmon KR, Abel J, Niewoehner DE: Aminophylline for acute exacerbations of chronic obstructive pulmonary disease. *Ann Intern Med* 107:305–309, 1987.
14. Anthonisen NR, Monfreda J, Warren CPW, Hershfeld ES, Harding GKM, Nelson NA: Antibiotic therapy in exacerbations of chronic obstructive pulmonary disease. *Ann Intern Med* 106:196, 1987.
15. Redl H, Schlag G: Pathophysiology of multi-organ failure (MOF)—Proposed mechanisms. *Clin Intensive Care* 1:66, 1990.
16. Fein A, Lippmann M, Holtzman H, et al: The risk factors, incidence and prognosis of the adult respiratory distress syndrome following septicemia. *Chest* 83:40–42, 1983.
17. Fowler AA, Hamman RF, Good JT, et al: Adult respiratory distress syndrome: risk with common predisposition. *Ann Intern Med* 98:593–597, 1983.
18. Brigham KL, Meyrick B, Berry LC, et al: Antioxidants protect cultured bovine lung endothelial cells from injury by endotoxin. *J Appl Physiol* 63:840–850, 1987.
19. Parsons PE, Worthen GS, Moore EE, et al: The association of circulating endotoxin with the development of the adult respiratory distress syndrome. *Am Rev Respir Dis* 140:294–301, 1989.
20. Border JR: Hypothesis: sepsis, multiple systems organ failure and the macrophage. *Arch Surg* 123:285–286, 1988.
21. Said SI, Foda HD: Pharmacologic modulation of lung injury. *Am Rev Respir Dis* 139:1553–1564, 1989.
22. Seidenfeld JJ, Pohl DF, Bell RD, et al: Incidence, site, and outcome of infections in patients with the adult respiratory distress syndrome. *Am Rev Respir Dis* 134:12–16, 1986.
23. Montgomery AB, Stager MA, Carrico C, et al: Causes of mortality in patients with the adult respiratory distress syndrome. *Am Rev Respir Dis* 132:485–489, 1985.
24. Hyers TM, Fowler AA: Adult respiratory distress syndrome: causes, morbidity, and mortality. *Fed Proc* 45:25–29,1986.
25. Bell RC, Coalson JJ, Smith JD, et al: Multi-organ system failure and infection in adult respiratory distress syndrome. *Ann Intern Med* 99:293–298, 1983.
26. Van Deventer SJH, ten Cate JW, Tytgat GNJ: Intestinal endotoxemia: clinical significance. *Gastroenterology* 94:825, 1988.

27. Deitch EA, Berg R, Specian R: Endotoxin promotes in the translocation of bacteria from the gut. *Arch Surg* 122:185, 1986.
28. Van Saene HKF, Stoutenbeek CP, Zandstra DF: Concept of selective decontamination of the digestive tract in the critically ill. In van Seane HKF, Stoutenbeek CP, Lawin P, et al (eds). *Infection Control by Selective Decontamination*. Springer-Verlag, Berlin, pp 88–94, 1989.
29. Vandenbroucke-Grands CM, Vandenbroucke JP: Effect of selective decontamination of the digestive tract on respiratory tract infections and mortality in the intensive care unit. *Lancet* ii:859–862, 1991.
30. Cook DJ, Laine LA, Guyalt GH, Raffin TA: Nosocomial pneumonia and the role of gastric pH: a meta-analysis. *Chest* 100:7–13, 1991.
31. Heyland D, Mandell ZA: Gastric colonization by Gram-negative bacilli and nosocomial pneumonia in the intensive care unit patient: Evidence for causation. *Chest* 101:187–193, 1992.
32. Eddlestone JM, Vohra A, Scott P, et al: A comparison of the frequency of stress ulceration and secondary pneumonia in sucralfate—or ranitidine—treated intensive care unit patients. *Crit Care Med* 19:1491–1496, 1991.
33. Vincent LJ, Roman A, de Backer D, Kahn RJ: Oxygen uptake/supply dependency: effects of a short-term dobutamine infusion. *Am Rev Respir Dis* 142: 2–7, 1990.
34. Bihari D, Smithies M, Gimson A, Tinker J: The effects of vasodilation with prostacyclin on oxygen delivery and uptake in critically ill patients. *N Engl J Med* 317:397–404, 1987.
35. Shoemaker WC, Appel PL, Kram HB, Waxman K, Lee TS: Prospective trial of supranormal values of survivors as therapeutic goals in high risk surgical patients. *Chest* 94:1176–1186, 1988.
36. Ziegler EJ, McCutchan AM, Fiererr J, et al: Treatment of Gram-negative bacteremia and shock with human antiserum to a mutant *Escherichia coli*. *N Engl J Med* 307:1225–1230, 1982.
37. Baumgartner JD, Glauser MP, McCutchan JA, et al: Prevention of Gram negative shock and death in surgical patients by antibody to endotoxin. *Lancet* ii:59–63, 1985.
38. Greenman RL, Schein RMH, Martin MA, et al: A controlled clinical trial of E5 murine monoclonal IgM antibody to endotoxin in the treatment of Gram-negative sepsis. *JAMA* 266:1097–1102, 1991.
39. Ziegler EJ, Fisher Jr CJ, Sprung CL, et al: Treatment of Gram-negative bacteremia and septic shock with HA-1A human monoclonal antibody against endotoxin—a randomized double blind, placebo-controlled trial. *N Engl J Med* 324:429–436, 1991.
40. Mathison JC, Wolfson D, Ulevith RJ: Participation of tumor necrosis factor in the mediation of Gram negative bacterial lipopolysaccharide-induced injury in rabbits. *J Clin Invest* 81:1925–1937, 1988.
41. Tracey KJ, Lowry SF, Cerami A: Cachetin/TNF-α in septic shock and septic adult respiratory distress sydnrome. *Am Rev Respir Dis* 138:1377–1379, 1988.
42. Stephens KE, Ishizaka A, Larrick JW, et al: Tumor necrosis factor causes increased pulmonary permeability and edema. *Am Rev Respir Dis* 147:1364–1370, 1988.
43. Beutler B, Milsark IW, Cerami AC: Passive immunization against cachectic tumor necrosis factor protects mice from lethal effects of endotoxin. *Science* 229:869–871, 1985.
44. Tracey KJ, Fong Y, Wesse DG, et al: Anti-cathectin/TNF monoclonal antibodies prevent septic shock during lethal bacteremia. *Nature* 330:662–664, 1987.
45. Metz CA, Sheagren JN: Ibuprofen in animal models of septic shock. *J Crit Care* 5:206, 1990.

46. Snapper JR, Hutchison AA, Ogletree ML, et al: Effects of cyclooxygenase inhibitors on the alterations in lung mechanics caused by endotoxemia in the unanesthetized sheep. *J Clin Invest* 72:63, 1983.
47. Balk RA, Jacobs RF, Tryka AF, et al: Effects of ibuprofen on neutrophil function and acute lung injury in canine endotoxin shock. *Crit Care Med* 16:1121, 1988.
48. Bernard GR, Reines HD, Metz CA, et al: Effects of a short course of ibuprofen in patients with severe sepsis. *Am Rev Respir Dis* 137:138, 1988.
49. Haupt MT, Justremski MS, Clemmer TP, Metz CA, Goris GB: Effect of ibuprofen in patients with severe sepsis: a randomized, double-blind, multicenter study. *Crit Care Med* 19:1339–1347, 1991.
50. Bernard GR, Reines HD, Halushka PV, et al: Prostacyclin and thromboxane A_2 formation is increased in human sepsis syndrome. Effect of cyclooxygenase inhibition. *Am Rev Respir Dis* 144:1095–1101, 1991.
51. Zopol WM, Snider MT, Hill JD, et al: Extracorporeal membrane oxygenation in severe acute respiratory failure. *JAMA,* 242:2193–2196, 1979.
52. Hull RD, Hirsh J, Carter CJ, et al: Pulmonary angiography, ventilation lung scanning, and venography for clinically suspected pulmonary embolism with abnormal perfusion lung scan. *Ann Intern Med* 98:891–899, 1983.
53. The PIOPED Investigators: Value of the ventilation/perfusion scan in acute pulmonary embolism. Results of the prospective investigation of pulmonary embolism diagnosis (PIOPED). *JAMA* 263:2753–2759, 1990.
54. Kelley MA, Carson JL, Palevsky HI, Schwartz S: Diagnosing pulmonary embolism: new facts and strategies. *Ann Intern Med* 114:300–306, 1991.
55. Hull RD, Raskob GE: Low-probability lung scan findings: a need for change. *Ann Intern Med* 114:142–144, 1991.
56. Bell WR, Meek AG: Guidelines for the use of thrombolytic agents. *N Engl J Med* 301:1266, 1979.
57. Genton E: Thrombolytic therapy of pulmonary thromboembolism. *Prog Cardiovasc Dis* 21:333, 1979.
58. Dalen JE: The case against fibrinolytic therapy. *J Cardiovasc Med* 5:798, 1980.
59. Gore JM, Thompson MJ, Becker RC: Rapid resolution of acute core pulmonale with recombinant tissue plasminogen activator. *Chest* 96:939, 1989.
60. Sprung CL, Caralis PV, Marcial EH, et al: The effects of high-dose corticosteroids in patients with septic shock: a prospective controlled study. *N Engl J Med* 311:1137–1143, 1984.
61. Veterans Administration Systems Sepsis Cooperative Study Group: Effect of high dose glucocorticoid therapy on mortality in patients with clinical signs of systemic sepsis. *N Engl J Med* 317:659–665, 1987.
62. Luce JM, Montgomery AB, Marks JD, et al: Ineffectiveness of high-dose methylprednisolone in preventing parenchymal lung injury and improving mortality in patients with septic shock. *Am Rev Respir Dis* 138:62–68, 1988.
63. Bernard GR, Luce JM, Sprung CL, et al: High-dose corticosteroids in patients with the adult respiratory distress syndrome. *N Engl J Med* 317:1565–1570, 1987.
64. Bone RC, Slotman G, Maunder R, et al: Randomized double-blind, multicenter study of prostaglandin E_1 in patients with the adult respiratory distress syndrome. *Chest* 96:114–119, 1989.
65. PIOPED Investigators: Tissue plasminogen activator for the treatment of acute pulmonary embolism. *Chest* 97:528, 1990.
66. Molloy WD, Leeky, Girling L, Schick U, Prewitt RM: Treatment of shock in a canine model of pulmonary embolism. *Am Rev Respir Dis* 130:870–874, 1984.
67. Brent BN, Mahler D, Verger HJ, et al: Augmentation of right ventricular performance in chronic obstructive pulmonary disease by terbutaline: a combined radionuclide and hemodynamic study. *Am J Cardiol* 50:313–319, 1982.

68. Ringsted CV, Eliasen K, Andersen JB, et al: Ventilation-perfusion distributions and central hemodynamics in chronic obstructive pulmonary disease: effects of terbutaline administration. *Chest* 96:976–983, 1989.
69. Fishman AP: Chronic cor pulmonale. *Am Rev Respir Dis* 114:775–794, 1976.
70. Mathur PN, Powles ACP, Pugsley SO, et al: Effect of digoxin on right ventricular function in severe chronic airflow obstruction. *Ann Intern Med* 95:283–288, 1981.
71. Brown SE, Pakron FJ, Milne N, et al: Effects of digoxin on exercise capacity and right ventricular function during exercise in chronic airflow obstruction. *Chest* 85:187–191, 1984.
72. Mathur PN, Powles ACP, Pubsley SO, et al: Effect of long-term administration of digoxin on exercise performance in chronic airflow obstruction. *Eur J Respir Dis* 66:273–283, 1985.
73. Kim YS, Aviado DM: Digitalis and the pulmonary circulation. *Am Heart J* 62:680–686, 1961.
74. Green LH, Smith TW: The use of digitalis in patients with pulmonary disease. *Ann Intern Med* 87:459–465, 1977.
75. Rubin LJ: Vasodilators and pulmonary hypertension: where do we go from here? *Am Rev Respir Dis* 135:288–293, 1987.
76. Brent BN, Berger HJ, Matthay RA, et al: Contrasting acute effects of vasodilators (nitroglycerin, nitroprusside, and hydralazine) on right ventricular performance in patients with chronic obstructive pulmonary disease and pulmonary hypertension: a combined radionuclide-hemodynamic study. *Am J Cardiol* 51:1682–1689, 1983.
77. Corriveau ML, Minh V-D, Dolan GF: Long-term effects of hydralazine on ventilation and blood gas values in patients with chronic obstructive pulmonary disease and pulmonary hypertension. *Am J Med* 83:886–892, 1987.
78. Corriveau ML, Rosen BJ, Keller CA, et al: Effect of posture, hydralazine, and nifedipine on hemodynamics, ventilation, and gas exchange in patients with chronic obstructive pulmonary disease. *Am Rev Respir Dis* 138:1494–1498, 1988.
79. Dal Nogare AR, Rubin LJ: The effects of hydralazine on exercise capacity in pulmonary hypertension secondary to chronic obstructive pulmonary disease. *Am Rev Respir Dis* 133:385–389, 1986.
80. Keller CA, Shepard JW, Chun DS, et al: Effects of hydralazine in hemodynamics, ventilation and gas exchange in patients with chronic obstructive pulmonary disease and pulmonary hypertension. *Am Rev Respir Dis* 130:606–611, 1984.
81. Rubin LJ, Peter RH: Hemodynamics at rest and during exercise after oral hydralazine in patients with cor pulmonale. *Am J Cardiol* 47:116–122, 1981.
82. Lupi-Herrera E, Seoane M, Verdejo J: Hemodynamic effect of hydralazine in advanced, stable chronic obstructive pulmonary disease with cor pulmonale: immediate and short-term evaluation at rest and during exercise. *Chest* 85:156–163, 1984.
83. McGoon MD, Seward JB, Vlietstra RE, et al: Hemodynamic response to intravenous hydralazine in patients with pulmonary hypertension. *Br Heart J* 50:579–585, 1983.
84. Packer M, Greenberg B, Massie B, et al: Deleterious effects of hydralazine in patients with pulmonary hypertension. *N Engl J Med* 1306:1326–1331, 1982.
85. Agostoni P, Doria E, Galli C, et al: Nifedipine reduces pulmonary pressure and vascular tone during short—but not long—term treatment of pulmonary hypertension in patients with chronic obstructive pulmonary disease. *Am Rev Respir Dis* 139:120–125, 1989.
86. Kennedy TP, Michael JR, Huang C-K, et al: Nifedipine inhibits hypoxic pulmonary vasoconstriction during rest and exercise in patients with chronic obstructive pulmonary disease. *Am Rev Respir Dis* 129:544–551, 1984.

87. Melot C, Hallemans R, Naeije R, et al: Deleterious effect of nifedipine on pulmonary gas exchange in chronic obstructive pulmonary disease. *Am Rev Respir Dis* 130:612–616, 1984.
88. Morley TF, Zappasodi SJ, Belli A, et al: Pulmonary vasodilator therapy for chronic obstructive pulmonary disease and cor pulmonale: treatment with nifedipine, nitroglycerin, and oxygen. *Chest* 92:71–76, 1987.
89. Simonneau G, Escourrou P, Duroux P, et al: Inhibition of hypoxic pulmonary vasoconstriction by nifedipine. *N Engl J Med* 304:1582–1585, 1981.
90. Sturani C, Bassein L, Schiavina M, et al: Oral nifedipine in chronic cor pulmonale secondary to severe chronic obstructive pulmonary disease (COPD): short- and long-term hemodynamic effects. *Chest* 84:135–142, 1983.
91. Brown ES, Linden GS, King RR, et al: Effects of verapamil on pulmonary hemodynamics during hypoxemia, at rest, and during exercise in patients with chronic obstructive pulmonary disease. *Thorax* 38:840–844, 1983.
92. Clozel JP, Delorme N, Battistella P, et al: Hemodynamic effects of intravenous diltiazem in hypoxic pulmonary hypertension. *Chest* 91:171–175, 1987.
93. Naeije R, Melot C, Mols P, Hallemans R: Reduction in pulmonary hypertension by prostaglandin E_1 in decompensated chronic obstructive pulmonary disease. *Acta Ther* 6:29, 1980.
94. Ziment I: Mucus in Bronchial Asthma. In Allergra L, Bragu PC (eds): *Bronchial Mucology and Related Disease.* Raven Press, New York, pp 127–140, 1990.
95. Clarke SW: Rationale of airway clearance. *Eur Respir J* 2:599–604, 1989.
96. Puchelle E, Zahm JM, Girard D, et al: Mucociliary transport in vivo and in vitro. Relations to sputum properties in chronic bronchitis. *Eur J Respir Dis* 61:254–264, 1980.
97. Lundgren JD, Shelhamer JH: Pathogenesis of airway mucus hypersecretion. *J Allergy Clin Immunol* 85:399–417, 1990.
98. Wanner A: Clinical aspects of mucociliary transport. *Am Rev Respir Dis* 115:73–125, 1977.
99. Sleigh MA, Blake JR, Liron N: The propulsion of mucus by cilia. *Am Rev Respir Dis* 137:726–741, 1988.
100. Annis P, Landa J, Lichtiger M: Effects of atropine on velocity of tracheal mucus in anesthetized patients. *Anesthesiology* 44:74–77, 1976.
101. Corssen G, Allen CR: Acetylcholine: its significance in controlling ciliary activity of human respiratory epithelium in vitro. *J Appl Physiol* 14:901–904, 1959.
102. Groth ML, Langenback EG, Foster WM: Influence of inhaled atropine on lung mucociliary function in humans. *Am Rev Respir Dis* 144:1042–1047, 1991.
103. Wick MM, Ingram RH: Bronchorrhea responsive to aerosolized atropine. *JAMA* 235:1356–1357, 1976.
104. Pavia D, Batement JRM, Sheahan NF, et al: Effect of ipratropium bromide on mucociliary clearance and pulmonary function in reversible airways obstruction. *Thorax* 34:501–507, 1979.
105. Matthys H, Hundenborn J, Daikeler G, Kohler D: Influence of 0.2 mg ipratropium bromide on mucociliary clearance in patients with chronic bronchitis. *Respiration* 48:329–339, 1985.
106. Foster WM, Langenback EG, Bergofsky EH: Acute effect of ipratropium bromide at therapeutic dose on mucus transport of adult asthmatics. *Eur J Resp Dis* 64(suppl 128):554–557, 1983.
107. Ruffine RE, Wolff RK, Dolorich MB, Rossman CR, Fitzgerald JD, Newhouse MT: Aerosol therapy with Sch 1000. Short-term mucociliary clearance in normal and bronchitic subjects and toxicology in normal subjects. *Chest* 73:501–506, 1978.
108. Sackner MA, Epstein S, Wanner A: Effects of beta adrenergic agonists aerosolized by freon propellant on tracheal mucous velocity and cardiac output. *Chest* 69:593–598, 1976.

109. Foster WM, Bergofsky EH, Bohning DE, Lippman M: Effect of adrenergic agents and their mode of action on mucociliary clearance. *J Appl Physiol* 41:146–152, 1976.
110. Clarke SW, Lopez-Vidriero MT: The effect of beta-2 agonist on the activity of human bronchial cilia in vitro. *J Physiol* 336:40–41, 1982.
111. Welsh MJ, Widdicombe JH, Nadel JA: Fluid transport across the canine tracheal epithelium. *J Appl Physiol* 49:905–909, 1980.
112. Serafini SM, Wanner A, Michaelson ED: Mucociliary transport in central and intermediate size airways: effect of aminophylline. *Bull Eur Physiopathol Respir* 12:415–422, 1976.
113. Sutton PP, Pavia D, Bateman JRM, et al: The effect of oral aminophylline on lung mucociliary clearance in man. *Chest* 80S:889–891, 1981.
114. Agnew JE, Bateman JRM, Sheahan NF, et al: Effect of oral corticosteroids in mucus clearance by cough and mucociliary transport in stable asthma. *Bull Eur Physiopathol Respir* 19:37–41, 1983.
115. Lundgren JD, Kaliner MA, Shelhamer JH: Mechanisms by which glucocorticosteroids inhibit secretion of mucus in asthmatic airways. *Am Rev Respir Dis* 141 (suppl): S52–S58, 1990.
116. Wiggins J, Elliott JA, Stevenson RD, Stockley RA: Effect of corticosteroids on sputum sol-phase protease inhibitors in chronic obstructive pulmonary disease. *Thorax* 37:652–656, 1982.
117. Marom Z, Shelhammer J, Alling D, et al: The effects of corticosteroids on mucous glycoprotein secretion from human airways in vitro. *Am Rev Respir Dis* 129:62–65, 1984.
118. Ziment I: Mucokinetic agents. In Ziment I (ed): *Respiratory Pharmacology and Therapeutics.* WB Saunders, Philadelphia, pp 60–104, 1978.
119. Pavia D, Agnew JE, Glassman JM, Sutton PP, Lopez-Vidriero MT, Soyka JP, et al: Effects of iodopropylidene glycerol on tracheobronchial clearance in stable, chronic bronchitic patients. *Eur J Respir Dis* 67:177–184, 1985.
120. Ziment I: Inorganic and organic iodides. In Braga PC, Allegra L (eds): *Drugs in Bronchial Mycology.* Raven Press, New York, 1989.
121. Repsher LM, Glassman JM, Soyka JP: Evaluation of iodopropylidene glycerol as adjunctive therapy in stable, chronic asthmatic patients on theophylline maintenance. *Today's Ther Trends* 1:77–89, 1983.
122. Prenner BM: Chronic respiratory disease complicated by mucus: results of a clinical evaluation of the mucolytic agent iodinated glycerol in a four-week, open trial of adult asthmatics. *Immunol Allergy Pract* 10:17–20, 1988.
123. Petty TL: The National Mucolytic Study. Results of a randomized, double-blind placebo-controlled, study of iodinated glycerol in chronic obstructive bronchitis. *Chest* 97:75–83, 1990.
124. Sanders RL. The composition of pulmonary surfactant. In Farrell PM (ed): *Lung Development: Biological and Clinical Perspectives.* Academic Press, New York, p 183, 1982.
125. Clements JA: Dependence of pressure-volume characteristics of lungs on intrinsic surface active material. *Am J Physiol* 187:592, 1956.
126. Pattle RE: Surface lining of the lung alveoli. *Physiol Rev* 45:48–79, 1965.
127. Von Neergaard K: New notions on a fundamental principle of respiratory mechanisms. The retractile force of the lungs, dependent on the surface tension in the alveoli (translated by Arnold R, Hahn H). In Comroe JH (ed). *Pulmonary and Respiratory Physiology.* Dowden, Hutchison, and Ross, Stroudsburg, PA, pp 214–234, 1976.
128. Avery ME, Mead J: Surface properties in relation to atelectasis and hyaline membrane disease. *Am J Dis Child* 97:517–523,1959.
129. Wright JR, Clements JA: Metabolism and turnover of lung surfactant. *Am Rev Respir Dis* 135:426–444, 1987.

130. Holm BA, Matalon S: Role of pulmonary surfactant in the development and treatment of adult respiratory distress syndrome. *Anesth Analg* 69:805–818, 1989.
131. Weaver TE: Surfactant proteins and SP-D. *Am J Respir Cell Mol Biol* 5:4–5, 1991.
132. Hollingsworth M, Gilfillan AM: The pharmacology of lung surfactant secretion. *Pharmacol Rev* 36:69–90, 1984.
133. Lachmann B, Hallman M, Bergmann KC: Respiratory failure following anti-lung serum: study on mechanisms associated with surfactant system damage. *Exp Lung Res* 12:163–180, 1987.
134. Berry D, Ikegami M, Jobe A: Respiratory distress and surfactant inhibition following vagotomy in rabbits. *J Appl Physiol* 61:1741–1748, 1986.
135. Holm BA, Notter RH, Seigle J, Matalon S: Pulmonary physiological and surfactant changes during injury and recovery from hyperoxia. *J Appl Physiol* 59:1402–1409, 1985.
136. Ikegami M, Jobe A, Jacobs H: A protein from airways of premature lambs that inhibits surfactant function. *J Appl Physiol* 57:1134–1142, 1984.
137. Seeger W, Stohr G, Wolf HRD: Alteration of surfactant function due to protein leakage: special interaction with fibrin monomer. *J Appl Physiol* 58:326–338, 1985.
138. Fuchimukai T, Fujiwara T, Takahashi A, Enhorning G: Artificial pulmonary surfactant inhibited by proteins. *J Appl Physiol* 62:429–437, 1987.
139. Ryan SF, Lian DF, Loomis-Bell AL, et al: Correlation of lung compliance and quantities of surfactant phospholipids after acute alveolar injury from *N*-nitroso-*N*-methylurethane in the dog. *Am Rev Respir Dis* 123:200–204, 1981.
140. Pison U, Oberatacke U, Brand M, Seeger W, Joka T, Bruch J, Schmit-Neuerburg KP: Altered pulmonary surfactant in uncomplicated and septicemia-complicated courses of acute respiratory failure. *J Trauma* 30:19–26, 1990.
141. Petty TL, Silvers GW, Paul GW, et al: Abnormalities in lung elastic properties and surfactant function in adult respiratory distress syndrome. *Chest* 75:571–574, 1979.
142. Hallman M, Spragg R, Harrell JH, et al: Evidence of lung surfactant abnormality in respiratory failure. *J Clin Invest* 70:673–683, 1982.
143. Holm BA, Notter RH, Finkelstein JN: Surface property changes from interactions of albumin with natural lung surfactant and extracted lung lipids. *Chem Phys Lipids* 38:287–298, 1985.
144. Holm BA, Notter RH: Effects of hemoglobin and cell membrane lipids on pulmonary surfactant activity. *J Appl Physiol* 63:1434–1442, 1987.
145. Holm BA, Enhorning GE, Notter RH: A biophysical mechanism by which plasma proteins inhibit surfactant activity. *Chem Phys Lipids* 49:49–55, 1988.
146. Merritt TA, Hallman M, Spragg R, Heldt GP, Gilliard N: Exogenous surfactant treatments for neonatal respiratory distress syndrome and their potential role in the adult respiratory distress syndrome. *Drugs* 38:591–611, 1989.
147. Matalon S, Holm BA, Notter RH: Mitigation of pulmonary hyperoxic injury by administration of exogenous surfactant. *J Appl Physiol* 62:756–761, 1987.
148. Loewen GM, Holm BA, Milanowski I, Wild LM, Matalon S: Alveolar hyperoxic injury in rabbit receiving exogenous surfactant. *J Appl Physiol* 66:1087–1092, 1988.
149. Kobayashi T, Kataoka H, Ueda T, Murakami S, Takada Y, Kokubo M: Effects of surfactant supplement and end-expiratory pressure in lung-lavaged rabbits. *J Appl Physiol* 57:995–1001, 1984.
150. Berggren P, Lachmann B, Curstedt T, Grossman G, Robertson B: Gas exchange and lung morphology after surfactant replacement in experimental adult respiratory distress syndrome induced by repeated lung lavage. *Acta Anaesthesiol Scand* 30:321–328, 1986.

151. Merit TA, Hallman M, Bloom BT: Prophylactic treatment of very premature infants with human surfactant. *N Engl J Med* 315:785–790, 1986.
152. Collaborative European Multicenter Study Group: Surfactant replacement therapy for severe neonatal respiratory distress syndrome: an international randomized clinical trial. *Pediatrics* 82:683–691, 1988.
153. Horbar JD, Soll SF, Sutherland JM et al: A multicenter, randomized, placebo-controlled trial of surfactant therapy for respiratory distress syndrome. *N Engl J Med* 320:959–965, 1989.
154. Corbet AJ, Goldman SA, Lombrady L, Mammel MA, Long WA: Decreased mortality in small premature infants treated at birth with a single dose of synthetic surfactant: a multicenter trial. *J Pediatr* 118:277–284,1991.
155. Long WA, Thompson T, Sundell H, Schumacher R, Volberg F, Guthrie R: Effects of two rescue doses of synthetic surfactant on mortality in 700–1300 gram infants with RDS. *J Pediatr* 118:595–605, 1991.
156. Richmann PS, Spragg RG, Merritt TA, Curstedt T: The adult respiratory distress syndrome: first trials with surfactant replacement. *Eur Respir J* 2(suppl):109–111, 1989.
157. Lachmann B: Animal models and clinical pilot studies of surfactant replacement in adult respiratory distress syndrome. *Eur Respir J* 2(suppl):98:103, 1989.
158. Weg J, Reines H, Balk R, et al: Safety and efficacy of an aerosolized surfactant (EXOSURF) in human sepsis-induced ARDS. *Chest* 100:137S, 1991.
159. Reines HD, Silverman H, Hurst J: Effects of two concentrations of nebulized surfactant (EXOSURF) in sepsis-induced adult respiratory distress syndrome (ARDS). *Crit Care Med* 20:S61, 1992.
160. Dusting GJ, Moneada S, Vane JR: Recirculation of prostacyclin in the dog. *Br J Pharmacol* 64:315–320, 1978.
161. Gillis CN, Pitt BR, Wiedemann HP, Hammond GL: Depressed prostaglandin E_1 and 5-hydroxytryptamine removal in patients with adult respiratory distress syndrome. *Am Rev Respir Dis* 134:739–744, 1986.
162. Cox JW, Andreadis NA, Bone RC, Maunder RJ, Pullen RH, Ursprung JJ, Vassar MJ: Pulmonary extraction and pharmacokinetics of prostaglandin E_1 during continuous intravenous infusion in patients with adult respiratory distress syndrome. *Am Rev Respir Dis* 137:5–12, 1988.
163. Dusting JD, Moncada S, Van J: Prostaglandins, their intermediates and precursors: cardiovascular actions and regulatory roles in normal and abnormal circulatory systems. *Prog Cardiovasc Dis* 21:405–430, 1979.
164. Metsa-Ketela T: Cyclic AMP-dependent and -independent effects of prostaglandins on the contraction-relaxation cycle of spontaneously beating isolated rat atria. *Acta Physiol Scand* 112:481–485, 1981.
165. Goldstein I, Malmsten C, Samuelsson B, Weissman G: Prostaglandins, thromboxanes and polymorphonuclear leukocytes. *Inflammation* 2:309, 1977.
166. Robert A: Cytoprotection by prostaglandins. *Gastroenterology* 77:761, 1979.
167. Araki H, Lefer A: Cytoprotective actions of prostacyclin during hypoxia in the isolated perfused cat liver. *Am J Physiol* 238:H176, 1980.
168. Sikujara O, Monden M, Toyoshima K, Okamura J, Kosaki G: Cytoprotective effect of prostaglandin I2 (prostacyclin) on ischaemia induced hepatic cell injury. *Transplantation* 36:238, 1983.
169. Whittle B, Moncada S, Vane JR: Comparison of the effects of prostacyclin, prostaglandin E1 and D2 on platelet aggregation of different species. *Prostaglandins* 16:373–388, 1978.
170. Sinzinger H, Reiter R: The intrafusion platelet rebound during and following PGE-infusion is faster and more intensive than that with PGI2. *Prostaglandins Leukotrienes Med* 13:281–288, 1984.
171. Rich S: Primary pulmonary hypertension. *Prog Cardiovasc Dis* 31:205–238, 1988.

172. Szczeklik J, Szczeklik A, Nizankowski R: Hemodynamic effects produced by prostacyclin in man. *Br Heart J* 44:254–258, 1980.
173. Guadagni DN, Ikram H, Maslowski AH: Haemodynamic effects of prostacyclin (PGI_2) in pulmonary hypertension. *Br Heart J* 45:385–388, 1981.
174. Rubin LJ, Groves BM, Reeves JT, Frosolono M, Handel F, Cata AE: Prostacyclin-induced acute pulmonary vasodilation in primary pulmonary hypertension. *Circulation* 66:334–338, 1982.
175. Higenbottam T, Wells F, Wheeldon D, Wallwork J: Long-term treatment of primary pulmonary hypertension with continuous intravenous epoprostenol (prostacyclin). *Lancet* ii:1046–1047, 1984.
176. Kaapa P, Koivisto M, Ylikorkala O, Kouvalainen K: Prostacyclin in the treatment of neonatal pulmonary hypertension. *J Pediatr* 107:951–953, 1985.
177. Groves BM, Rubin LJ, Frosolono MF, Cato AE, Reeves JT: A comparison of the acute hemodynamic effects of prostacyclin and hydralazine in primary pulmonary hypertension. *Am Heart J* 110:1200–1204, 1985.
178. Barst RJ: Pharmacologically induced pulmonary vasodilation in children and young adults with primary pulmonary hypertension. *Chest* 89:497–503, 1986.
179. Rubin LJ, Mendoza J, Hood M, McGoon M, Barst R, Williams WB, Diehl JH, Crow J, Long W: Treatment of primary pulmonary hypertension with continuous intravenous prostacyclin (epoprostenol). *Ann Intern Med* 112:485–491, 1990.
180. Packer M: Vasodilator therapy for primary pulmonary hypertension: limitations and hazards. *Ann Intern Med* 103:258–270, 1985.
181. Packer M: Is it ethical to administer vasodilator drugs to patients with primary pulmonary hypertension? *Chest* 95:1173–1175, 1989.
182. Long W, Barst R, Fishman AP, et al: Acute hemodynamic effects of prostacyclin in 65 primary pulmonary hypertension patients. *J Crit Care* 1:127–128, 1986.
183. Long WA, Rubin LJ: Prostacyclin and PGE_1 treatment of pulmonary hypertension. *Am Rev Respir Dis* 136:773–776, 1987.
184. Palevsky HI, Long W, Crow J, Fishman AP: Prostacyclin and acetylcholine as screening agents. *Circulation* 82:2018–2026, 1990.
185. Reeves JT, Groves BM, Turkevich D: The case for treatment of selected patients with primary pulmonary hypertension. *Am Rev Respir Dis* 134:342–346, 1986.
186. Rich S, Brundage BH, Levy PS: The effect of vasodilator therapy on the clinical outcome of patients with primary pulmonary hypertension. *Circulation* 71:1191–1196, 1985.
187. Rozkovec A, Stradling JR, Shepherd G, MacDermot J, Oakley CM, Dollery CT: Prediction of favourable responses to long term vasodilator treatment of pulmonary hypertension by short term administration of epoprostenol (prostacyclin) or nifedipine. *Br Heart J* 59:696–705, 1988.
188. Watkins WD, Peterson MB, Crone RK, Shannon DC, Levine L: Prostacyclin and prostaglandin E_1 for severe idiopathic pulmonary artery hypertension (letter). *Lancet* 2:1083, 1980.
189. Swan PK, Tibballs J, Duncan AW: Prostaglandin E_1 in primary pulmonary hypertension. *Crit Care Med* 14:72–73, 1986.
190. Vandenbossche JL, Melot C, Naeije R: Prostaglandin E_1 in primary pulmonary hypertension. Acta Ther 6:44, 1980.
191. Lambert RJ, Corrigan PE, Caldwell EJ: The use of PGE_1 to improve the safety of vasodilators in pulmonary hypertension. *Chest* 89:459S, 1986.
192. Halpern SM, Shah PK, Lehrman S, Goldberg HS, Jasper AC, Koerner SK: Prostaglandin E_1 as a screening vasodilator in primary pulmonary hypertension. *Chest* 92:686–691, 1987.
193. Burrows B, Earle RH: Course and prognosis of chronic obstructive lung disease: a prospective study of 200 patients. *N Engl J Med* 280:397–404, 1969.

194. Ishizaki T, Miyabo S, Mifune J, et al: OP-1206, a prostaglandin E_1 derivative: effects of oral administration to patients with chronic lung disease. *Chest* 85:383–386, 1984.
195. Jones K, Higenbottam TW, Wallwork J: Pulmonary vasodilation with prostacyclin in primary and secondary pulmonary hypertension. *Chest* 96:784–788, 1989.
196. Zapol WMC, Snider MT: Pulmonary hypertension in severe acute respiratory failure. *N Engl J Med* 296:476–480, 1977.
197. Smith ME, Gunther R, Zaiss C, et al: Prostaglandin infusion and endotoxin-induced lung injury. *Arch Surg* 117:175–180, 1982.
198. Slotman GJ, Machiedo GW, Casey KF, Lyons MJ: Histologic and hemodynamic effects of prostacyclin and prostaglandin E1 following oleic acid infusion. *Surgery* 92:93–100, 1982.
199. Radermacher P, Santak B, Wust HJ, Tarnow J, Falke KJ: Prostacyclin for the treatment of pulmonary hypertension in the adult respiratory distress syndrome: effects on pulmonary capillary pressure and ventilation—perfusion distributions. *Anesthesiology* 72:238–244, 1990.
200. Appel PL, Shoemaker WC: Hemodynamic and oxygen transport effects of prostaglandin E_1 in patients with adult respiratory distress syndrome. *Crit Care Med* 12:528–529, 1984.
201. Tokioka H, Kobayashi O, Ohta Y, Wakabayashi T, Kosaka F: The acute effects of prostaglandin E_1 on the pulmonary circulation and oxygen delivery in patients with adult respiratory distress syndrome. *Intensive Care Med* 11:61–64, 1985.
202. Shoemaker WC, Appel PL: Effects of prostaglandin E_1 in adult respiratory distress syndrome. *Surgery* 99:275–283, 1986.
203. Holcroft JW, Vassar MJ, Weber CJ: Prostaglandin E_1 and survival in patients with the adult respiratory distress syndrome. *Ann Surg* 203:371–378, 1986.
204. Lugliani R, Whipp BJ, Wasserman K: Doxapram hydrochloride: a respiratory stimulant for patients with primary alveolar hypoventilation. *Chest* 76:414–419, 1979.
205. Moser KM, Luchsinger PC, Adamason JS, et al: Respiratory stimulation with intravenous doxapram in respiratory failure. *N Engl J Med* 288:427–431, 1973.
206. Dowell AR, Heyman A, Sieker HO, Tripathy K: Effect of aminophylline on respiratory center sensitivity in Cheyne-Stokes respiration and in pulmonary emphysema. *N Engl J Med* 273:1447–1453, 1965.
207. Eldridge FL, Millhorn DE, Waldrop TG, et al: Mechanism of respiratory effects of methylxanthines. *Respir Physiol* 53:239–261, 1983.
208. Sanders JS, Berman TM, Bartlett MM, et al: Increased hypoxic ventilatory drive due to administration of aminophylline in normal men. *Chest* 78:279–282, 1980.
209. Gerhardt T, McCarthy J, Bancalari E: Effects of aminophylline on respiratory center and reflex activity in premature infants with apneas. *Pediatr Res* 17:188–191, 1983.
210. Aranda JV, Turman T: Methylxanthines in apnea of prematurity. *Clin Perinatol* 6:87–108, 1979.
211. Guilleminault C, Vanden Hoed J, Mitler: Clinical overview of the sleep apnea syndrome. In Guilleminault C, Dement WC (eds): *Sleep Apnea Syndromes.* Alan R. Liss, New York, pp 1–11, 1978.
212. Delaunois L, Delwiche JP, Lulling J: Effect of medroxyprogesterone on ventilatory control and pulmonary gas exchange in chronic obstructive patients. *Respiration* 47:107–113, 1985.
213. Schoene RB, Pierson DJ, Lakshminarayan S, et al: Effect of medroxyprogesterone acetate on respiratory drives and occlusion pressure. *Bull Eur Physiopathol Respir* 16:645–653, 1980.
214. Skatrud JB, Dempsey JA, Bhansali P, et al: Determinants of chronic carbon dioxide retention and its correction in humans. *J Clin Invest* 65:813–821, 1980.

215. Skatrud JB, Dempsey JA, Kaiser DG: Ventilatory response to medroxyprogesterone acetate in normal subjects: time course and mechanism. *J Appl Physiol* 44:939–944, 1978.
216. Sutton Jr FD, Zwillich CW, Creagh CE, et al: Progesterone for outpatient treatment of Pickwickian syndrome. *Ann Intern Med* 83:476–479, 1975.
217. Tyler JM: The effect of progesterone on the respiration of patients with emphysema and hypercapnea. *J Clin Invest* 39:34–41, 1960.
218. Strohl KP, Hensley MJ, Saunders NA, et al: Progesterone administration and progressive sleep apneas. *JAMA* 245:1230–1232, 1981.
219. Bromnell LG, West P, Sweatman P, et al: Protriptyline in obstructive sleep apnea. *N Engl J Med* 307:1037–1042, 1982.
220. Conway WA, Zorick F, Piccione P, et al: Protriptyline in the treatment of sleep apnea. *Thorax* 37:49–53, 1982.
221. Smith PL, Haponik EF, Allen RM, et al: The effects of protriptyline in sleep-disordered breathing. *Am Rev Respir Dis* 127:8–13, 1983.
222. Bonora M, St. John WM, Bledsoe TA: Differential elevation by protriptyline and depression by diazepam of upper airway respiratory motor activity. *Am Rev Respir Dis* 131:41–45, 1985.
223. White DP, Zwillich CW, Pickett CK, et al: Central sleep apnea: improvement with acetazolamide therapy. *Arch Intern Med* 142:1816–1819, 1982.
224. Sharp J, Druz W, D'Souza V, et al: Effect of metabolic acidosis and alkalosis upon sleep apnea. *Am Rev Respir Dis* 125(suppl):233, 1982.

CHAPTER 6

Pediatrics[a]

Children develop and grow, and their response to drug therapy is conditioned by age, size, and stage of development. It is axiomatic that the change in body size associated with growth is a factor in determining dosage and response. However, even when the effect of size is accommodated, age and level of maturity exert a profound effect on response to pharmacotherapy. The influence of developmental factors is modulated, and usually amplified, by the imposition of critical illness, multiple organ system failure, heredity, and coadministration of other drugs. In infants and small children, vagaries of drug delivery systems and administration techniques assume significance (1–5). This chapter provides a review of selected aspects of pediatric clinical pharmacology. The pharmacology of individual agents is reviewed in greater detail in other chapters. The purpose here is to describe specific features that distinguish pharmacologic responses of children from those of adults, and to indicate, when possible, which observed pharmacologic differences are likely to result in important clinical differences.

[a]Daniel A. Notterman, M.D., contributed the opening text and Figures 6.1 and 6.2 in this chapter to *The Pharmacologic Approach to the Critically Ill Patient*, Third Edition. The other material in this chapter was contributed by the following: Tables 6.1–6.4 and 6.6 were contributed by Daniel A. Notterman, M.D., F.A.A.P., F.C.C.M.; Table 6.5 was contributed by Arno L. Zaritsky, M.D.; Table 6.7 was contributed by Rodolfo I. Godinez, M.D., Ph.D., Marye H. Godinez, M.D., and Russell C. Raphaely, M.D.

Age-related differences in response are both pharmacokinetic and pharmacodynamic in origin (6–9). The pharmacokinetic description concerns the relationship, over time, between drug *dosage* and drug concentration. The pharmacodynamic description concerns the relationship between this concentration and the resulting *response*. Narrowly construed, "pharmacodynamics" means "sensitivity" and applies to the relationship between unbound drug concentration (theoretically at the site of action; in practice, in the plasma) and magnitude of effect. Broadly conceived, pharmacodynamics comprises all of the biochemical and physiologic effects of a substance (8). Sensitivity is graphically represented in several ways (8), most often as a plot of the log of drug concentration versus intensity of pharmacologic response. Figure 6.1, described in more detail in a subsequent section, is from a study by Driscoll and associates (10) and displays the pharmacodynamic relationship between dopamine concentration and the resulting inotropic effect in puppy ventricles from animals of different ages. In some instances, immaturity is associated with enhanced sensitivity to a pharmacologic effect. For example, as indicated in Figure 6.2, the concentration of vecuronium necessary to induce a 50% depression of twitch tension is less in infants (mean age 6.6 months) than it is in children (mean age 41.4 months) or adults.

A fundamental requirement for pharmacodynamic analysis is that there be precise pharmacokinetic information regarding the drug of interest *in the population in question*. Such is gradually becoming available in the pediatric age group.

PHARMACODYNAMIC VARIATION

Pharmacodynamic differences between the responses of pediatric patients and adult patients will be considered in the context of (*a*) effects that are unique in children, (*b*) adverse effects, and (*c*) therapeutically desired effects. This last category will focus on the catecholamines.

UNIQUE EFFECTS

Drugs may have unique effects in children. Examples include substances that disturb patterns of growth and differentiation

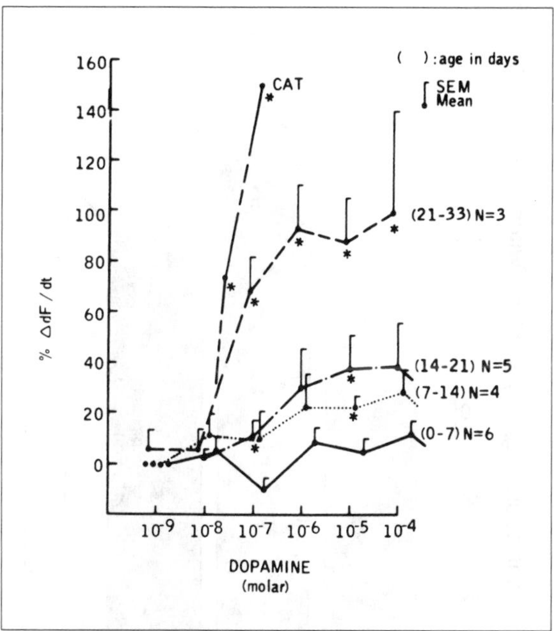

FIGURE 6.1. Inotropic (%ΔdF / dt) dose-response curves of puppy ventricles and adult cat ventricle treated with dopamine. There is an increasing inotropic responsiveness with age of isolated puppy ventricle to dopamine * P < .05 using puppies 0–7 days old as control. (From Driscoll DJ, Gillette PC, Ezrailson EG, et al: Inotropic response of the neonatal canine myocardium to dopamine. *Pediatr Res* 12:42, 1978.)

that occur only during particular phases of life (11). Notable in this regard are teratogens, which have unique adverse effects on the fetus (4, 7, 11–13). To a certain extent, children share this special vulnerability with the fetus until growth and development cease at maturity. Thus, the tetracyclines affect bone growth in the fetus and newborn infant (14), as well as development of the teeth in children less than 6 years of age (15–16). Corticosteroids, among their other adverse effects, suppress the linear growth of children (17), an effect that cannot occur in adults.

Cartilage toxicity is a concern with nalidixic acid (18) and related fluoroquinoline antibiotics such as ciprofloxacin and

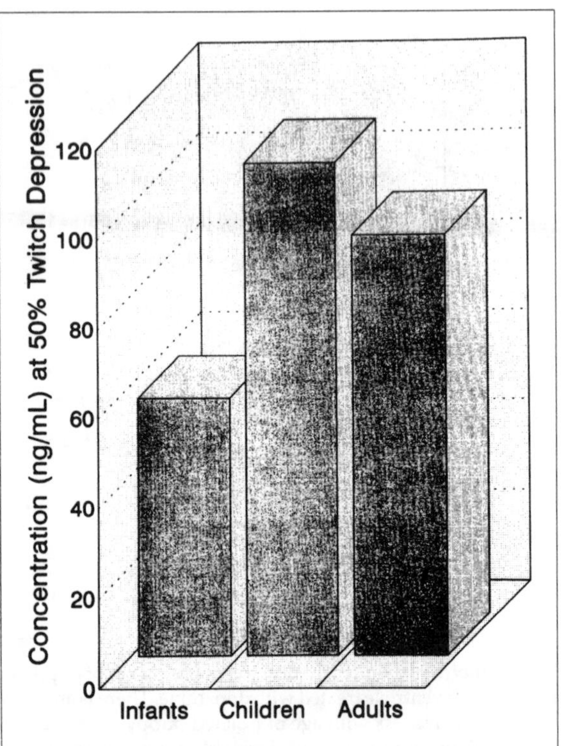

FIGURE 6.2. Effect of age upon pharmacodynamic response to vecuronium. The concentration of vecuronium needed to achieve 50% depression of twitch tension is lower in the infant than in older children or adults. This implies a pharmacodynamic increase in sensitivity to the drug. (Adapted from data in Fisher DM, Castagnoli K, Miller RD: Vecuronium kinetics and dynamics in anesthetized infants and children. *Clin Pharmacol Ther* 37:402, 1985.)

norfloxacin (19, 20). These newly developed quinoline derivatives should be avoided in children until age 17, when skeletal growth is presumed complete (19, 20).

ADVERSE EFFECTS

Increased Occurrence or Sensitivity. Metoclopramide and other dopamine antagonists such as prochlorperazine (Compazine), haloperidol, and chlorpromazine have a variety of potential critical care indications (21–24). These drugs produce acute dystonic reactions much more frequently in children and adolescents than in adults (25–27). A pharmacokinetic basis for this increase in dystonic reactions has been examined and rejected (25). The increase in CNS sensitivity to a variety of dopamine antagonists might be caused by the greater concentration of dopamine-2 receptors in the brains of young subjects (28).

Verapamil, a calcium entry blocking agent, is used to treat supraventricular tachycardia and other atrial dysrhythmias in children (29–31). There are clinical reports of infants developing acute severe cardiorespiratory failure following administration of the drug (32–34). For this reason, verapamil should not be administered to individuals less than 1 year of age (33–35). Fortunately, adenosine, which has been recently introduced for treatment of supraventricular tachycardia, has been shown to be safe and effective in infants and children. The initial dosage employed is 50 μg/kg. The dosage is increased by 50 μg/kg and the dose repeated in 30 seconds until the dysrhythmia resolves (36, 37).

In infants, elastic and resistive properties of the lung entail optimal efficiency at high respiratory rates with low tidal volumes (38). Thus, the resting respiratory rate is higher, and the infant responds to the need for hyperventilation by increasing rate in preference to tidal volume (38). The need to maintain rapid respiratory rates implies greater sensitivity to respiratory depressants. Indeed, some years ago, Way and associates (39) demonstrated that, compared with adults, infants required one-third the dose of morphine (on a weight-normalized basis) for comparable depression in CO_2 sensitivity. Pharmacokinetic factors were not excluded, and further work on the effect of depressant drugs on the immature respiratory system would be useful.

Valproic acid is a broad-spectrum anticonvulsant, but its use is limited by concern regarding hepatic toxicity. There is evidence that the incidence of toxicity is increased in children younger than 2 years of age and is rare over the age of 10 years (40). Paradoxical excitement and hyperactivity very frequently complicate therapy with barbiturates (41, 42). This problem often requires termination of therapy and is more frequent in young children. Of greater concern are reports that indicate that long-term treatment of children with phenobarbital may adversely affect intelligence (43). While the potential effects of phenobarbital upon behavior and intelligence are of concern during chronic management, they are not relevant during acute therapy and do not contraindicate treatment with these drugs in the critical care unit.

Continuous intravenous infusion of sedative-hypnotics and analgesics is employed in critically ill children for control of movement, pain, and anxiety. Midazolam, a benzodiazepine with a short half-life, and fentanyl, an opioid, have been extensively employed for this purpose in pediatric intensive care units (44). Recently, reports of serious movement and cognitive disorders following cessation of infusions with these compounds have been of concern (45). It is likely that these abnormalities represent an abstinence syndrome. It is not known whether induction of such a syndrome occurs with greater facility in children than adults. However, these reports indicate a need for caution before adopting into pediatric practice new therapeutic strategies, such as long-term, continuous intravenous infusion of drugs of this type (46).

Decreased Occurrence or Sensitivity. Children enjoy relative protection from the adverse effects of several drugs. In most cases, the mechanism responsible for the relative immunity of youth has not been determined.

Several drugs cause hepatic injury less frequently in children than in adults. These include isoniazid (35, 47–50), halothane (51–56), and acetaminophen (57–62).

Therapy with isoniazid (INH) is associated with asymptomatic increases in hepatic enzymes in 10–20% of adults (47, 48). In children 9–14 years of age, 17% had elevations of serum glutamic-oxaloacetic transaminase (SGOT) or glutamic-pyruvic transaminase (SGPT), similar to the proportion in adults (50). INH hepatitis, a potentially fatal disorder, develops in some individuals receiving the drug. The risk of developing INH hepatitis increases with age: 0 per 1000 in patients less than 20 years of age; 3 per 1000 for those 20–34 years of age; 12 per 1000 for those 35–49 years old; 23 per 1000 for those 50–65 years of age; and 8 per 1000 for those older than 65 years (34). Despite occasional reports of INH hepatitis in children (50), usually when INH and rifampin are coadministered (49), the incidence is still extremely low, and measurement of SGOT is not routinely performed in children receiving INH alone. Neither the mechanism of INH hepatitis nor the reason for the relative protection of youth has been elucidated.

Although there are isolated case reports to the contrary (52, 56), halothane hepatotoxicity appears to be extremely rare in children, even following multiple exposures to the drug, which increases risk in adults (56). Again, the mechanism of protection is unknown.

Acetaminophen produces marked elevation (>1000 IU / liter) of SGOT following ingestion of a substantial overdose (>150 mg/kg) (60). Without administration of an antidote, such as *N*-acetylcysteine (61), severe hepatitis occurs in 10% of adults, with an associated mortality of 10–20% (58). Of individuals with potentially toxic acetaminophen levels, 5.5% of those less than 12 years of age had SGOT levels above 1000 IU/liter, while 29% of those older than 12 years had an increase of this magnitude (60). The protection conferred by young age has been related to ingestion of relatively small quantities of drug and to early emesis (60, 61). This fact is not the only explanation, since severe hepatotoxicity in children is rare even in the presence of levels associated with severe injury to adults (60). Children younger than about 9 years of age conjugate acetaminophen with sulfate as well as glucuronate (62). It is suggested that this additional pathway of detoxification reduces flux through the mixed-function oxidase pathway implicated in acetaminophen hepatotoxicity (60, 62), or that children have increased availability of glutathione, used to detoxify acetaminophen metabolites (60). These explanations remain speculative. Cases of severe acetaminophen toxicity and death have occurred in children (57, 59). Thus, children who ingest a potentially toxic quantity should be fully evaluated and treated with *N*-acetylcysteine if the concentration of acetaminophen exceeds the "probable risk" line of the Rumack nomogram (61) or if more than 150 mg/kg have been ingested and a serum level cannot be determined within 16 hours of ingestion (60).

Aminoglycoside ototoxicity and nephrotoxicity are probably less common in infants and children than in adults (63–66). There is experimental and clinical evidence that the kidney of the infant or child is more tolerant of aminoglycoside exposure (63, 64). Enzymuria, a marker of renal tubular injury, is less in infants and children following treatment with an aminoglycoside, and there is less renal accumulation of these drugs in infants (64). In an analysis of controlled studies, the incidence of cochlear and vestibular toxicity was not found to be greater in infants receiving aminoglycosides than in control subjects (65). The relatively low incidence of aminoglycoside toxicity in infants and children should not be taken as evidence that these drugs are innocuous (65). The usual precautions for minimizing aminoglycoside toxicity, including therapeutic drug monitoring when appropriate, are indicated.

Infants tolerate higher serum concentrations of digoxin than do older children or adults (67–69), although some investigators dispute this observation (70). Lessened susceptibility to glycoside-induced arrhythmias may be a result of decreased norepinephrine content and sympathetic innervation of ventricular myocardium (69–72), increased vagal tone (73), and/or a healthier myocardium without superimposed coronary artery disease (72).

Three other points should be mentioned regarding digoxin. *First,* the observation that infants tolerate higher concentrations of digoxin without manifesting toxicity does not mean that they require higher concentrations in order to achieve therapeutic benefit. In fact, no therapeutic advantage accrues to maintaining serum digoxin levels greater than those also associated with therapeutic efficacy (1–2 ng/ml) in adults (69, 74–76). Infants with relatively high and relatively low digoxin levels have comparable shortening of systolic time intervals (76, 77). An average level of 1.3 ng/ml provides adequate cardiac functional improvement in infants with congestive heart failure (69, 75). *Second,* when normalized by weight, the dose of digoxin needed to achieve a particular digoxin concentration is larger in infants than in adults (69, 74, 75). This fact represents a true pharmacokinetic difference between the two populations and is reflected in different dosage requirements (69, 74). As discussed, this pharmacokinetic observation does not mean that infants are less sensitive to the drug. *Third,* the discovery of an endogenous digoxin-like substance that interacts with digoxin assays employing antibody systems (78, 79) means that older information concerning digoxin pharmacokinetics and dosage in infants and patients with hepatic or renal failure may need revision.

Because of their size, children need and are able to tolerate smaller volumes of intravenous fluid than do adults. Obviously, drug dosage requirements differ between adults and children. When administering drugs, the clinician must be aware of potential drug toxicities, interactions, and adverse affects in all patients. When treating a pediatric patient, the clinician must ensure that the drug dosage is appropriate for the size and age of the child. While there are innumerable differences between the pediatric and adult patients, this chapter highlights some of the more important differences and provides a framework of dosing information for the pediatric patient:

1. Maximum drug concentrations for intravenous infusions in infants and children (Table 6.1)
2. A formula to calculate creatinine clearance in children (Table 6.2)
3. Fraction of drug dose excreted in urine in patients with normal renal function (Table 6.3)
4. Plasma half-lives of oxidating drugs in newborns and adults (Table 6.4)
5. Preparation of inotrope infusions in children (Table 6.5)
6. Dosage of neuromuscular blocking drugs in children (Table 6.6)

Pediatric patients with respiratory distress are increasingly treated with surfactant therapy. This relatively new treatment is also addressed in this chapter:

7. Recommended dose of surfactants in clinical use (Table 6.7)

TABLE 6.1. Maximum Drug Concentration for Intravenous Infusions in Infants and Children[a]

Drug	*Concentration*
Antibiotics	
Acyclovir	7 mg/ml
Amikacin	6 mg/ml
Amphotericin B	0.1 mg/ml
β-Lactams[b]	50–100 mg/ml
Chloramphenicol	100 mg/ml
Clindamycin	12 mg/ml
Co-Trimoxazole[c]	1 mg/15 ml
Erythromycin lactobionate	5 mg/ml
Gentamicin	2 mg/ml
Imipenem/Cilastatin	5 mg/ml
Kanamycin	6 mg/ml
Metronidazole	8 mg/ml
Penicillin G	50,000–100,000 U/ml
Tobramycin	2 mg/ml
Vancomycin	5 mg/ml
Vidarabine	0.7 mg/ml
Neuromuscular Blocking Agents	
Atracurium	10 mg/ml
Pancuronium	1–2 mg/ml
Vecuronium	1 mg/ml
Inotropes and Pressors	
Dobutamine	5 mg/ml
Dopamine	3.2 mg/ml
Epinephrine	100 mg/ml
Norepinephrine	4 mg/ml
Other Cardiovascular Drugs	
Bretylium Tosylate	10 mg/ml
Lidocaine	0.2–1.2 mg/ml
Methyldopate	10 mg/ml
Nitroprusside	100–200 μg/ml
Procainamide	2-4 mg/ml
Miscellaneous	
Aminophylline	25 mg/ml
Cimetidine	6 mg/ml
Diphenhydramine	50 mg/ml
Ethacrynate	2 mg/ml
Magnesium	200 mg/ml
Ranitidine	2 mg/ml

[a] From Ford DC, Leist ER, Phelkps SJ: *Guidelines for Administration of Intravenous Medications to Pediatric Patients*, ed 3. American Society of Hospital Pharmacists, Inc., Bethesda, MD, 1988; Lipkin F: Personal communication, 1992.
[b] β-Lactams, penicillin derivatives and cephalosporins.
[c] Co-trimoxazole is trimethoprim/sulfamethoxazole.

TABLE 6.2. Method for Calculating Cl_{cr} in Children Aged 1 Week to 21 Years[a,b]

Cl_{cr} (ml/min/1.73 m^2) = length (cm) × k/P_{cr} (mg dl)

Age	*k*
Infant (1–52 weeks)	0.45
Child (1–13 years)	0.55
Adolescent (14–21 years)	
Male	0.7
Female	0.55

[a] Based on Schwartz and associates (80–82).
[b] This method is valid for individuals without severe muscle wasting and with stable plasma creatinine (P_{cr}) values.

TABLE 6.3. Fraction of Dose Excreted Unchanged in Urine (*f*) with Normal Renal Function[a]

Antibiotics	*f*
Acyclovir[b]	0.8
Aminoglycosides[b]	1.0
Ampicillin[b]	0.8
Amphotericin	0
Erythromycin	0.1
Cefazolin[b]	0.8
Cefoperazone	0.3
Cefotaxime	0.5
Cefoxitin[b]	0.9
Ceftazidime[b]	0.9
Ceftriaxone	0.5
Cefuroxime[b]	0.9
Chloramphenicol	0
Clindamycin	0.1
Ganciclovir[b]	1.0
Imipenem/Cilastin[b]	0.7
Methicillin[b]	0.9
Metronidazole	0.1
Nafcillin	<0.2
Oxacillin[b]	0.8
Penicillin[b]	0.9
Rifampin	0
Sulfamethoxazole[b]	0.9
Trimethoprim[b]	0.7
Vancomycin[b]	1.0
Miscellaneous	*f*
Acetaminophen	0
Atenolol[b]	0.9
Atricurium	0
Cimetidine[b]	0.6
Digoxin[b]	0.7
Lithium[b]	1.0
Lorazepam	0
Midazolam	0
Pancuronium[b]	0.7
Ranitidine[b]	0.7
Vecuronium	0.2

[a] Adapted from Rowland M, Tozer TN: *Clinical Pharmacokinetics.* Lea & Febiger, Philadelphia, 1980.

[b] Indicates that dosage reduction may be necessary with clinically significant renal dysfunction. Individual product information should be consulted.

TABLE 6.4. Calculation of Half-life for a Proposed Drug with the Same Clearance as Inulin (Glomerular Filtration) or *p*-Aminohippuric Acid (PAH) (Tubular Secretion) in an Infant (1.5 months old) and Adult[a,b]

Weight (kg)	*ECW*		*Inulin*		*PAH*	
	% of Weight	*Total Volume (ml)*	*Clearance (ml/min)*	$t_{1/2}$ *(min)*	*Clearance (ml/min)*	$t_{1/2}$ *(min)*
4.5	32	1,440	10	100	25	40
70.0	18	12,600	130	67	650	13

[a] From Rane A, Wilson JT: Clinical pharmacokinetics in infants and children. In Gibaldi M, Prescott L (eds): *Handbook of Clinical Pharmacokinetics.* ADIS Health Science Press, New York, 1983.

[b] The drug distributes in the extracellular water space (ECW). Calculation is based on $t_{1/2} = 0.693 \times V_d \times Cl^{-1}$.

TABLE 6.5. Preparation of Inotrope Infusions in Children

Inotrope	*Preparation*	*Dose*
Epinephrine Norepinephrine Isoproterenol	0.6 × body weight (kg) is the number of milligrams added to diluent to make final volume of 100 ml	1 ml/h delivers 0.1 μg/kg/min
Dopamine Dobutamine Amrinone[a]	6 × body weight (kg) is the number of milligrams added to diluent to make final volume of 100 ml	1 ml/h delivers 1 μg/kg/min

[a] A loading dose of 3–4.5 mg/kg should precede the continuous infusion; the loading dose should be given as repeated 1–1.5 mg/kg infusions over several minutes with careful monitoring of blood pressure.

TABLE 6.6. Dosage of Neuromuscular Blocking Drugs in Children

Drug	*Dosage (mg/kg)*
Succinylcholine	
Newborns, infants	2
Children to adults	0.6–1
Pancuronium	
Newborns	0.02–0.04
2–4 weeks	0.06–0.08
>4 weeks	0.1
Continuous infusion[a]	0.1 mg/kg/h
Atricurium[b]	
All ages	0.4–0.5 mg/kg
Vecuronium[b]	
All ages[c]	0.08–1.0 mg/kg
Continuous infusion[a]	0.1 mg/kg/h

[a] Titrate.
[b] Not examined in neonates.
[c] Duration of action prolonged in infants.

TABLE 6.7. Recommended Dose of Surfactants in Clinical Use

Trade Name	*Type*
Surfactant TA	Modified Natural
Infrasurf	Natural
Curosurf	Natural
	Natural
ALEC	Artificial
HDL	Artificial
Exosurf	Artificial

[a]DPPC, dipalmitoyl phosphatidyl choline; PG, phosphatidyl glycerol.

REFERENCES

1. Gould T, Roberts RJ: Therapeutic problems arising from the intravenous route for drug administration. *J Pediatr* 95:465, 1979.
2. Leff RD, Roberts RJ: Methods of intravenous drug administration in the pediatric patient. *J Pediatr* 98:631, 1981.
3. Nelson JD: *Pocketbook of Pediatric Antimicrobial Therapy,* ed 7. Williams & Wilkins, Baltimore, 1987.
4. Roberts RJ: *Drug Therapy in Infants.* WB Saunders, Philadelphia, 1984.
5. Roberts RJ: Intravenous administration of medications in pediatric patients: problems and solutions. *Pediatr Clin North Am* 28:23, 1986.
6. Barthels H: Drug therapy in childhood: what has been done and what has to be done. *Pediatr Pharmacol* 3:31, 1983.
7. Boreus LO: *Principles of Pediatric Pharmacology.* Churchill Livingstone, New York, 1982.
8. Ross EM, Gilman AG: Pharmacodynamics: mechanisms of drug action and the relationship between drug concentration and effect. In Gilman AG, Goodman LS, Roll TW, Murad F (eds): *The Pharmacological Basis of Therapeutics,* ed 7. Macmillan, New York, 1985.
9. Rowland M, Tozer TN: *Clinical Pharmacokinetics.* Lea & Febiger, Philadelphia, 1980.
10. Driscoll DJ, Gillette PC, Ezrailson EG, et al: Inotropic response of the neonatal canine myocardium to dopamine. *Pediatr Res* 12:42, 1978.
11. Lowrey GH: *Growth and Development of Children,* ed 7. Year Book, Chicago, 1978.
12. McBride WG: Thalidomide and congenital abnormalities. *Lancet* 2:1358, 1961.
13. Shaywitz SE, Caparulo BK, Hodgson ES: Developmental language disability as a consequence of prenatal exposure to ethanol. *Pediatrics* 68:850, 1981.
14. Cohlan SQ, Bevelander G, Tiamsic T: Growth inhibition of prematures receiving tetracycline: clinical and laboratory investigation. *Am J Dis Child* 105:453, 1963.
15. Grossman ER, Walchek A, Freedman H, et al: Tetracycline and permanent teeth: the relation between dose and tooth color. *Pediatrics* 47:567, 1971.
16. Yaffe SJ, Bierman CW, Cann HM, et al: Requiem for tetracyclines. *Pediatrics* 55:142, 1975.
17. Leob JN: Corticosteroids and growth. *N Engl J Med* 295:547, 1976.
18. Tatsumi H, Senda H, Yatera S, et al: Toxicological studies on pipemidic acid. V. Effect on diarthrodial joints of experimental animals. *J Toxicol Sci* 3:357, 1978.
19. Hooper DC, Wolfson JS: The fluoroquinolones: pharmacology, clinical uses and toxicities in humans. *Antimicrob Agents Chemother* 28:716, 1985.
20. Shawn DH, McGuigan MA: Poisoning from dermal absorption of promethazine. *Can Med Assoc J* 130:1460, 1984.

Source	Dose
Minced bovine lung	100 mg phospholipid/kg body weight
Calf lung lavage	100 mg phospholipid/kg body weight
Minced porcine lung	200 mg phospholipid/kg body weight
Human amniotic fluid	60 mg phospholipid/kg body weight
DPPC:PG in saline[a]	50–100 mg/treatment
DPPC with high density lipoprotein	30 mg DPPC/dose
DPPC, hexadecanol, tyloxapol	67.5 mg DPPC/kg body weight

21. Kittinger JW, Sandler RS, Heizer WD: Efficacy of metoclopramide as an adjunct to duodenal placement of small bore feeding tubes: a randomized, placebo-controlled, double-blind study. *J Parenter Enteral Nutr* 11:33, 1987.
22. Metoclopramide for gastroesophageal reflux. *Med Lett Drugs Ther* 27:21, 1985.
23. Ricci DA, Saltzman MB, Meyer C, et al: Effect of metoclopramide in diabetic gastroparesis. *J Clin Gastroenterol* 7:25, 1985.
24. Whately K, Turner Jr WW, Dey M, et al: When does metoclopramide facilitate transpyloric intubation? *J Parenter Enteral Nutr* 8:679, 1984.
25. Bateman DN, Croft AW, Nicholson E, et al: Dystonic reactions and the pharmacokinetics of metoclopramide in children. *Br J Clin Pharmacol* 15:557, 1983.
26. Bennett EJ, Ignacio A, Patel K, et al: Tubocurarine and the neonate. *Br J Anaesthesiol* 48:687, 1976.
27. Terrin BN, McWilliams NB, Maurer HM: Side effects of metoclopramide as an antiemetic in childhood cancer chemotherapy. *J Pediatr* 104:138, 1984.
28. Wong DF, Wagner HN, Dannals RF, et al: Effects of age on dopamine and serotonin receptors measured by positron tomography of the living human brain. *Science* 226:1393, 1984.
29. Greco R, Musto B, Arienzo V: Treatment of paroxysmal supraventricular tachycardia in infancy with digitalis, adenosine-5-triphosphate, and verapamil: a comparative study. *Circulation* 66:504, 1982.
30. Porter CJ, Garson A, Gillette PC: Verapamil: an effective calcium blocking agent for pediatric patients. *Pediatrics* 71:748, 1983.
31. Singh BN, Nademanee K, Baky SH: Calcium antagonists. Clinical use in the treatment of arrhythmias. *Drugs* 25:125, 1983.
32. Epstein ML, Kiel EA, Victorica BE: Cardiac decompensation following verapamil therapy in infants with supraventricular tachycardia. *Pediatrics* 75:737, 1983.
33. Garson A: Medicolegal problems in the management of cardiac arrhythmias in children. *Pediatrics* 79:84, 1987.
34. Radford D: Side effects of verapamil in infants. *Arch Dis Child* 58:465, 1983.
35. Food and Drug Administration: *FDA Drug Bull* 8:11, 1978.
36. Till J, Shinebourne EA, Rigby ML, et al: Efficacy and safety of adenosine in the treatment of supraventricular tachycardia in infants and children. *Br Heart J* 62:204, 1989.
37. Overholt ED, Rheuban KS, Gutgesell HP, et al: Usefulness of adenosine for arrhythmias in infants and children. *Am J Cardiol* 61:336, 1988.
38. Polgar G, Weng TR: The functional development of the respiratory system. *Am Rev Respir Dis* 120:625, 1979.
39. Way WL, Costley EC, Way EL: Respiratory sensitivity of the newborn infant to meperidine and morphine. *Clin Pharmacol Ther* 6:454, 1962.

40. Dreifuss FE, Langer DH, Molinbe KA, Maxwell JE: Valproic acid hepatic fatalities. *Neurology* 39:201, 1989.
41. American Academy of Pediatrics. Behavioral and cognitive effects of anticonvulsant therapy. Committee on Drugs. *Pediatrics* 76:644, 1985.
42. Herranz JL, Armijo JA, Arteaga-R: Clinical side effects of phenobarbital, primidone, phenytoin, carbamazepine, and valproate during monotherapy in children. *Epilepsia* 29:794, 1988.
43. Farwell JR, Lee YJ, Hirtz, DG, et al: Phenobarbital for febrile seizures—effects on intelligence and on seizure recurrence. *N Engl J Med* 322:364, 1990.
44. Hartwig S, Roth B, Theisohn M: Clinical experience with continuous intravenous sedation using midazolam and fentanyl in the paediatric intensive care unit. *Eur J Pediatr* 150:784, 1991.
45. Bergman I, Steeves M, Burckart G, Thompson A: Reversible neurologic abnormalities associated with prolonged intravenous midazolam and fentanyl administration. *J Pediatr* 119: 644, 1991.
46. Kauffman RE: Fentanyl, fads, and folly: who will adopt the therapeutic orphans? *J Pediatr* 119:588, 1991.
47. Bailey WC, Weill H, DeRoven, et al: The effect of isoniazid on transaminase levels. *Ann Intern Med* 81:200, 1974.
48. Drugs for tuberculosis. *Med Lett Drugs Ther* 24:17, 1982.
49. O'Brien RJ, Long MW, Cross FS, et al: Hepatotoxicity from isoniazid and rifampin among children treated for tuberculosis. *Pediatrics* 72:491, 1983.
50. Spyridis P, Sinaniotis C, Papadea I, et al: Isoniazid liver injury during chemoprophylaxis in children. *Arch Dis Child* 94:65, 1979.
51. Brown Jr BR: Halothane hepatitis revisited. *N Engl J Med* 313:1347, 1985.
52. Carney FT, Van Dyke RA: Halothane hepatitis: a critical review. *Anesth Analg* 51:135, 1972.
53. Farrell G, Prendergast D, Murray M: Halothane hepatitis. Detection of a constitutional susceptibility factor. *N Engl J Med* 313;1310, 1985.
54. Marshall BE, Wollman H: General anesthetics. In Gilman AG, Goodman LS, Roll TW, Murad F (eds): *The Pharmacological Basis of Therapeutics*, ed 7. Macmillan, New York, 1985.
55. McLain GE, Sipes IG, Brown Jr BR: An animal model of halothane hepatotoxicity: roles of enzyme induction and hypoxia. *Anesthesiology* 91:321, 1979.
56. Warner LO, Beach TP, Garvin JP: Halothane and children. The first quarter century. *Anesth Analg* 63:838, 1984.
57. Arena JM, Rourk Jr MH, Sibrack CD: Acetaminophen: report of an unusual poisoning. *Pediatrics* 61:68, 1978.
58. Flower RJ, Moncada S, Vane JR: Analgesic-antipyretics and anti-inflammatory agents; drugs used in the treatment of gout. In Gilman AG, Goodman LS, Roll TW, Murad F (eds): *The Pharmacological Basis of Therapeutics*, ed 7. Macmillan, New York, 1985.
59. Nogen AG, Bremner JE: Acetaminophen overdosage in a young child. *J Pediatr* 92:832, 1978.
60. Rumack BH: Acetaminophen overdose in young children. *Am J Dis Child* 138:428, 1984.
61. Rumack BH, Peterson RC, Koch G, et al: Acetaminophen overdose. *Arch Intern Med* 141:380, 1981.
62. Tenenbein M: Pediatric toxicology: current controversies and recent advances related to nephrotoxicity in the premature newborn. Clinical and recent advances. *Curr Probl Pediatr* 16:185, 1986.
63. Cowan RH, Jukkola AF, Arant BS: Pathophysiologic evidence of gentamicin nephrotoxicity in neonatal puppies. *Pediatr Res* 14:1204, 1980.

64. Heimann G: Renal toxicity of aminoglycosides in the neonatal period. *Pediatr Pharmacol* 3:251, 1983.
65. McCracken Jr GH: Aminoglycoside toxicity in infants and children. *Am J Med* 80:172, 1986.
66. Rajchgot P, Prosber CG, Soldins S, et al: Aminoglycoside related nephrotoxicity in the premature newborn. *Clin Pharmacol Ther* 35:394, 1984.
67. Goldbloom RB, Goldbloom A: Boric acid poisoning, *J Pediatr* 43:631, 1953.
68. O'Mally K, Coleman EN, Doig WB, et al: Plasma digoxin levels in infants. *Arch Dis Child* 48:99, 1973.
69. Park MK: Use of digoxin in infants and children with specific emphasis on dosage. *J Pediatr* 108:871, 1986.
70. Halkin H, Radomsky M, Blieden L, et al: Steady state serum digoxin concentration in relation to digitalis toxicity in neonates and infants. *Pediatrics* 61:184, 1978.
71. Friedman WF, Pool PE, Jacobiwitz D, et al: Sympathetic innervation of the developing rabbit heart. Biochemical and histochemical comparisons of fetal, neonatal, and adult myocardium. *Circ Res* 23:25, 1968.
72. Kelliher GJ, Roberts J: Effect of age on the cardiotoxic action of digitalis. *J Pharmacol Exp Ther* 197:10, 1976.
73. Perloff WH: Physiology of the heart and circulation. In Swedlow DB, Raphaely RC (eds): *Cardiovascular Problems in Pediatric Critical Care.* Churchill Livingstone, New York, 1986.
74. Morselli PL, Franco-Morselli R, Bossi L: Clinical pharmacokinetics in newborns and infants. *Clin Pharmacokinet* 5:485, 1980.
75. Park MK, Ludden T, Arom KV, et al: Myocardial vs serum digoxin concentrations in infants and adults. *Am J Dis Child* 136:418, 1982.
76. Pinsky WW, Jacobsen JR, Gillette PC, et al: Dosage of digoxin in premature infants. *J Pediatr* 96:639, 1976.
77. Sandor GGS, Bloom KR, Izukawa T, et al: Noninvasive assessment of left ventricular function related to serum digoxin levels in neonates. *Pediatrics* 65:541, 1980.
78. Valdes Jr R: Endogenous digoxin-like immunoreactive factors: impact on digoxin measurement and potential physiological implications. *Clin Chem* 31:1985, 1985.
79. Valdes Jr R, Graves SW, Brown BA: Endogenous substance in newborn infants causing false-positive digoxin measurements. *J Pediatr* 152:947, 1983.
80. Schwartz GJ, Feld LG, Langford DJ: A simple estimate of glomerular filtration rate in full term infants during the first year of life. *J Pediatr* 104:849, 1984.
81. Schwartz GJ, Haycock GB, Edelmann Jr CM, et al: A simple estimate of glomerular filtration rate in children derived from body length and plasma creatinine. *Pediatrics* 58:259, 1976.
82. Schwartz GJ, Haycock GB, Gauthier B: A simple estimate of glomerular filtration rate in adolescent boys. *J Pediatr* 106:522, 1985.

CHAPTER

7

Special Problems: Sedation, Analgesia, Paralytic Therapy[a]

Patients in the intensive care unit (ICU) are frequently monitored via invasive routes such as indwelling catheters. Many patients require mechanical ventilation. Such invasive procedures can cause any patient discomfort and / or agitation. Therefore, the use of sedatives, analgesics, and muscle relaxants is common in the ICU. The severity of the patient's illness can affect the amount of drug needed. Patients with higher severity of illness index scores require less drug to achieve deeper levels of sedation than patients with less severe illness. The duration of action for a drug must be considered when choosing the appropriate drug for the ICU patient. This chapter includes several detailed tables that provide a wide range of information on sedatives, analgesics, and muscle relaxants:

1. Dose and cost of most commonly used neuromuscular blocking drugs in mechanically ventilated patients (Table 7.1)

[a]The material in this chapter was contributed by the following: Tables 7.1, 7.2, 7.4, 7.6, 7.8, and 7.10 were contributed by David J. Cullen, M.D., M.S., Luca M. Bigatello, M.D., and Harold J. DeMonaco, M.S.; Table 7.3 was contributed by David J. Greenblatt, M.D.; Table 7.5 was contributed by Frank Balestrieri, D.D.S., M.D., F.C.C.P., and Sherry Fisher, R.N.; Tables 7.7 and 7.9 were contributed by Neelakantan Sunder, M.B.B.S., and J. A. Jeevendra Martyn, M.D., F.F.A.R.C.S.; Tables 7.11–7.16 were contributed by Jeffrey S. Kelly, M.D., and Drew A. MacGregor, M.D.

2. Scoring system to access sedation in ICU patients (Table 7.2)
3. Characteristics of intravenous benzodiazepenes used in critically ill patients (Table 7.3)
4. Most common sedative drugs used during mechanical ventilation (Table 7.4)
5. Classification and dosage of some narcotic agonists/antagonists (Table 7.5)
6. Use of opioids in adult ICU patients (Table 7.6)
7. Clinical pharmacology of neuromuscular blockers (Table 7.7)
8. Muscle relaxant dosage and duration of effect (Table 7.8)
9. Commonly used antibiotics and their interactions with nondepolarizing muscle relaxants (Table 7.9)
10. Interactions between disease and muscle relaxants (Table 7.10)
11. Adverse effects of succinylcholine (Table 7.11)
12. Conditions associated with succinylcholine-induced hyperkalemia (Table 7.12)
13. Classification, recommended dosage, and usual clinical effects of nondepolarizing muscle relaxants (Table 7.13)
14. Side effects of nondepolarizing neuromuscular blocking agents (Table 7.14)
15. Conditions associated with altered responsiveness to nondepolarizing neuromuscular blocking agents (Table 7.15)
16. Metabolism and clearance of nondepolarizing neuromuscular blocking drugs (Table 7.16)

TABLE 7.1. Dose and Cost of Most Commonly Used Neuromuscular Blocking Drugs in Mechanically Ventilated Patients

Drug	*Maintenance Dose*[a]	*Cost/Day*[b] ($)
Sedative/hypnotic		
Phenobarbital	15–90 mg q6–8h	3.25
Pentobarbital	100–200 mg q6–8h	12.50
Thiopental	25–200 mg/h	15.00
Propofol	50–300 mg/h	300.00
Anxiolytics		
Diazepam	5–10 mg i.v. q6h	1.50
Lorazepam	2–4 mg i.v. q6h	70.00
Midazolam	2.5–25 mg/h	550.00
Narcotics		
Morphine	5–50 mg/h	17.00
Fentanyl	50–500 μg/h	17.25
Alfentanil	250–2500 μg/h	210.00
Sufentanil	10–100 μg/h	430.00
Neuromuscular blockers		
d-Tubocurarine	2–10 mg/h	19.00
Pancuronium	1–3 mg/h	38.00
Metocurine	1–5 mg/h	56.00
Vecuronium	2–4 mg/h	170.00
Atracurium	20–30 mg/h	293.00

[a] The maintenance dose listed is the usual dose range for a 70-kg patient.
[b] Institutional costs are approximated and represent the acquisition cost for a 24-hour supply of the maximum dose listed.

TABLE 7.2. Scoring System for Assessment of Sedation in ICU Patients

Level	*Response*
1	Anxious and agitated or restless
2	Cooperative, oriented, tranquil
3	Responds to commands only
4	Asleep but brisk response to glabellar tap or loud auditory stimulus
5	sleep, sluggish response to glabellar tap or loud auditory stimulus
6	No response

TABLE 7.3. Characteristics of Benzodiazepines Used Intravenously in Critical Care Medicine[a]

Parent Drug	*Metabolite of Potential Importance*	*Benzodiazepine Receptor* K_i (nM)
Diazepam		9.57
	Desmethyldiazepam	5.58
Lorazepam		1.64
Midazolam		0.44
	1-Hydroxymidazolam	2.23

[a] See Refs. 1 and 2.

TABLE 7.4. Most Commonly Used Drugs and Method of Administration for Sedation during Mechanical Ventilation[a]

Drug	*Method of Administration*	*Frequency of Reported Use (%)*
Morphine	Intermittent i.v.	95
Lorazepam	Intermittent i.v.	86
Midazolam	Intermittent i.v.	81
Diazepam	Intermittent i.v.	78
Pancuronium	Intermittent i.v.	82
Vecuronium	Intermittent i.v.	60
Atracurium	Continuous infusion	17

[a] Adapted from Hansen-Flaschen JH, Brazxinsky S, Basile C, et al: Use of sedating and neuromuscular blocking agents in patients requiring mechanical ventilation for respiratory failure: a national survey. *JAMA* 266:2870–2875, 1991. Copyright 1991, American Medical Association.

Lipid Solubility Index (vs. Diazepam)	*Usual Range of Elimination $t_{1/2}$ (h)*
1.00	20–70
0.79	36–90
0.48	10–20
1.54	1–4
0.71	

TABLE 7.5. Classification and Dosage of Some Narcotic Agonists and Antagonists

Drug (Trade Name)	*Dose (in 70-kg adult)*	
	i.v. (mg)	*i.m./s.c. (mg)*
Natural alkaloids of opium		
Morphine	2–10 (titrate)	5–10
Codeine	30–60	60–120
Semisynthetic derivatives		
Hydromorphone (Dilaudid)	0.5–1 (titrate)	2
Oxymorphone (Numorphan)	0.5 (titrate)	1
Synthetic derivatives		
Meperidine (Demerol, etc.)	25–100 (titrate)	50–100
Methadone (Dolophine, etc.)	2–5 (titrate)	2–10
Pentazocine (Talwin)	10–30 (titrate)	30
Fentanyl (Sublimaze)	0.05–0.1 (titrate)	0.1
Narcotic antagonists		
Naloxone (Narcan)	0.2–0.4	0.4
Nalorphine (Nalline)	5–10	
Levallorphan (Lorfan)	1	

TABLE 7.6. Use of Opioids in Adult ICU Patients

	Postoperative Analgesia
	Continuous Infusion
Morphine	5 mg/h, up to 20–30 mg/h
Meperidine	Not reported
Fentanyl	50–100 μg/h
Alfentanil	500–1500 μg/h
Sufentanil	Not reported
Comments	Very large individual variations Tachyphylaxis Respiratory depression Most patients are intubated

Dose Interval (h)	Comparative Narcotic Potency
2–4	1
2–4	0.1
3–4	5
3–4	10
2–4	0.1
2–4	1.2
3–4	0.25
½–2	150
½–¾	
prn	
prn	

Postoperative Analgesia	
PCA	*Epidural*
e.g., boluses of 1–2 mg at lockout intervals of 6–10 min	Preservative-free: 0.25–1 mg/h
Equivalent doses, no advantage over morphine	Preservative-free form not available in U.S.
	3–10 μg/ml at 5–10 ml/h
Too potent not ideal for PCA	Not frequently used in U.S.
Too potent not ideal for PCA	Not frequently used in U.S.
Very large individual variations	In most instances epidural opioids are more effective when mixed with local anesthetics: 0.075%–0.125% bupivacaine

TABLE 7.7. Clinical Pharmacology of Neuromuscular Blockers

Drug	*ED_{95} (mg/kg)*	*Intubating Dose (mg/kg)*
Succinylcholine	0.2	1
d-Tubocurarine	0.5	0.5–0.6
Metocurine	0.28	0.3
Gallamine	3	3–4
Pancuronium	0.07	0.1
Pipecuronium	0.05	0.05–0.1
Atracurium	0.3	0.05–0.6
Vecuronium	0.07	0.1
Doxacurium	0.03	0.03–0.04
Mivacurium	0.08	0.15–0.2

TABLE 7.8. Muscle Relaxants

Relaxant	*Intubating Dose (mg/kg)*	*Duration of Clinical Effect (min)*
Depolarizing:		
Succinylcholine	1–2	10–20
Nondepolarizing:		
d-Tubocurarine	0.6	60–90
Metocurine	0.4	60–90
Pancuronium	0.1	60–90
Atracurium	0.4	30–60
Vecuronium	0.08	30–60
Mivacurium	0.15	15–20

Time to Recovery (min)	Route of Elimination
10–15	Plasma cholinesterase
80–100	Kidney; liver
80–100	Kidney
100–180	Kidney
80–100	Kidney
80–100	Kidney
30–60	Hofman elimination
30–60	Liver; kidney
80–100	Kidney
15–20	Plasma cholinesterase

TABLE 7.9. Commonly Used Antibiotics and Their Interactions with NDMR[a]

Polymyxin	Most potent of the antibiotics to have an effect on the neuromuscular junction. Blocks ACh receptor ion channel.	
Aminoglycosides	Neomycin	• Decreases acetylcholine release
	Gentamicin Kanamycin Amikacin	• Lowers sensitivity of the postjunctional membrane to acetylcholine
Tobramycin	May also have a direct effect on the muscle.	
Lincomycin	Blocks ion channels and also has a direct depressant action on contractility of the muscle.	
Clindamycin	Direct action on the muscle and may also block ACh receptor ion channel.	

[a]NDMR, nondepolarizing muscle relaxants; ACh, acetylcholine.

TABLE 7.10. Disease-Muscle Relaxant Interactions

Disease	*Types of Relaxant Interactions and Clinical Implications*
Myasthenia gravis	• Resistance to depolarizing drugs. • Extreme sensitivity to nondepolarizers (*d*-tubocurarine test). The weakness responds to anticholinesterase.
Myasthenic syndrome (Eaton-Lambert syndrome)	• Marked sensitivity to nondepolarizing relaxants. Block not readily reversed with neostigmine. In contrast to myasthenia gravis, the response to fast rates of stimulation is a progressive increase in twitch amplitude to as much as six times the initial height. • Release sensitivity to an average clinical dose of depolarizing relaxant.
Thyrotoxic myopathy	• Decreased response to succinylcholine (pseudocholinesterase levels are at the upper limit of normal or increased). • Increased sensitivity to decamethonium. • Normal *d*-tubocurarine requirement.
Amyotropic lateral sclerosis, syringomyelia, and poliomyelitis	• Defective neuromuscular transmission and nerve conduction. • Exaggerated response to nondepolarizers.
von Recklinghausen's disease	• Variable response. Some subjects show prolonged responses to both nondepolarizing and depolarizing relaxants. Others, like myasthenics, are sensitive to *d*-tubocurarine and resistant to succinylcholine.
Myotonic syndrome Myotonia dystrophica Myotonia congenita Paramyotonia	• Generalized muscle spasm (myotonic response) occurs after depolarizing agents. Myotonia is alleviated by quinine and procainamide.

Condition	Response
Muscular dystrophy Obscure congenital myopathies Familial periodic paralysis Steroid myopathy Myxedema myopathy Alcoholic myopathy Diabetic myopathy	Unpredictable response to relaxants, their use is better avoided.
Polymyositis Dermatomyositis Systemic lupus erythematosus Polyarteritis nodosa	Muscle weakness and fatigability. Respond to neostigmine, hence the term "myasthenic state."
Hypokalemia Hyperkalemia Traumatized patients Burn patients Muscle-wasting disease Lower motor neuron lesions with hemiplegia Muscular dystrophy Denervation and spinal cord transection Multiple sclerosis Tetanus Denervation	Theoretically increased sensitivity to nondepolarizing relaxants. Theoretically increased sensitivity to depolarizing relaxants and decreased sensitivity to nondepolarizing relaxants.
Primary muscle disease or myopathy	High incidence of malignant hyperpyrexia in these patients and susceptible relatives. Usually, the myopathy is mild or subclinical. Squints, hernias, and minor orthopaedic problems are often found in affected families. Malignant hyperpyrexia muscle is more sensitive to caffeine-induced rigor than normal muscle.

[a] From Ali HH, Savarese JJ: Monitoring of neuromuscular function. *Anesthesiology* 45:216–249, 1976.

TABLE 7.11. Adverse Effects of Succinylcholine

Cardiac arrhythmias
Skeletal muscle myalgias
Sustained skeletal muscle contraction
Myoglobinemia
Hyperkalemia
Increased intraocular pressure
Increased intragastric pressure
Increased intracranial pressure
Malignant hyperthermia
Allergic reactions

TABLE 7.13. Classification, Recommended Doses, and Usual Clinical Effects of Nondepolarizing Relaxants

	Short-Acting	*Intermediate-Acting*	
	Mivacurium	*Atracurium*	*Vecuronium*
Structure	BZ-ISO[b]	BZ-ISO	Steroid
ED_{95} (mg/kg)	0.08	0.20–0.25	0.05
Intubation dose (mg/kg)	0.15–0.20	0.40–0.50	0.10
Onset intubating conditions (min)	2–3	3–4	3–4
Intubation dose duration (min)	12–20	20–40	20–40
Onset rapid intubation (sec)[c]	60–90	90	90
Duration rapid intubation (min)[c]	20–25	50–60	50–60
Infusion rate (µg/kg/min)	5–15	5–9	1–2
Cost	Moderate	High	High

[a] Manufacturer specifically recommends against ICU administration.
[b] BZ-ISO, benzyl isoquinolinium.
[c] "Priming" followed by 3 times the ED_{95} (see text).
[d] NA, not applicable. Use in this fashion limited by accentuated histamine release (see text).

TABLE 7.14. Side Effect Profiles of Nondepolarizing Neuromuscular Blocking Drugs

Drug	*Cardiac Muscarinic Effects*
Mivacurium	NS[a]
Atracurium	NS
Vecuronium	NS
d-Tubocurarine	Mild-modest blockade
Metocurine	NS
Pancuronium	Modest blockade
Pipecuronium	NS
Doxacurium	NS

[a] NS, not significant.

TABLE 7.12. Conditions Associated with Succinylcholine-induced Hyperkalemia

Upper motor neuron lesions
Lower motor neuron lesions
Muscle denervation
Trauma/severe tissue damage
Muscle immobilization and atrophy
Thermal burns
Muscular dystrophy
Clostridial infections
? Severe prolonged infections (>1 week)
? Anterior horn cell disease
? Diffuse CNS insult (head injury, aneurysmal rupture, encephalitis)

?, Possible.

		Long-Acting		
d-Tubocurarine	*Metocurine*	*Pancuronium*	*Pipecuronium*[a]	*Doxacurium*
BZ-ISO	BZ-ISO	Steroid	Steroid	BZ-ISO
0.50	0.28	0.07	0.05	0.025–0.030
0.50–0.60	0.40	0.10	0.10	0.05–0.075
3–5	3–5	3–5	3–5	4–6
60–90	60–90	90–120	90–120	120–150
NA[d]	NA[d]	90–120	90–120	120–150
NA[d]	NA[d]	150–200	150–200	>200
NA	NA	NA	NA	NA
Low	Moderate	Very low	Very high	Very high

Sympathetic Nicotinic Effects	*Histamine Release*
NS	Slight-modest
NS	Slight-modest
NS	NS
Moderate blockade	Moderate
Mild blockade	Modest
NS	NS
NS	NS
NS	NS

TABLE 7.15. Conditions Associated with Altered Responsiveness to Nondepolarizing Neuromuscular Blocking Agents

Increased Sensitivity to	
Condition	*Drug Therapy*
Hypothermia	Inhalation anesthetics
Hypokalemia	Local anesthetics
Hypocalcemia	Aminoglycosides
Hypermagnesemia	Clindamycin
Acidosis	Polymyxin
Myasthenia gravis	Calcium channel blockers
Myasthenia syndrome	Procainamide
Paraplegia	Quinidine
Neurofibromatosis	Magnesium
Amyotrophic lateral sclerosis	Trimethaphan
Poliomyelitis	Cyclophosphamide
Neonates[a]	Cyclosporine
? Myotonia	Furosemide
? Muscular dystrophy	Dantrolene
	? Lithium
Increased Resistance to	
Condition	*Drug Therapy*
Hemiplegia	Corticosteroids
Thermal burns	Carbamazepine
Peripheral neuropathies	Phenytoin
Peripheral nerve transection	? Aminophylline/theophylline
Hyperkalemia	? Azathioprine
Hypercalcemia	? Nondepolarizing relaxants (chronic)
Clostridial infections	
Cirrhosis with ascites	

[a]Sensitivity effects are offset by neonates' increased volume of distribution.

TABLE 7.16. Metabolism and Clearance of Nondepolarizing Neuromuscular Blocking Drugs

Drug	*% Renal Excretion*	*% Biliary Excretion*	*% Hepatic Metabolism*	*% Plasma Hydrolysis*	*Active Metabolites*	*Duration in Renal Disease*	*Duration in Hepatic Disease*
Mivacurium	5	NS[a]	NS	95[b]	No	Minimal increase	Mild to modest increase
Atracurium	5–10	NS	NS	90–95[d]	Laudanosine[e]	No change	No change
Vecuronium	50	35–50	15–30	None	3-Hydroxyvecuronium[f]	Minimal increase	Mild to modest increase
d-Tubocurarine	45	10–40	NS	None	No	Modest increase	? Mild to modest increase
Metocurine	46–58	<2	NS	None	No	Moderate increase	No change to mild increase
Pancuronium	85	10–15	10–15	None	3-Hydroxypancuronium[ga]	Modest increase	Mild to modest increase
Pipecuronium	70	20	10	None	No	Modest increase	?
Doxacurium	70	Present (significance unknown)	?	Minimal	? None	Modest increase	? No change to slight increase

[a] NS, not significant.
[b] Plasma pseudocholinesterase.
[c] Only when significant (>70%) decreases in plasma pseudocholinesterase activity occur.
[d] Nonspecific plasma esterases plus Hofmann degradation.
[e] ? CNS stimulation.
[f] 60% potency of parent compound.
[g] 33–50% potency of parent compound.

REFERENCES

1. Greenblatt DJ, Shader RI: Pharmacokinetics of antianxiety agents. In Meltzer HY (ed): *Psychopharmacology: The Third Generation of Progress*. Raven Press, New York, pp 1377–1386, 1987.
2. Arendt RM, Greenblatt DJ, Liebisch DC, Luu MD, Paul SM: Determinants of benzodiazepine brain uptake: lipophilicity versus binding affinity. *Psychopharmacology* 93:72–76, 1987.

CHAPTER

8

Cardiovascular Medications[a]

There is a wide armamentarium of available medications to treat the wide spectrum of cardiovascular disorders. This chapter focuses first on antihypertensive therapy and then shifts toward disorders of cardiac pacing. Hypertension may be treated by several therapies. Nutritional approaches may help, but if pharmacologic intervention is indicated, there are a variety of drug classes: diuretics, sympatholytics, vasodilators, calcium channel blockers, and converting-enzyme inhibitors. Pacing disturbances are also treatable by an assortment of drugs: calcium channel blockers, sympatholytics, vagotonic agents, sympathomimetics, antiarrhythmics, vasodilator agents, inotropic medications, and plasminogen activators, just to name a few. This chapter provides an overview of available drugs to treat cardiovascular disorders:

1. Antihypertensive therapies (Table 8.1)
2. Properties of oral β-adrenergic receptor-blocking drugs (Table 8.2)
3. Clinical settings influencing use of β-blockers (Table 8.3)

---

[a]The material in this chapter was contributed by the following: Tables 8.1–8.9 were contributed by Michael G. Ziegler, M.D., and Pablo F. Ruiz-Ramon, M.D.; Tables 8.10 and 8.11 were contributed by Paul M. Heerdt, M.D., Ph.D., and Robert M. Forstot, M.D.; Tables 8.12–8.15 were contributed by Robert D. Colucci, Pharm.D., F.C.P., F.C.C.M., and John C. Somberg, M.D., F.C.P.; Tables 8.16, Figure 8.1, and "Clinical Indications" text were contributed by Joseph E. Parrillo, M.D.; Figure 8.2 and Table 8.17 were contributed by Arno L. Zaritzky, M.D.; Tables 8.18 and 8.19 were contributed by Allan S. Jaffe, M.D.

4. Properties of oral calcium channel blockers used to treat hypertension (Table 8.4)
5. Properties of oral angiotensin-converting enzyme (ACE) inhibitors used to treat hypertension (Table 8.5)
6. Effects of combination antihypertensive therapy (Table 8.6)
7. Causes of hypertensive crisis (Table 8.7)
8. Parenteral drugs for hypertensive emergencies (Table 8.8)
9. Oral drugs for hypertensive urgencies (Table 8.9)
10. Properties of drugs used to treat supraventricular tachycardia (Table 8.10)
11. Properties of drugs used to treat bradycardia (Table 8.11)
12. Antiarrhythmic agents (Table 8.12)
13. Properties of β-adrenergic-blocking drugs (Table 8.13)
14. Guidelines for implantation of permanent cardiac pacemakers (Table 8.14)
15. Indications for temporary pacing (Table 8.15)
16. Ability of different vasodilators to shift ventricular function toward normal (Fig. 8.1)
17. Vasodilators and their principal site of action (Table 8.16)
18. Relationship between catecholamine concentration and its effect (Fig. 8.2)
19. Prescribing infusions of inotropic agents: Deriving concentrations (Table 8.17)
20. Doses of plasminogen activators for use in patients with acute myocardial infarction (Table 8.18)
21. Contraindications to thrombolytic therapy (Table 8.19)

CLINICAL INDICATIONS FOR VASODILATOR THERAPY

The following are the clinical situations in which vasodilator therapy is beneficial:

- In acute heart failure, in combination with diuretics and digitalis, vasodilator therapy will reduce filling pressures and usually improve cardiac output. In chronic heart failure, enalapril and (to a somewhat lesser degree) hydralazine/isosorbide dinitrate have been shown to improve long-term mortality.

- In acute cardiogenic pulmonary edema, vasodilator therapy with acute vasodilation can rapidly reduce high filling pressures and reverse symptoms. Vasodilators can be used in conjunction with supplemental oxygen, rotating tourniquets, morphine, and intravenous diuretics.
- In acute or chronic mitral regurgitation, aortic regurgitation, or ventricular septal defect, vasodilator-induced decreases in systemic vascular resistance (SVR) increase forward (systemic) CO. Vasodilators are usually employed in these situations as a temporizing measure to allow time to prepare the patient for cardiac surgery.
- Intravenous nitroglycerin has been shown to reduce infarct size and improve mortality in acute myocardial infarction. Nitrate therapy is useful in treating stable and unstable angina. Vasodilators such as nitroprusside can reduce myocardial oxygen consumption in patients with persistent chest pain who are hypertensive.
- In patients with cardiogenic shock, vasodilator therapy combined with inotropic drugs (e.g., dopamine or dobutamine) or intraaortic balloon counterpulsation can produce substantial hemodynamic improvement. Once stabilized, such patients can be considered for revascularization.
- As reviewed in other chapters of this book, vasodilators are highly useful to treat hypertension, malignant hypertension, and dissecting aortic aneurysms (in conjunction with β-blockade) and possibly may be useful in some patients with primary pulmonary hypertension.

TABLE 8.1. Antihypertensive Therapies

- Nutritional therapies
  - Weight loss
  - Sodium restriction
  - Ethanol restriction
  - Potassium
  - Calcium
- Diuretics
  - Thiazides
  - Loop diuretics
  - Potassium-sparing diuretics
- Sympatholytics
  - α-Adrenergic receptor blockers
    - Phenoxybenzamine
    - Phentolamine
    - Prazosin
    - Terazosin
    - Doxazosin
  - β-Adrenergic receptor blockers
    - Atenolol
    - Metoprolol
    - Nadolol
    - Propranolol
    - Timolol
    - Acebutolol
    - Labetalol
    - Penbutolol
    - Betaxolol
    - Dilevalol
    - Carteolol
    - Esmolol
  - α_2-Adrenergic receptor agonists
    - Clonidine
    - Guanabenz
    - Methyldopa
    - Guanfacine
- Vasodilators
  - Diazoxide
  - Hydralazine
  - Minoxidil
  - Nitroprusside
  - Nitroglycerin
- Calcium channel blockers
  - Nifedipine
  - Diltiazem
  - Verapamil
  - Nicardipine
  - Felodipine

TABLE 8.1. (*Continued*)

Converting-enzyme inhibitors
Captopril
Enalapril
Lisinopril
Fosinopril
Benazapril
Ramipril

TABLE 8.2. Properties of Oral β-Adrenergic Receptor-Blocking Drugs

Generic Name *Brand Name*	*Propranolol* *Inderal*	*Atenolol* *Tenormin*	*Metoprolol* *Lopressor*	*Nadolol* *Corgard*	*Pindolol* *Visken*
Oral bioavailability (%)	30	40	50	30	90
Dose in hypertension (mg)	80–640	50–100	100–450	80–320	15–60
Variation in plasma levels between patients	20×[a]	4×	10×	7×	4×
Protein-bound (%)	93	<5	12	30	60
Half-life (h)	3–6	6–9	3–4	14–24	3–4
Fat solubility	+	0	+	0	+
Eliminated by	Liver	Kidney	Liver	Kidney	Kidney and liver
Membrane-stabilizing effect	++	0	±	0	+
Cardioselectivity	0	+	+	0	0
Intrinsic sympathomimetic activity	0	0	0	0	++
Active metabolites	+	0	0	0	0
Potency (relative)	10	10	10	10	60

[a] ×, fold increase; +, increased or present; ++, markedly increased; ±, little to none; 0, none or absent.

TABLE 8.3. Clinical Settings That Influence the Use of β-Adrenergic Receptor Blockers (β-Blockers)

Clinical Setting
Bronchospasm
Angina pectoris
Heart failure
Cardiac conduction defects
Bradycardia
Raynaud's phenomenon and peripheral vascular disease
Insulin-dependent diabetes mellitus
Pheochromocytoma
Renal insufficiency
Depression
Clonidine

Timolol Blocardren	*Acebutolol Sectral*	*Labetalol Trandate*	*Carteolol Cartrol*	*Betaxolol Kerlone*	*Penbutolol Levatol*	*Dilevalol Unicard*
75	40	25	85	90	>95	30
20–60	200–1200	200–2400	2.5–10	5–40	10–80	200–800
7×	7×	7×	3×	2×	5×	2×
10	25	50	25	50	95	75
3–4	3–13	6–8	6	14–22	26	8–12
0	0	+	0	+	+	+
Liver	Kidney and liver	Kidney and liver	Kidney	Liver and kidney	Kidney	Kidney and liver
0	+	+	0	±	±	0
0	+	0	0	+	0	0
±	+	0	+	0	+	+(β_2)
0	+	0	+	0	0	0
60	5	2	100	90	50	10

Consideration in β-Blocker Use
Avoid β-blockers. Drugs with intrinsic sympathomimetic activity (ISA) such as pindolol and dilevalol or drugs with β_1 selectivity can be used in low doses with close monitoring.
Drugs with ISA are usually contraindicated. Labetalol may be useful in variant angina. Use other β-blockers with caution. Drugs with a short half-life need to be given frequently.
β-blockers are usually contraindicated.
β-blockers are usually contraindicated; however, those with intrinsic sympathomimetic activity can be tried with close monitoring.
β-blockers with ISA affect heart rate to a lesser extent.
Avoid β-blockers if possible. Drugs with ISA and β_1 selectivity are better.
β_1-selective drugs and those with ISA favored.
Avoid all β-blockers, except with concurrent α-blocker use.
Use lower doses of renally excreted agents. Drugs with active metabolites may accumulate.
Avoid β-blockers if possible.
Enhanced rebound phenomenon with clonidine withdrawal.

TABLE 8.4. Properties of Oral Calcium Channel Blockers Used in Treating Hypertension

Generic Name *Brand Name*	*Verapamil* *Calan, Isoptin*	*Diltiazem* *Cardizem*	*Nifedipine* *Adalat, Procardia*	*Nicardipine* *Cardene*	*Isradipine* *Dynacirc*	*Felodipine* *Plendil*
Chemical class	P[a]	B	D	D	D	D
Daily dose (mg)	120–480	120–360	30–180	60–120	5–20	5–20
Bioavailability	20–25%	40%	45–70%	10–30%	15–20%	20%
Half-life (h)	5–18	3–4.5	2–5	8.6	8	11–16
Protein binding	85%	80%	95%	98%	95%	>99%
Elimination	Hepatic	Renal and hepatic	Hepatic	Hepatic	Hepatic	Hepatic
Active metabolites	+	+	0	0	0	0
Peripheral vasodilation	↑↑	↑↑	↑↑↑	↑↑↑	↑↑↑	↑↑↑
Heart rate	↔	↔	↑*/↔+	↑*/↔+	↔	↑*/↔+
Myocardial contractility	↓	↓	↔	↔	↔	↔
Coronary vasodilation	↑	↑	↑↑	↑↑	↑↑	↑↑
AV conduction	↓↓	↓	↔	↔	↔	↔
Cardiac output	↔	↔	↑*/↔+	↑*	↔	↔
Myocardial O_2 demand	↓	↓	↓	↓	↓	↓

[a] P, phenylalkylamine; B, benzothiazepine; D, dihydropyridine; +, chronic use; *, acute use.

TABLE 8.5. Properties of Oral ACE Inhibitors Used in Treating Hypertension

Generic Name *Brand Name*	*Captopril* *Capoten*	*Enalapril* *Vasotec*	*Lisinopril* *Zestril,* *Prinivil*	*Fosinopril* *Monopril*	*Ramipril* *Altace*	*Benazapril* *Lotensin*
Zinc ligand	Sulfhydryl	Carboxyl	Carboxyl	Phosphinyl	Carboxyl	Carboxyl
Prodrug	No	Yes	No	Yes	Yes	Yes
Daily dose (mg)	25–150	5–20	20–40	10–40	2.5–20	5–40
Bioavailability (%)	70	40	25	30	60	28
Route of elimination	Kidney	Kidney	Kidney	Kidney and liver	Kidney	Kidney
Terminal half-life (h)	2	11	12	12	110	21
Onset of action (h)	0.5–1	1–2	2–4	2–6	1–2	1–2

TABLE 8.6. Effects of Combination Antihypertensive Therapy

	Salt Restriction	*Thiazides*	*α-Blockers*	*β-Blockers*	*α_2-Agonists*	*Vasodilators*	*Calcium Channel Blockers*	*ACE Inhibitor*
Salt restriction	0[a]	+	+	+	+	+	0	+
Thiazides	+	0	+	+	+	+	0	++
α-Blockers	+	+	0	+/0	0	?	+	+
β-Blockers	+	+	+/0	0	–	+	+/–*	0
α_2-Agonists	+	+	0	–	0	+	+	+
Vasodilators	+	+	?	+	+	0	0	++
Calcium channel blockers	0	0	+	+/–*	+	0	0	+
ACE inhibitors	+	++	+	0	+	++	+	0

[a]0, no additive effect; +, additive effect; ++, strong additive effect; –, adverse effect; *, do not combine two drugs that depress AV node conduction/myocardial contractility.

TABLE 8.7. Causes of Hypertensive Crisis

Vasospasm
Exacerbation of essential hypertension
Scleroderma
Vasculitis
Preeclampsia and eclampsia
↑ Renin release
Renal artery stenosis
Acute glomerulonephritis
Renal parenchymal diseases
Cholesterol embolization syndrome
Renin-secreting tumors
↑ Central sympathetic activity
Stroke
Head trauma
Clonidine withdrawal
Spinal cord dysreflexia
CNS drugs
↑ Peripheral sympathetic activity
Pheochromocytoma
Monoamine oxidase inhibitor and tyramine ingestion
Sympathomimetic drugs
Extensive burns, trauma, and pain

TABLE 8.8. Parenteral Drugs for Hypertensive Emergencies

Drug	*Dose*	*Onset*
Sodium nitroprusside	0.25–8 μg/kg/min i.v. infusion	Seconds
Nitroglycerin	5–100 μg/min i.v. infusion	1–2 min
Diazoxide	50–150 mg i.v. bolus, may repeat q5–10 min up to 600 mg *or* 15–30 mg/min infusion	1–2 min
Trimethaphan	0.5–5 mg/min i.v. infusion	1–5 min
Hydralazine	10–20 mg i.v. 10–50 mg i.m.	10–30 min
Phentolamine	5–15 mg i.v. q5–15min	1–2 min
Labetalol	2 mg/min i.v. or 20 mg i.v. bolus, then 20–80 mg at 10 min (300 mg/max)	5–10 min
Methyldopa	250–500 mg i.v.	30–60 min
Enalaprilat	1.25–5 mg q6h	15 min
Nicardipine	5 mg/h increase by 1–2 mg/h q15min up to 15 mg/h	5–15 min

[a]MAO, monoamine oxidase.

Duration	Recommended for	Avoid in
3–5 min	Hypertensive encephalopathy, cerebral infarction, cerebral hemorrhage, left ventricular failure, aortic dissection, eclampsia, burns	Renal failure
5–10 min	Myocardial ischemia, postcoronary bypass surgery.	
10 h	Substitute when nitroprusside not available	Myocardial ischemia and infarction, aortic dissection, pregnancy
10 min	Aortic dissection	Myocardial ischemia, renal insufficiency, pregnancy
2–4 h	Eclampsia, post-op hypertension	Left ventricular failure, myocardial ischemia, mycocardial infarction, aortic dissection, intracranial processes
3–10 min	Pheochromocytoma, recreational drugs, MAO[a] inhibitors and tyramine, spinal cord dysreflexia	
3–6 h	Eclampsia, spinal cord dysreflexia, intracranial process when nitroprusside not available	Heart failure
6–12 h	Eclampsia, perioperative hypertension	Myocardial ischemia, myocardial infarction, aortic dissection
12–24 h	Scleroderma crisis, left ventricular failure, renovascular hypertension, acute glomerulonephritis	Pregnancy
4–6 h	(Still being evaluated)	

TABLE 8.9. Oral Drugs for Hypertensive Urgencies

Drug	*Dose*	*Onset*
Nifedipine	10–20 mg	5–15 min
Clonidine	0.2 mg, then 0.1 mg/h (max 0.8 mg)	0.5–2 h
Captopril	6.5–25 mg	15 min
Prazosin	1–2 mg, repeat after 1 h	15–30 min
Minoxidil	2.5–10 mg q4–6h	0.5–1 h

TABLE 8.10. Dose, Kinetics, and Side Effects of Drugs Used to Treat Supraventricular Tachycardia

	Dosage (Adult)
Intrinsic action	
Calcium channel blockers	
Verapamil	*Bolus:* 2.5–10 mg i.v. over 2 min; may repeat in 30 min *Infusion (short-term):* 0.005 mg/kg/min, up to total of 1 mg/min
Diltiazem	*Bolus:* 0.25 mg/kg over 2 min; may repeat in 15 min: 0.35 mg/kg over 2 min. *Infusion:* 5–15 mg/h
Adenosine	Rapid i.v. bolus 6 mg; repeat 12 mg in 1–2 min
Sympatholytic action	
β-blockers	
Esmolol	*Loading:* 500 μg/kg over 4 min *Infusion:* 50–300 μg/kg/min
Propranolol	*Bolus:* 15–45 μg/kg (1–3 mg) slowly (1 mg/min); may repeat in 3 min
Vagotonic action	
Digoxin	*Loading:* 0.75–1.0 mg i.v. in 3 divided doses over 12–24 h
Anticholinesterase	
Edrophonium	10–20 mg i.v. bolus (single dose) for heart rate control
α_1-agonist	
Phenylephrine	*Bolus:* 50–100 μg i.v. *Infusion:* 50 μg/min titrated to effect

Duration	Comments
3–5 h	Oral, buccal, or sublingual administration have similar effects. Causes tachycardia.
6–8 h	Sedating.
4–6 h	Avoid in pregnancy and compromised renal perfusion. May abruptly decrease blood pressure.
8 h	Useful in catecholamine excess states. Watch for orthostatic hypotension.
12–16 h	Causes tachycardia.

Elimination	Side Effects
Hepatic $t_{1/2}$ = 4 h	Hypotension, AV block, myocardial depression, constipation
Hepatic $t_{1/2}$ = 4–6 h	Hypotension, flushing, AV block, constipation, pruritus
Plasma/endothelial cells $t_{1/2}$ 1–3 sec	Dyspnea, flushing, chest pain, transient AV block/asystole, bronchospasm
Plasma hydrolysis $t_{1/2}$ = 9 min Hepatic $t_{1/2}$ = 4 h	Bradycardia, hypotension, myocardial depression, bronchospasm
Renal $t_{1/2}$ = 36–48 h	Nausea, arrhythmias, AV block
66% renal 33% hepatic $t_{1/2}$ = 110 min	Cholinergic crisis, bronchoconstriction, bradycardia, AV block, muscle weakness
Hepatic $t_{1/2}$ = 2–3 h (although clinical duration of action is short)	Bradycardia, hypertension, cardiac failure

TABLE 8.11. Dose, Kinetics, and Side Effects of Drugs Used to Treat Bradycardia

	Dosage (Adult)
Vagolytic	
Antimuscarinic	
Atropine	*Bolus:* 0.4–1.0 mg i.v.
Sympathomimetic	
Direct	
Isoproterenol	*Infusion:* 1–5 μg/min i.v.
Indirect	
Ephedrine	*Bolus:* 5–25 mg i.v.

[a] COMT, catechol-*o*-methyltransferase.

TABLE 8.12. Antiarrhythmic Agents[a]

Drug	*Indication*	*Route*
Class Ia		
Quinidine	AF, PSVT VT, WPW[b]	i.v. Oral
Procainamide	AF, VT, WPW	i.v. Oral
Disopyramide	AF, VT	Oral
Class Ib		
Lidocaine	VT, VF, PVC	i.v.
Mexiletine	VT	Oral
Tocainide	VT	Oral
Class Ic		
Encainide	VT	Oral
Flecainide	VT	Oral
Propafenone	VT	Oral
Moricizine	VT	Oral
Class II		
Propranolol	SVT, VT, PVC, digoxin toxicity	i.v. Oral
Esmolol	ST, SVT	i.v.

Elimination	Side Effects
50% hepatic 50% renal $t_{1/2}$ = 4 h	Paradoxical bradycardia (with low doses), drying of secretions, mental status changes/sedation, central anticholinergic syndrome, mydriasis/cycloplegia
Hepatic (COMT)[a] $t_{1/2}$ = 2 min	Tachycardia, tachyarrhythmia, flushing, myocardial ischemia
60% hepatic—MAO 40% renal unchanged $t_{1/2}$ = 3–6 h	Tachycardia, hypertension, tachyphylaxis

Dosing[c] (mg/day)	Adverse Effects
6–10 mg/kg (infusion) (QG) 648–972 (QP) 550–825 (QS) 600–1200 (RR)	Hypotension, GI, thrombocytopenia, cinchonism
(QS) 1200–1800 (SR)	
5–15 mg/kg, LD 2–6 mg/min, MD	GI, CNS, lupus fever, hematological, anticholinergic effects
2000–5000 (SR)	
400–800 (RR)	Anticholinergic effects, CHF
400–800 (SR)	
1–2 mg/kg, LD (may repeat × 1)	CNS, GI
1–4 mg/min, MD	CNS, blood dyscrasia
600–1200	GI, CNS
1200–1800	GI, CNS, pulmonary agranulocytosis
75–200	GI, CNS,
200–400	CHF, GI, CNS, blurred vision
450–900	GI, blurred vision, dizziness
600–900	Dizziness, nausea, rash, seizures
1–3 mg (may repeat × 1) 30–120 (RR)	CHF, bradycardia, hypotension, CNS, fatigue
120–160 (SR)	
500 µg/kg/min for 1 min, followed by 50 µg/kg/min for 4 min, then titrate with repeat LD 50–300 µg/kg/min MD	CHF, CNS, lupus-like syndrome, hypotension, bradycardia bronchospasm

TABLE 8.12. *(Continued)*

Drug	*Indication*	*Route*
Class III		
Amiodarone	VT	Oral
Bretylium	VT, VF	i.v.
Sotalol	VT	p.o.
Class IV		
Verapamil	AF, PSVT	i.v.
		Oral
Diltiazem	AF, PSVT	i.v.
		Oral
Miscellaneous		
Adenosine	SVT, PSVT,	i.v.
Digoxin	AF, PSVT	i.v.
		p.o.
Magnesium	VT, VF	i.v.

[a] All doses and indications are based on current standards of practice that are subject to change, and all recommendations should be verified before being clinically implemented.
[b] AF, atrial fibrillation; PSVT, paroxysmal supraventricular tachycardia; VT, ventricular tachycardia; VF, ventricular fibrillation; PVC, premature ventricular contraction; CHF,

TABLE 8.13. Selected Properties of β-Adrenergic-Blocking Drugs

Drug	*Relative β_1 Selectivity*	*ISA*[a]	*MSA*
Acebutolol	+	+	+
Atenolol	+	−	−
Esmolol	+	−	−
Metoprolol	+	−	−
Nadolol	−	−	−
Pinadolol	−	++	+
Propranolol	−	−	++
Sotalol	−	−	−
Timolol	−	−	−

[a] ISA, intrinsic sympathomimetic activity; MSA, membrane-stabilizing activity.

Dosing[c] (mg/day)	Adverse Effects
800–1600 (21 days LD) 600–800 MD (30 days, LD) 400 MD	CNS, GI, thyroid, pulmonary fibrosis, liver, corneal deposits
5–10 mg/kg, LD may repeat as needed 5–10 mg/kg q6–8h or 1–2 mg/min MD	GI, orthostatic hypotension, CNS
320–640	Bradycardia, hypotension, CHF, CNS, fatigue
5–10 mg (may repeat after 15–30 min)	Hypotension, CHF, bradycardia, vertigo, constipation
240–480 (RR) 120–480 (SR)	
0.25 mg/kg × 2 min LD 0.35 mg/kg × 2 min (2nd LD optional) 5–15 mg/h, MD	Hypotension, GI, liver
120–360 (RR)	
6 mg (may repeat up to 12 mg)	Flushing, dizziness, bradycardia, syncope
0.4–1 LD 0.125–0.375 MD	GI, CNS, arrhythmias
0.750–1.25 LD 0.125–0.375 MD	
1–2 g LD 0.5–1 g/h MD	Hypotension, CNS hypothermia, myocardial depression

congestive heart failure; WPW, Wolff-Parkinson-White; LD, loading dose; MD, maintenance dose; ST, sinus tachycardia; RR, regular release; SR, sustained release; QG, quinidine gluconate; QP, quinidine polygalactoronate.

[c] Total dosing for 1 day, unless otherwise noted.

Absorption (%)	Bioavailability (%)	Elimination Half-life	Major Route Elimination
70	50	3–4 h	Renal
50	40	6–9 h	Renal
—	—	9–10 min	Hepatic
90	50	3–4 h	Hepatic
30	30	14–24 h	Renal
90	90	3–4 h	Renal, hepatic
90	30	3–4 h	Hepatic
70	60	8–10 h	Renal
90	75	4–5 h	Renal, hepatic

TABLE 8.14. Guidelines for Implantation of Cardiac Pacemakers (Permanent)

Class I (agreement exists for permanent pacemaker insertion)
- AV block
  - Complete with symptoms
  - 2nd degree type II (Mobitz)—symptomatic
  - Pauses greater than 3 sec
- Periinfarction period
  - Complete heart block
  - New bifascicular block (RBBB and LAH)[a] with Mobitz II SSS
  - SSS and syncope

Class II (experts disagree on pacemaker indication)
- AV block
  - Complete heart block asymptomatic or HR > 40/min
    - Mobitz II asymptomatic
- Periinfarction period
  - AV node block (complete without symptoms)
  - Isolated bifascicular block (RBBB and LAH, LBBB)

Class III (agreement against pacemaker implantation)
- AV block
  - 1st degree
  - 2nd degree AV block type I (supra His)
- Periinfarction period:
  - Isolated left anterior hemiblock
  - 1st degree AV block
- Sick sinus syndrome
  - Asymptomatic

[a] RBBB, right bundle branch block; LAH, left anterior hemiblock; HR, heart rate; SSS, sick sinus syndrome; LBBB, left bundle branch block.

TABLE 8.15. Indications for Temporary Pacing

SA node dysfunction
- Sick sinus syndrome—symptomatic with syncope

AV node disease
- Acute complete heart block
- Type II (Mobitz II) with symptoms
- Symptomatic pauses greater than 3 sec

Periinfarction period
- Acute Mobitz II
- Acute RBBB and LAH[a]
- Acute trifascicular block (1st degree AV block with RBBB and LAH or 1st degree and LBBB)
- Isolated acute LBBB[b]

[a] RBBB, right bundle branch block; LAH, left anterior hemiblock; LBBB, left bundle branch block.
[b] Disagreement exists among experts.

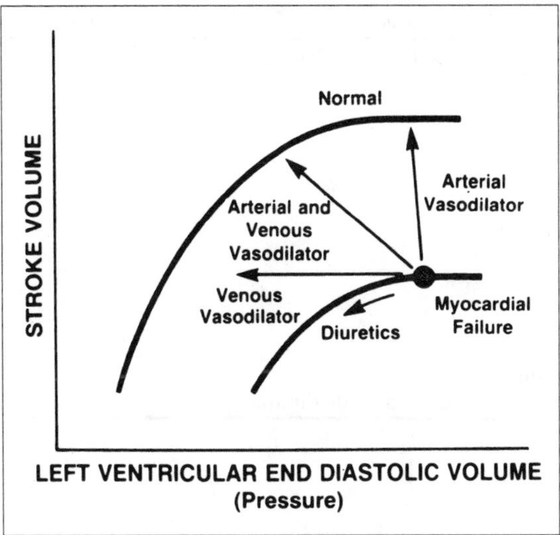

FIGURE 8.1. Ability of different types of vasodilators to shift depressed ventricular function curve toward normal. Arterial vasodilators produce an increase in stroke volume with few or no changes in preload. Venous vasodilators produce a reduction in end-diastolic volume with little or no change in stroke volume. Vasodilators with both arterial and venous effects improve stroke volume and reduce filling pressures. An inotropic agent, along with a vasodilator, would shift the depressed curve even closer toward normal. At low levels of end-diastolic volume (on the slope rather than the plateau of the ventricular function curve), vasodilators may cause decreases in stroke volume and / or end-diastolic volume, resulting in decreased cardiac performance and hypotension.

TABLE 8.16. Vasodilators Classified by Their Principal Site of Action

Arterial and venous vasodilators—"balanced vasodilators"
Nitroprusside
Phentolamine
Prazosin
Captopril
Enalapril
Lisinopril
Nifedipine
Verapamil
Diltiazem
Arterial vasodilators
Hydralazine
Minoxidil
Venous vasodilators
Nitrates (nitroglycerin, isosorbide dinitrate)

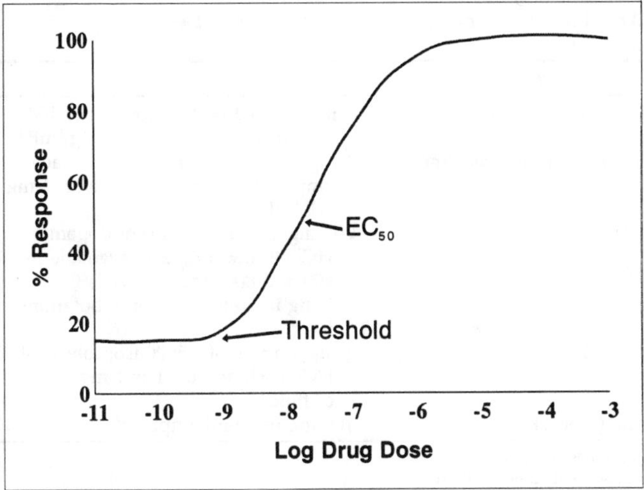

FIGURE 8.2. Typical relationship between log (catecholamine concentration) and effect. *EC_{50}*, drug concentration associated with 50% maximal drug response. *Threshold*, the concentration that produces a noticeable effect.

TABLE 8.17. Prescribing Infusions of Inotropic Agents: Deriving Concentrations

Inotrope	*How Supplied*
Epinephrine (adrenaline chloride)	1-mg (1 ml) dosette ampules of 1:1000 EPI; also in 30-ml vial of 1 mg/ml[a–c]
Norepinephrine (noradrenaline)	4-mg ampule of NE bitartrate; each ampule has 4 ml of fluid with 1 mg NE/ml[a–c]
Dopamine	200-mg ampules (5 ml) of dopamine HCl (40 mg/ml); also available in 400 and 800 mg, 5-ml vials[a,b]
Dobutamine	250 mg in 20-ml vials of dobutamine HCl[a,b]
Isoproterenol	1-mg ampule of 1:5000 isoproterenol HCl; each ampule has 1 mg/5 ml of fluid[a]
Amrinone (Inocor)	100 mg in 20-ml ampules[d]

[a] Protect ampules from light.
[b] Avoid use with alkaline solutions.
[c] EPI, epinephrine; NE, norepinephrine.
[d] Do not mix in dextrose-containing solutions.

Diluent	*Concentration*
250 ml of either D_5W or 0.9% NaCl	4 μg/ml
500 ml of either D_5W, or NaCl or 0.45% NaCl	8 μg/ml
250 ml of D_5W or 0.9% NaCl	800 μg/ml
250 ml of either D_5W or 0.9% NaCl	1000 μg/ml
250 ml of either D_5W or 0.9% NaCl	4 μg/ml
20 ml of 0.9% NaCl or 0.45% NaCl	2.5 mg/ml

TABLE 8.18. Conventional Doses of Plasminogen Activators for Patients with Acute Myocardial Infarction

Agent	*Dosing*
t-PA[a]	
"Conventional"	100 mg or 1 mg/kg for those ≤65 kg, over 3 h with 10% of the dose given as an initial bolus
"Front-loaded"	100 mg over 1.5 h with a 15-mg initial bolus
SK	1,500,000 U over 1 h
APSAC	30 mg over 2–5 min
UK	2,000,000 U over 1 h
scu-PA	80 mg over 1 h with 20 mg given as an initial bolus

[a] t-PA, tissue plasminogen activator; SK, streptokinase; APSAC, acylated streptokinase/plasminogen complexes; UK, urokinase; scu-PA, single-chain urokinase-like plasminogen activator.

TABLE 8.19. Contraindications to Thrombolytic Therapy

Absolute contraindications
- Active bleeding
- Cerebrovascular accident within 2 months or active intracerebral process

Major relative contraindications
- Major recent surgery, organ biopsy, or invasive vascular procedure within 10 days
- Active malignancy
- Recent serious trauma, including prolonged cardiopulmonary resuscitation
- Severe hypertension (systolic ≥ 180 mm Hg or diastolic ≥ 110 mm Hg)

Other relative contraindications
- Chronic or acute renal failure
- Endocarditis
- Pregnancy or immediate postpartum state
- Age (75 yr or older)
- Diabetic hemorrhagic retinopathy
- Chronic therapeutic anticoagulation
- Inflammatory bowel disease
- Cutaneous ulcerations
- Chronic liver disease
- Disorders of hemostasis
- History of cerebrovascular accident

CHAPTER 9

Neurologic/Psychiatric Medications[a]

Neurologic emergencies frequently are treatable with pharmacologic agents. Acute seizures, stroke, subarachnoid hemorrhage, and other brain disorders are addressed in this lengthy chapter. In treating seizure patients, drug interactions must be duly noted. This area of concern is addressed in several of this chapter's tables:

1. Common causes of seizures in critically ill patients (Table 9.1)
2. Interactions with phenytoin (Table 9.2)
3. Interactions with phenobarbital (Table 9.3)
4. Dosing parameters for benzodiazepines (Table 9.4)
5. Interactions with diazepam (Table 9.5)
6. Interactions with carbamazepine (Table 9.6)
7. Interactions with valproic acid (Table 9.7)
8. Physiologic changes during status epilepticus (Table 9.8)

[a]The material in this chapter was contributed by the following: Tables 9.1–9.10 were contributed by Brian Litt, M.D., and Gregory L. Krauss, M.D.; Tables 9.11–9.17 and Figures 9.1 and 9.2 were contributed by Barney J. Stern, M.D., and Michael N. Diringer, M.D.; Tables 9.18–9.23 were contributed by Jeffrey S. Kelly, M.D., and Drew A. MacGregor, M.D.; Table 9.24 was contributed by Howard D. Weiss, M.D.; Table 9.25 was contributed by Edwin H. Cassem, M.D., C. Raymond Lake, M.D., Ph.D., and William F. Boyer, M.D.; Figures 9.3–9.7 and Tables 9.26 and 9.27 were contributed by Donald S. Prough, M.D., and Douglas S. Dewitt, Ph.D.

9. Treatment protocol for status epilepticus (Table 9.9)
10. Guidelines for use of pentobarbital in patients with status epilepticus (Table 9.10)
11. Selected conditions associated with ischemic stroke (Table 9.11)
12. Causes of nontraumatic intracerebral hemorrhage (Table 9.12)
13. Management of cardiogenic embolic stroke (Fig. 9.1)
14. Management of arterial disease causing an acute ischemic event (Fig. 9.2)
15. Management of obtunded patients with suspected intracerebral hematoma (Table 9.13)
16. Acute blood pressure management in patients with intracerebral hematoma (Table 9.14)
17. Causes of subarachnoid hemorrhage (Table 9.15)
18. Early management of patients with subarachnoid hemorrhage (Table 9.16)
19. Prophylactic therapies for vasospasm (Table 9.17)
20. End-organ responses to cholinergic stimulation (Table 9.18)
21. Cholinomimetic and anticholinergic actions and agents (Table 9.19)
22. Anticholinesterase agents (Table 9.20)
23. Clinical uses of cholinesterase inhibitors (Table 9.21)
24. Comparison of antimuscarinic agents (Table 9.22)
25. Clinical uses and side effects of commonly used cholinergic drugs (Table 9.23)
26. Diagnostic criteria for neuroleptic malignant syndrome (Table 9.24)
27. Medications with psychiatric side effects (Table 9.25)
28. Response of cerebral blood flow to changes in $PaCO_2$ (Fig. 9.3)
29. Response of cerebral blood flow to changes in mean arterial pressure (Fig. 9.4)
30. Cerebral autoregulation is impaired by coexistent cerebral vasodilatory stimuli (Fig. 9.5)
31. Relationship between intracranial volume and intracranial pressure (Fig. 9.6)
32. Causes of intracranial hypertension (Table 9.26)

33. Strategies to control intracranial pressure (Table 9.27)
34. Strategies to control intracranial pressure based on intracranial compartments (Fig. 9.7)

TABLE 9.1. Common Causes of Seizures in Critically Ill Patients

Condition	*Examples*
Mechanical brain injury	Trauma, neurosurgery, SAH/ICH[a]
Hypoxic/ischemic insult	Stroke, hemorrhage, shock, cardiac arrest, cerebral edema
CNS infection	Meningitis, encephalitis (especially herpes simplex), abscess, sepsis
Metabolic disorders	Electrolyte abnormalities (low Na, low Mg, high Ca), hepatic failure, renal failure, hypo- or hyperglycemia, very rare genetic disorders
Drug sensitivity/toxicity	Theophylline, phenothiazines, alcohol, cocaine
Idiopathic epilepsy	Absence, complex partial
Seizure-prone states	Alcohol abuse, eclampsia, drug withdrawal
Electric shock	Lightning, electroconvulsive therapy
Tumor	Primary brain, metastases, other

[a]SAH, subarachnoid hemorrhage; ICH, intracranial hemorrhage; CNS, central nervous system.

TABLE 9.2. Phenytoin Interactions[a]

Action Increased by	*Action Decreased by*	*Increases Action of*	*Decreases Action of*
AEDs[b]			
Pentobarbital	Phenobarbital	Phenobarbital	Phenobarbital
Valproic acid	Valproic acid	Valproic acid	Valproic acid
Carbamazepine	Carbamazepine		Carbamazepine
Primidone	Primidone	Primidone	
Clonazepam	Clonazepam		Clonazepam
Diazepam	Diazepam		
Ethosuximide			
Methsuximide			
Felbamate			
Other drugs			
Acute alcohol intake	Antacids with calcium		Antipyrine
Calcium carbimide	Chronic alcohol abuse		Corticosteroids
Cimetidine	Dioxide		Coumarin
Chloramphenicol	Folate		Digitoxin
Chlordiazepoxide	Molindone HCl with calcium		Doxycycline
Chlorpheniramine	Pyridoxine		Estrogens
Clofibrate	Reserpine		Furosemide
Dicoumarol			Haloperidol
Disulfiram			Nortriptyline

Estrogens	Oral contraceptives
Furosemide	Phenylbutazone
Halothane	Pyridoxine
Imipramine	Quinidine
Isoniazid	Rifampin
Methylphenidate	Theophylline
Nortriptyline	Vitamin D
Pheneturide	
Phenothiazines	
Phenylbutazone	
Phenyramidol	
Propoxyphene	
Salicylates	
Sulfonamides	
Tolbutamide	
Trazodone	
Warfarin	

[a] Data taken from Refs. 1–3.
[b] AEDs, antiepileptic drugs.

TABLE 9.3. Phenobarbital Drug Interactions[a]

Action Increased by	*Action Decreased by*	*Increases Action of*	*Decreases Action of*
AEDs[b]			
Phenytoin	Phenytoin	Phenytoin	Phenytoin
Methsuximide		Methsuximide	
Valproate			Valproate
			Clonazepam
			Carbamazepine
Other drugs			
Amitriptyline	Ammonium chloride		Alprenolol
Antihistamines	Dicoumarol		Aminopyrine
Corticosteroids	Folate		Bishydroxycoumarin
Imipramine	Phenylbutazone		Chloramphenicol
MAO inhibitors	Pyridoxine		Chlorpromazine
Narcotics			Dexamethasone
Propoxyphene			Digitoxin
Rauwolfia alkaloids (e.g., reserpine)			Dipyrone
Tranquilizers			Doxycycline
			Griseofulvin
			Isoniazid
			Metoprolol
			Oral contraceptives
			Phenylbutazone
			Propranolol
			Quinine
			Tricyclic antidepressants
			Vitamin D
			Warfarin

[a] Data taken from Refs. 1 and 4.
[b] AEDs, antiepileptic drugs; MAO, monoamine oxidase.

TABLE 9.4. Benzodiazepines: Parameters and Administration[a]

Parameter	*Diazepam*	*Lorazepam*	*Midazolam*
V_d (liter/kg)[2,3]	1.0–2.0	1.0	2.5
Lipid solution[2,3]	Very	Yes	Very
Protein-bound[2,3]	95%	90%	97%
Metabolism/liver[2,3]	95%	90%	95%
Alkaline urine increases excretion	No	No	No
Half-life clearance[3–6]	36 h	18 h	2.8 h
Anticonvulsant	20–30 min	4–12 h	?
Onset effect[8,9]	½–2 min	3–5 min	1–2.5 min
Time to peak level[1–3,8,9]			
i.v.	8 min	23 min	30 min
i.m.	30–60 min	90 min	45 min
p.o.	30–90 min	90–120 min	N/A
prn	65 min (mean)	Unclear	Unclear
Dilute[1,3]	No	Yes	Optional
Bolus dose[6,7,10]	5 mg	2 mg	1 mg
Rate of administration[3,6,7,10]	2 mg/min	1 mg/min	1/2–1 mg/min
Time between boluses[6,7,10]	2–5 min	2–5 min	2–5 min
Maximum dose (nontolerant)[5,6,10]	0.25 mg/kg	0.1 mg/kg	0.08 mg/kg
Continuous infusion[5,6,11]	Yes	Yes	Yes Efficacy not studied

TABLE 9.4. *(Continued)*

Parameter	*Diazepam*	*Lorazepam*	*Midazolam*
Fluid	All i.v. fluids (may precipitate in NaCl solutions at high concentrations)	All i.v. fluids	All i.v. fluids
Suggested concentration[5, 11–13]	20 mg/250 ml i.v. fluids	?	50 mg/250 ml (may be less concentrated)
Bolus before infusion[6, 12, 13]	0.25 mg/kg	?	0.1–0.3 mg/kg
Rate of infusion[1, 6, 12, 13]	2 mg/kg/24 h	?	0.05–0.40 mg/kg/h
Remix preparation[14]	q 6–8h at > 1.0 mg/ml q24h < 1.0 mg/ml	?	24h

[a]Table notes, by reference number: 1, 5; 2, 6; 3, 2; 4, 7; 5, 8; 6, 9; 7, 10; 8, 11; 9, 12; 10, 13; 11, 14; 12, 15; 13, 16; 14, Johns Hopkins Hospital Pharmacy Protocol.

TABLE 9.5. Diazepam Interactions[a]

Action Increased by	*GI Absorption Decreased by*	*Action Decreased by*	*Decreases Action of*
Valproic acid	Metoclopramide	Aminophylline	Levodopa
Digoxin			
Disulfiram	Ethanol		
Cimetidine	Antacids		
Ethanol	Theophylline		
Cimetidine			

[a]Data taken from Refs. 17–23.

TABLE 9.6. Carbamazepine Interactions[a]

Action Increased by	*Action Decreased by*	*Increases Action of*	*Decreases Action of*
AEDs[b]			
Valproic acid		Valproic acid	Valproic acid
Felbamate[c]			
	Phenytoin	Phenytoin	Phenytoin
	Primidone	Primidone	
	Clonazepam		Clonazepam
	Phenobarbital		
			Ethosuxamide
Other drugs			
Calcium channel blockers			Doxycycline
Cimetidine			Haloperidol
Erythromycin			Oral contraceptives
Isoniazid			Theophylline
Lithium			Warfarin
Propoxyphene			
Triacetyloleandomycin			

[a] Adapted from Refs. 1, 2, 7, and 24.
[b] AEDs, antiepileptic drugs.
[c] Serum level decreased, but epoxide level increases.

...lproic Acid Interactions[a]

Action Increased by	Action Decreased by
AEDs[b]	
Phenytoin	Phenytoin
Carbamazepine	
Felbamate	
	Phenobarbital
Other drugs	
Dicumarol	
Phenylbutazone	
Salicylates	

[a] Adapted from Refs. 1, 2, and 7.
[b] AEDs, antiepileptic drugs; MAO, monamine oxidase.

TABLE 9.8. Physiologic Changes during Status Epilepticus[a]

Measure	0–30 min
Blood pressure	Up
PaO_2	Down
$PaCO_2$	Up
Serum pH	Down
Temperature	Up
Autonomic activity	Up
Lung fluids	Up
Serum K^+	Up
Serum CPK[b]	Normal
Cerebral blood flow	Up (900%)
Cerebral O_2 consumption	Up (300%)

[a] Adapted from Refs. 25 and 26.
[b] CPK, creatinine phosphokinase; ICP, intracranial pressure.

Increases Action of	*Decreases Action of*
Phenytoin Carbamazepine	Phenytoin Carbamazepine
Clonazepam Barbiturates Primidone Ethosuximide	
CNS depressants MAO inhibitors Antidepressants	

> 30 min	*Complication*
Down	Shock
Down	Hypoxia
Varies	ICP
Varies	Acidosis
Up	Fever
Up	Arrhythmias
Up	Atelectasis
Up	Arrhythmias
Up	Renal failure
Up (200%)	Hemorrhage
Up (300%)	Neuronal death

TABLE 9.9. Protocol for Treatment of Status Epilepticus

Time (min)	*Intervention*
0	Recognition Airway, breathing, circulation History, trauma survey Establish intravenous access Oxygen
5	Send blood sample for lab tests Dextrose 50% 50 ml i.v. Naloxone 2 mg i.v. Thiamine 100 mg i.v.
10	Benzodiazepines[a] Phenytoin load
30	Phenobarbital or benzodiazepine infusion (midazolam or diazepam) EEG monitoring (if not yet begun)
60	Pentobarbital coma
80	General anesthesia neuromuscular blockade

[a] Treatment with benzodiazepines should be initiated as rapidly as possible after addressing earlier items in the protocol, and always by 10 minutes, if possible.

TABLE 9.10. Pentobarbital-induced Anesthesia in Refractory Generalized Tonic-Clonic Status Epilepticus[a]

General guidelines for pentobarbital infusion
- Loading dose:[b] 5–20 mg/kg i.v. at infusion rate 25 mg/min
- Initial maintenance 2.5 mg/kg/h
- For breakthough seizures, 59-mg bolus and increase maintenance by 0.5–1 mg/kg/h
- Begin tapering 24 h after last seizure
- Tapering rate (q4–6h) 1.0 mg/kg/h if pentobarbital level >50 mg/liter or 0.5 mg/kg/h if pentobarbital level <50 mg/liter
- For seizures during tapering, 50-mg pentobarbital bolus; increase maintenance to closest preseizure dose

General guidelines for patient management
- Endotracheal intubation; assisted ventilation
- Continuous BP monitoring (arterial line)
- Hemodynamic monitoring (Swan-Ganz) optional
- Hypotension[c]: fluids and dopamine up to 12 μg/kg/min
- Prophylaxis of decubiti and venous thombosis
- Daily CBC
- Maintenance of high therapeutic AED serum concentrations
- Obtain serum at least once daily
- EEG monitoring
- Baseline
- Continuous for the first 2–6 h of anesthesia
- Ten-min strips every 30–60 min for duration of treatment

[a]From Osorio I, Reed RC: Treatment of refractory generalized tonic-clonic status epilepticus with pentobarbital anesthesia after high-dose phenytoin. *Epilepsia* 30:464–471, 1989.

[b]Separation of the cardiorespiratory complications of refractory generalized tonic-clonic status epilepticus from effects of pentobarbital may be difficult.

[c]In most patients, 5 mg/kg was effective for induction of anesthesia.

[d]Defined as decrease in systolic blood pressure by 10 mm Hg, as compared with preanesthetic BP. Decrease or discontinue pentobarbital temporarily if dopamine requirements exceed 12 μg/kg/min.

TABLE 9.11. Selected Conditions Associated with Ischemic Stroke

- Cardiogenic emboli
  - Atrial fibrillation
  - Recent myocardial infarction
  - Cardiac thrombus
  - Akinetic ventricular segment
  - Dilated cardiomyopathy
  - Valvular disease
  - Prosthetic heart valve
  - Patent foramen ovale
  - Atrial septal defect
  - Atrial septal aneurysm
  - Infective endocarditis
  - Nonbacterial thrombotic endocarditis
  - Left atrial spontaneous echo contrast
  - Myxoma
- Large artery disease
  - Atherosclerosis
  - Dissection
  - Fibromuscular dysplasia
  - Takayasu's disease
  - Moyamoya disease
  - Radiation-induced damage
- Small artery disease
  - Microatheroma
  - Lipohyalinosis
  - Inflammation
    - Sterile
    - Infectious
- Systemic and hematologic conditions
  - Polycythemia
  - Sickle cell disease
  - Hypercoagulable states
    - Malignancy
    - Pregnancy
    - Inflammatory bowel disease
    - Nephrotic syndrome
    - Antiphospholipid syndrome
    - Protein S and C deficiencies
    - Antithrombin III deficiency
    - Dysfibrinogenemia
- Miscellaneous conditions
  - Migraine
  - Drug use and abuse
    - Cocaine (including "crack")
    - Alcohol
    - *l*-Asparaginase
    - Birth control pills
    - Sympathomimetics

TABLE 9.12. Causes of Nontraumatic Intracerebral Hemorrhage

Vascular
Hypertension
Vascular malformation
Saccular aneurysm
Arteritis
Amyloid angiopathy
Surgical
Carotid endarterectomy
Postcraniotomy
Sympathomimetic drugs
Cocaine hydrochloride
"Crack" cocaine
Methylphenidate
Phenylpropanolamine
Amphetamine
Coagulopathy
Endogenous
Anticoagulants
Thrombolytic drugs
Infection
Meningitis
Encephalitis
Miscellaneous
Hemorrhage into tumor
Venous occlusion
Severe migraine
Exposure to cold

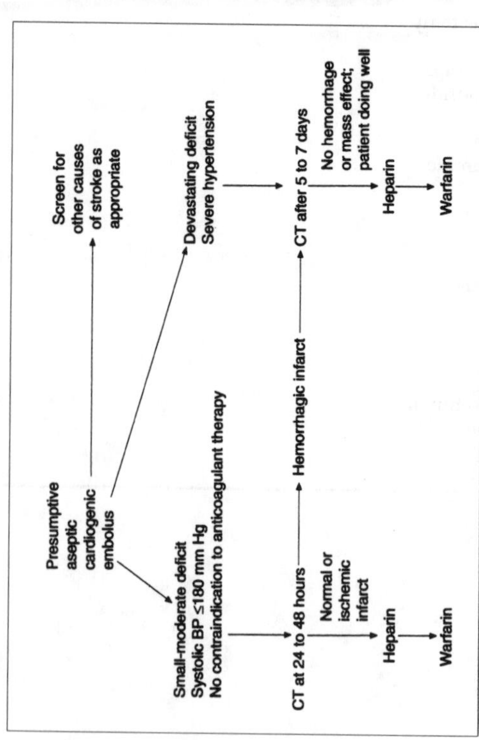

FIGURE 9.1. Management of cardiogenic embolic stroke.

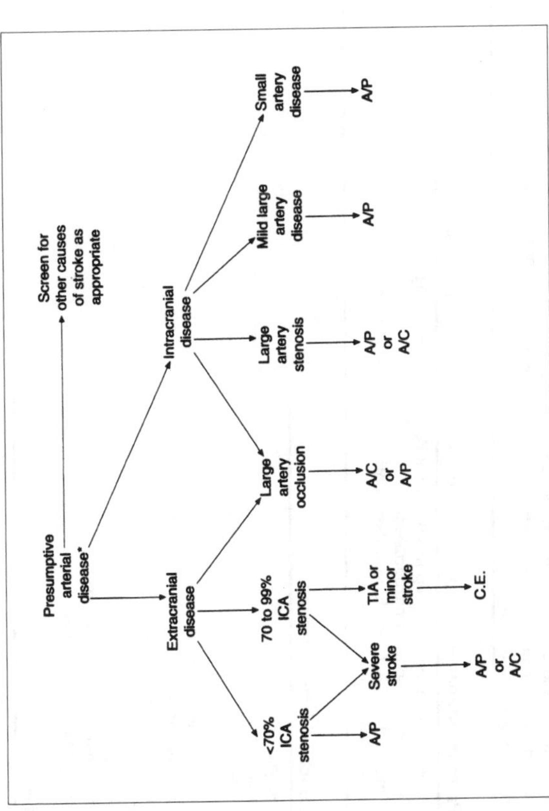

FIGURE 9.2. Management of arterial disease causing an acute ischemic event. *A/P*, antiplatelet therapy; *A/C*, anticoagulant therapy; *C.E.*, carotid endarterectomy; *ICA*, internal carotid artery; *, consider A/C if patient is deteriorating.

TABLE 9.13. Initial Management of Obtunded Patients with Suspected Intracerebral Hematoma

1. Assess level of consciousness, airway reflexes, blood pressure, and neurologic exam
2. If Glasgow Coma Score is ≤8, intubate and premedicate with thiopental 1–3 mg/kg i.v. and rapid-acting paralytic agent
3. Hyperventilate to $PaCO_2$ 25–30 mm Hg and administer mannitol 0.25–1.0 g/kg i.v.
4. Treat severe hypertension and reduce mean arterial blood pressure to 125–135 mm Hg (see Table 9.14)
5. Nonenhanced CT scan and neurosurgical evaluation

TABLE 9.14. Acute Blood Pressure Management in Patients with Intracerebral Hematomas

1. Avoid rapid "normalization" of mean arterial BP; keep mean arterial BP at 125–135 mm Hg
2. Avoid cerebral venodilators (nitrates and sodium nitroprusside)
3. Administer labetalol in 5–20 mg i.v. boluses to reach goal, then continue periodic boluses or infusion
4. If refractory, add hydralazine in 2.5–10 mg i.v. boluses

TABLE 9.15. Causes of Subarachnoid Hemorrhage

Saccular aneurysm
Vascular malformation
Moyamoya disease
Head trauma
Extension of intracerebral hematoma
Spinal vascular malformation
Ruptured superficial cortical artery
Angiopathy
Venous thrombosis
Coagulopathy (endogenous or iatrogenic)
Infection (meningitis, encephalitis)
Toxins
Idiopathic hemorrhage

TABLE 9.16. Early Management of Patients with Subarachnoid Hemorrhage

1. Assess level of consciousness and airway reflexes
2. Treat hypertension to patient's normal BP; if unknown, keep mean arterial BP at 100–110 mm Hg
3. CT scan (nonenhanced)
4. Lumbar puncture only if CT is negative
5. Selective four-vessel angiography; general anesthesia for agitated uncooperative patients
6. Monitor electrocardiogram
7. Normal saline at somewhat above maintenance requirements
8. Load with phenytoin 18–20 mg/kg i.v.
9. Dexamethasone 4 mg q6h i.v. or p.o. (optional)
10. Avoid excessive stimulation; sedate agitated patients with i.v. midazolam 1–3 mg, fentanyl 25–100 μg, or morphine 1–2 mg; titrate to effect; avoid long-acting agents
11. Prepare for surgery as soon as possible (most patients)

TABLE 9.17. Prophylactic Therapies for Vasospasm

1. Volume expansion with isotonic saline ± colloids
2. Nimodipine 60 mg orally q4h
3. Mechanical removal of subarachnoid blood at surgery
4. Intrathecal tissue plasminogen activator at surgery (experimental)

TABLE 9.18. End-Organ Responses to Cholinergic Stimulation

Tissue	*Response*
Heart	Decreased heart rate, decreased contractility, decreased conduction velocity, AV block
Lung	Bronchoconstriction, increased secretions
Adrenal medulla	Secretion of epinephrine and norepinephrine
Exocrine glands (pancreas, salivary, and lacrimal glands)	Increased secretions
Gastrointestinal tract	Increased motility and tone, relaxation of pylorus and gastroesophageal sphincter, relaxation of cecal valve and other sphincters, increased secretions, gallbladder contraction
Bladder	Relaxation of internal sphincter (micturition)
Sweat glands	Increased secretion
Male reproductive system	Erection
Eye	Contraction of iris (miosis), contraction of ciliary muscle for accommodation-convergence

TABLE 9.19. Cholinomimetic and Anticholinergic Actions and Agents

Mechanism of Action	*Drug or Other Agent*	*Effect*
Mimics effect of ACh[a]	Methacholine, nicotine	Cholinomimetic
	Succinylcholine	Muscle paralysis
Causes release of ACh	Black widow spider venom	Initially cholinomimetic
Inhibits enzymatic destruction of ACh	Anticholinesterase drugs	Cholinomimetic
Prevents ACh synthesis	Hemicholinium	Blocks ACh reuptake with eventual depletion of ACh
Prevents ACh release	Botulinum toxin	Anticholinergic
Blocks ACh receptors	Atropine	Anticholinergic
	d-Tubocurarine	Muscle paralysis
	Hexamethonium	Sympathetic blockade

[a] ACh, acetylcholine.

TABLE 9.20. Anticholinesterase Agents

Reversible	*Irreversible*
Physostigmine	"Nerve gases" (tabun, sarin, soman)
Neostigmine	Insecticides
Edrophonium	malathion, parathion, fenthion
Pyridostigmine	paraoxon (diazinon)
Demecarium	TEPP, others
Ambenonium	Echothiophate

TABLE 9.21. Clinical Uses of Cholinesterase Inhibitors

Drug	*Uses*	*Usual Dose*	*Duration*
Edrophonium	Myasthenia gravis	2–8 mg i.v. test	5–10 min
	Reversal of competitive neuromuscular blockade	30–50 mg i.v.	
Physostigmine	Glaucoma	Topical drops	2–6 h
	TCA overdose[a]	2–12 mg i.v.	10–20 min
Pyridostigmine	Myasthenia gravis	60–120 mg p.o.	3–6 h
		2–4 mg i.v.	2–4 h
	Reversal of competitive neuromuscular blockade	10–20 mg i.v.	
Neostigmine	Myasthenia gravis	15 mg p.o.	2–4 h
	Reversal of competitive neuromuscular blockade	2.5–5 mg i.v.	

[a]TCA, tricyclic antidepressant.

TABLE 9.22. Comparison of Antimuscarinic Agents

Drug	*Cardiovascular Effects*	*CNS Effects*	*Primary Uses*	*Other Uses*
Atropine	+++	+	Bradycardia	Decrease bronchial secretions
Scopolamine	++	+++	Motion sickness	Amnestic agent (anesthesia)
Propantheline	+	±	Incontinence	
Glycopyrrolate	+	0	Antisialogogue	Adjunct for neuromuscular blockade reversal

TABLE 9.23. Clinical Uses and Side Effects of Commonly Used Cholinergic Drugs

Drug	*Clinical Uses*
Choline esters	
Methacholine	Supraventricular tachycardia, methachol challenge
Carbachol	Stimulation of bladder and GI tract
Bethanechol	Stimulation of bladder and GI tract
Choline alkaloids	
Pilocarpine	Glaucoma
Aceclidine	Topical treatment of glaucoma
Metoclopramide	Antiemetic, treatment of gastroparesis
Anticholinesterases	
Physostigmine	Glaucoma, atropine intoxication, tricyclic antidepressant poisoning
Neostigmine	Reversal of nondepolarizing paralytics, treatment of gastroparesis and bladder atony
Pyridostigmine	Reversal of nondepolarizing paralytics, myasthenia gravis
Edrophonium	Differentiation of myasthenic crises, reversal of nondepolarizing paralytics; PSVT[a]
Echothiophate	Glaucoma
AChE regenerators	
Pralidoxime	Organophosphate poisoning, anticholinesterase overdose
Antimuscarinics	
Atropine	Symptomatic bradycardias, rarely used as mydriatic, cholinesterase-inhibitor poisoning
Scopolamine	Anesthesia (amnestic), antinausea (motion sickness)
Propantheline	Delays gastric emptying, augments bladder control
Glycopyrrolate	Anesthesia (antisialogogue)

[a]PSVT, paroxysmal supraventricular tachycardia; AChE, acetylcholinesterase.

Side Effects	*Notes*
Bradycardia, heart block, hypotension, syncope	Used in pulmonary function testing
Abdominal cramps, urinary urgency, bradycardia, hypotension	Relatively long duration
Fewer cardiovascular effects	Long duration of activity
Diaphoresis, salivation	
	Not available in U.S.
Dystonic reactions, extrapyramidal symptoms	
Confusion, nausea, bradycardia, hypotension	Tertiary amine
Severe bradycardia, arrhythmias, increased oral and bronchial secretions	Quaternary amine
Bradycardia, oropharyngeal and bronchial secretions	Fewer arrhythmias than with neostigmine
Less bradycardia than with other agents	
May prolong neuromuscular blockade of succinylcholine	Irreversible, with long duration of action
High dose may cause cholinergic blockade	Used in conjunction with atropine (see text)
Tachycardia, central anti-ACh syndrome	Tertiary amine
Dry mouth, sedation	Tertiary amine
Urinary retention	Few CNS effects (quaternary amine)
Dry mouth	Quaternary amine

TABLE 9.24. Diagnostic Criteria for Neuroleptic Malignant Syndrome

- Appropriate clinical setting
  - Neuroleptic use
    - Phenothiazines
    - Butyrophenones
    - Thioxanthenes
  - Dopamine-blocking drugs
    - Metoclopramide
  - Discontinuation of antiparkinsonian medications
- Mandatory clinical features (100% of cases)
  - High fevers
  - Marked rigidity
- Frequent accompanying features
  - Autonomic dysfunction
    - Tachycardia
    - Diaphoresis
    - Labile blood pressure
  - Extrapyramidal dysfunction
    - Tremulousness
    - Involuntary movements
    - Catatonic akinesia
  - Abnormal mental status
    - Mutism
    - Agitation
    - Stupor/coma
  - Laboratory abnormalities
    - Elevated creatinine phosphokinase
    - Leukocytosis
    - Dehydration

TABLE 9.25. Medications with Psychiatric Side Effects

Drug	*Anxiety*	*Despondency*	*Delirium or Psychosis*
Analgesics + antiinflammatories (nonsteroidal)			
Morphine + congeners		+	+
Meperidine, especially normeperidine		+	+
Pentazocine		+	+
Salicylates (severe abuse)			+
Acetaminophen			+
Fenoprofen	+	+	+
Indomethacin		+	+
Naproxen		+	
Phenylbutazone		+	
Propoxyphene		+	
Tolmetin sodium			+
Zomepirac sodium		+	+
Ibuprofen		+	+
Sulindac		+	+
Anticonvulsants			
Barbiturates	+	+	+
Hydantoins		+	+
Primidone		+	+
Sodium valproate		+	+
Succinimides (ethosuximide, phensuximide, methsuximide)	+	+	+
Antibiotics, antifungals, antihelminthics			
Ampicillin		+	
Sulfonamides		+	
Cephalosporins			+
Chloroquine			+
Ciprofloxacin			+
Clotrimazole		+	+
Cycloserine		+	+
Dapsone		+	+
Ethionamide		+	
Griseofulvin		+	
Isoniazid			+
Mefloquine		+	
Metronidazole		+	
Nitrofurantoin		+	
Nalidixic acid		+	
Ofloxacin			+
para-Aminosalicylic acid			+
Quinacrine			+
Streptomycin		+	

TABLE 9.25. (*Continued*)

Drug	*Anxiety*	*Despondency*	*Delirium or Psychosis*
Ketoconazole	+		
Aminoglycosides		+	+
Amodiaquine		+	+
Amphotericin B		+	+
Chloramphenicol		+	+
Colistin sulfate		+	+
Ethambutol HCl		+	+
Rifampin		+	+
Tetracycline		+	+
Ticarcillin		+	+
Trimethoprim-sulfamethoxazole		+	+
Tobramycin		+	+
Flucytosine		+	+
Thiabendazole			+
Anticholinergics (numerous drugs)	+	+	+
Antihistamines			
Cimetidine	+	+	+
Promethazine		+	+
Ranitidine	+	+	+
Antineoplastics			
Chlorambucil			+
Cyclosporine			+
Fluorouracil		+	+
Aminoglutethimide		+	+
Vinblastine		+	
Vincristine		+	+
Azathioprine		+	
Asparaginase		+	
Bleomycin		+	
Mithramycin		+	
Trimethoprim		+	
Azacitidine		+	+
Cytarabine (high dose)		+	+
Dacarbazine		+	+
Methenamine		+	+
Methotrexate (high dose)		+	+
Procarbazine		+	+
Tamoxifen		+	+
Interferon		+	+
Interleukin-2	+	+	+
Ifosfamide			+
Etoposide		+	
Antivirals			
Acyclovir	+	+	+
Azidothymidine (AZT)	+	+	+

TABLE 9.25. *(Continued)*

Drug	*Anxiety*	*Despondency*	*Delirium or Psychosis*
Didanosine			+
Foscarnet			+
Gancyclovir			+
Suramin		+	
Endocrine			
Adrenocorticosteroids (including ACTH)	+	+	+
Anabolic steroids	+	+	+
Clomiphene			+
Erythropoietin			+
Estrogens	+	+	+
Oral hypoglycemics			+
Thyroid	+	+	+
Sympatholytics (e.g., methysergide)	+	+	
Sympathomimetics (including theophylline preparations)			
Vitamins			
A	+		+
B complex	+	+	
D		+	
Folic acid			+
Other			
Aminocaproic acid			+
Baclofen	+		
Bupropion			+
Cyclobenzaprine			+
Diethyltoluamide (DEET)			+
Diphenoxylate	+		
Disulfiram		+	+
Metrizamide	+		+
Orphenadrine		+	
Pravastatin		+	
Halothane		+	
Coumarin		+	
Metoclopramide	+	+	+
Antiparkinsonians			
Anticholinergic (e.g., procyclidine)	+	+	+
Amantadine	+	+	+
Bromocriptine	+	+	+
Pergolide	+	+	+
Carbidopa	+	+	+
Levodopa	+	+	+
Cardiovascular			
Antiarrhythmics			
Amiodarone			+

TABLE 9.25. (*Continued*)

Drug	*Anxiety*	*Despondency*	*Delirium or Psychosis*
Lidocaine	+	+	+
Procainamide		+	+
Disopyramide	+	+	+
Mexiletine	+	+	+
Quinidine			+
Digitalis			+
Antihypertensives			
Captopril	+		+
Carbonic anhydrase inhibitors			+
Ethacrynic acid			+
Furosemide		+	+
Hydrochlorothiazide		+	+
Spironolactone			+
β-Blockers		+	+
Ganglionic blockers (mecamylamine, pentolinium, trimethaphan)			+
Rauwolfia alkaloids	+	+	+
Guanethidine		+	+
Methyldopa		+	+
Hydralazine	+	+	+
Clonidine	+	+	+
Prazosin		+	+
Calcium blockers			
Diltiazem		+	+
Nifedipine	+	+	+
Verapamil			+

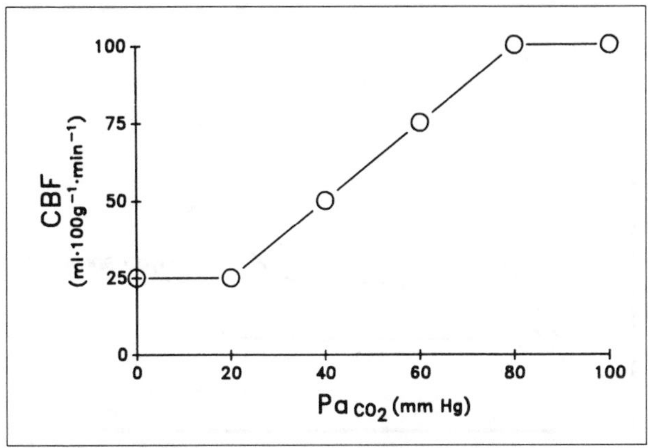

FIGURE 9.3. Response of cerebral blood flow (*CBF*) to changes in $PaCO_2$. As $PaCO_2$ is acutely decreased from 40 to 20 mm Hg, CBF is halved.

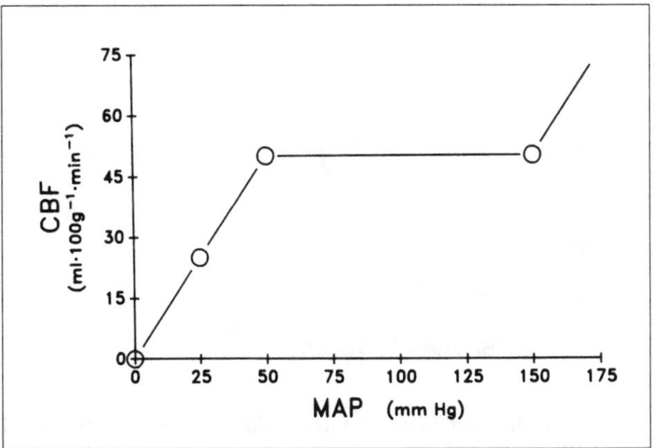

FIGURE 9.4. Response of cerebral blood flow (*CBF*) to changes in mean arterial pressure (*MAP*). Under normal circumstances, pressure autoregulation results in a nearly constant CBF over a MAP range from 60 to approximately 150 mm Hg.

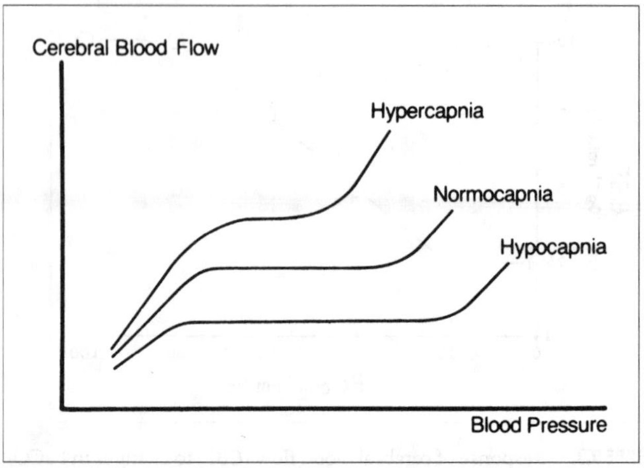

FIGURE 9.5. Cerebral autoregulation is impaired by coexistent cerebral vasodilatory stimuli. In the presence of hypercapnia, cerebral blood flow is higher and the upper limit of autoregulation is shifted to a lower mean blood pressure.

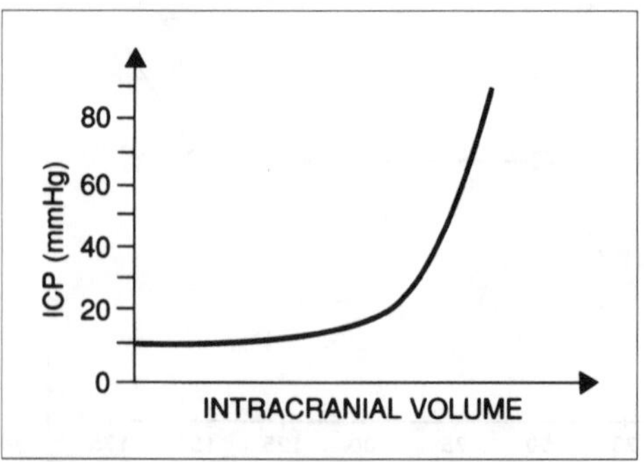

FIGURE 9.6. Relationship between intracranial volume and intracranial pressure (*ICP*). As the volume of one compartment (tissue, cerebrospinal fluid, or blood) increases, compensation initially is adequate; however, once a critical volume is obtained, intracranial pressure rapidly increases.

TABLE 9.26. Causes of Intracranial Hypertension

Cause	*Mechanism*
Intracranial mass lesions	Local expansion
Brain edema	Increased brain volume
Cellular (cytotoxic)	Cellular swelling secondary to hypoxia or ischemia
Vasogenic	Breakdown of blood-brain barrier with interstitial protein accumulation
Interstitial (hydrocephalic)	Block of CSF (reabsorption)
Brain engorgement (hyperemia)	Increased cerebral blood volume
Hypercarbia	Increased extracellular $[H^+]$
Hypoxia	Mechanism undetermined (adenosine?)
Hypertension	Impaired autoregulation
Improper head positioning	Obstruction of cerebral venous drainage

TABLE 9.27. Strategies for Controlling ICP [a]

Strategy	*Mechanism*
Endotracheal intubation	Prevention of hypoxia and hypercarbia
Neuromuscular blockade[a]	Prevention of coughing and straining
Passive hyperventilation[a]	Reduction of CBF[b] and cerebral blood volume
Fluid restriction[a]	Limitation of cerebral edema
Head positioning[a]	Facilitation of cerebral venous drainage
Osmotic diuresis	Reduction of brain water
Sedation/narcosis[a]	Reduction of $CMRO_2$, limitation of CBF response to noxious stimuli
Fever control	Limitation of $CMRO_2$
Barbiturates[c]	Reduction of $CMRO_2$, CBF, ICP
Glucocorticoids[c]	Limitation of cerebral edema
Decompressive craniectomy[a]	Increase space for brain expansion

[a] Controversial.
[b] CBF, cerebral blood flow; $CMRO_2$, cerebral metabolic rate for oxygen; ICP, intracranial pressure.
[c] Little or no demonstrable benefit.

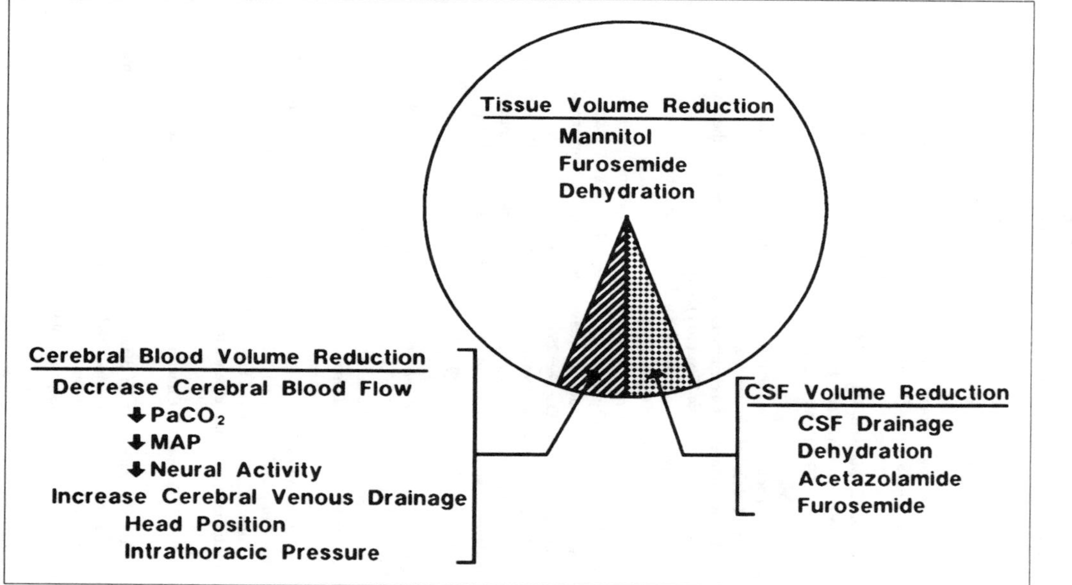

FIGURE 9.7. Strategies for reducing intracranial pressure based on the intracranial compartments: tissue volume, cerebrospinal fluid (*CSF*) volume, or cerebral blood volume (*MAP*, mean arterial pressure). The therapy of intracranial hypertension must either decrease the volume of the component that caused the original increase in intracranial pressure or decrease the volume of one of the other components.

REFERENCES

1. Engel Jr J: *Seizures and Epilepsy.* FA Davis, Philadelphia, 1989.
2. *Physicians Desk Reference (PDR) 1992:* Medical Economics Data, a division of Medical Economics Company, Inc, Montvale NJ, 1992.
3. Kutt H: Phenytoin: interactions with other drugs. In Levy RH, Dreifuss FE, Mattson RH, Meldrum BS, Penry JK (eds): *Antiepileptic Drugs,* ed 3. Raven Press, New York, 1989.
4. Kutt H: Phenobarbital: interactions with other drugs. In Levy RH, Dreifuss FE, Mattson RH, Meldrum BS, Penry JK (eds): *Antiepileptic Drugs,* ed 3. Raven Press, New York, 1989.
5. Levy RH, Dreifuss FE, Mattson RH, Meldrum BS, Penry JK (eds): *Antiepileptic Drugs,* ed 3. Raven Press, New York, 1989.
6. Gillman AG, Goodman LS, Gilman A: *The Pharmacologic Basis of Therapeutics.* Macmillan, New York, 1990.
7. McEvoy GK (ed): *American Hospital Formulary Service (AHFS) Drug Information 1990:* American Society of Hospital Pharmacists, Bethesda, MD, 1990.
8. Treiman DM: Pharmacokinetics and clinical use of benzodiazepines in the management of status epilepticus. *Epilepsia* 30(suppl 2):S4-S10, 1989.
9. Kuman A, Bleck TP: Intravenous midazolam for the treatment of refractory status epilepticus. *Crit Care Med* 20(4):483–488, 1992.
10. Leppik IE: Status epilepticus: the next decade. *Neurology* 40(suppl 2):4–9, 1990.
11. Greenblatt DJ, Ehrenberg BL, Gunderman J, Scavone JM, Tai NT, Harmatz JS, Shader RI: Kinetic and dynamic study of intravenous lorazepam: comparison with intravenous diazepam. *J Pharm Exp Ther* 250(1):134–139, 1989.
12. Greenblatt DJ, Ehrenberg BL, Gunderman J, Locniskar A, Scavone JM, Harmatz JS, Shader RI: Pharmacokinetic and electroencephalographic study of intravenous diazepam, midazolam and placebo. *Clin Pharmacol Ther* 45:356–365, 1989.
13. DeLorenzo RJ: Status epilepticus: concepts in diagnosis and treatment. *Semin Neurol* 10(4):396–405, 1990.
14. King J: *King's Guide to Parenteral Admixtures.* Pacemarq, Inc., St. Louis, 1992.
15. Delgado-Escueta AV, Enrile-Bacsal F: Combination therapy for status epilepticus: intravenous diazepam and phenytoin. *Adv Neurol* 34:477–485, 1983.
16. Bell DS, Bertino Jr JS: Constant diazepam infusion in the treatment of continuous seizure activity. *Drug Intell Clin Pharmacol* 18:965–970, 1984.
17. Schmidt D: Benzodiazepines. In Levy RH, Dreifuss FE, Mattson RH, Meldrum BS, Penry JK (eds): *Antiepileptic Drugs,* ed 3. Raven Press, New York, 1989.
18. MacLeod SM, Giles HG, Patzalek G, Thiessen JJ, Sellers EM: Diazepam actions and plasma concentrations following ethanol ingestion. *Eur J Clin Pharmacol* 11:345–349, 1977.
19. Klotz U, Anttila VJ, Reimann I: Cimetidine/diazepam interaction. *Lancet* ii:699, 1979.
20. Kulkarni SK, Jog MV: Facilitation of diazepam action by anticonvulsant agents against picrotoxin induced convulsions. *Psychopharmacology* 81:332–334, 1983.
21. Czuczwar SJ, Turski WA, Ikonomidou C, Turski L: Aminophylline and CGS 8216 reverse the protective action of diazepam against electroconvulsions in mice. *Epilepsia* 26(6):693–696, 1985.
22. Dhillon S, Richens A: Valproic acid and diazepam interaction in vivo. *Br J Clin Pharmacol* 13:553–560, 1982.
23. Marrosu F, Marchi A, De Martino MR, Saba G, Gessa GL: Aminophylline antagonizes diazepam-induced anesthesia and EEG changes in humans. *Psychopharmacology* 85:69–70, 1985.

24. Pitlick WH, Levy RH: Carbamazepine: interactions with other drugs. In Levy RH, Dreifuss FE, Mattson RH, Meldrum BS, Penry JK (eds): *Antiepileptic Drugs*, ed 3. Raven Press, New York, 1989.
25. Riela AR, Sires BP, Penry JK: Transient magnetic resonance imaging abnormalities during partial status epilepticus. 6:143–145, 1991.
26. Fisher RS: Emergency treatment for status epilepticus. *J Crit Illness* 2(4):27–38, 1987.

CHAPTER 10

Gastrointestinal Medications[a]

In the critical care setting, a large number of drugs are used for the management of gastrointestinal (GI) disorders. An in-depth knowledge of clinical pharmacology of these drugs is crucial for the effective management of critically ill patients. A vast array of GI disorders is encountered in the acutely ill patient, ranging from stress gastritis and bleeding ulcers to impaired gastric emptying and copious diarrhea. Frequent development of multiorgan failure, sepsis, and cardiopulmonary complications make careful selection of appropriate drug, optimal dosing, and close monitoring of drug interactions an essential part of the management of critically ill patients.

The purpose of this chapter is to provide the intensive care physician with a concise, succinct description of drugs commonly used for GI disorders in critically ill patients with frequent concomitant multiorgan system problems.

DRUGS FOR STRESS ULCERS, ACID PEPTIC DISEASE, AND GASTROESOPHAGEAL REFLUX

Gastric mucosal erosions are commonly seen in intensive care unit (ICU) patients. Severe trauma, burn injury, major surgical procedures, sepsis, serious medical illnesses, CNS disease, and

[a]Sudhir K. Dutta, M.D., and Rajat Sood, M.D., contributed this chapter to *The Pharmacologic Approach to the Critically Ill Patient,* Third Edition. Table 10.3 was contributed by Gary P. Zaloga, M.D., F.A.C.P.

drug overdose frequently are associated with stress-induced gastritis (1, 2). Acute hemorrhagic gastritis generally is seen 3–7 days after the initial injury. Development of stress gastritis is associated with persistent low intraluminal gastric pH in the majority of critically ill patients (3). Correction of intraluminal acidic pH in the stomach has been recommended for prevention of hemorrhage from stress gastritis. A large number of pharmacologic compounds are used to keep gastric pH higher than 5.0 to protect gastric mucosa from acid-induced injury in the critically ill patient.

ANTACIDS

Mechanism of Action. Antacids are basic salts of aluminum, magnesium, or calcium that neutralize acid in the gastric lumen and help to maintain an intraluminal gastric pH of 5.0 or higher. Antacids at this pH are also known to inhibit the proteolytic activity of pepsin. In addition, they have a local astringent effect and can increase the lower esophageal sphincter pressure to some degree. Most commonly used antacids have few systemic effects and do not cause systemic alkalosis. The various antacid preparations are compared on the basis of their acid neutralizing capacity. Acid neutralizing capacity of an antacid is defined as the quantity of 1 N HCl in mEq that can be brought to pH 3.5 in 15 minutes.

Route of Administration, Frequency, and Dosage. Antacids generally are administered orally or through a gastrostomy tube. The usual doses of an antacid in stress gastritis in critically ill patients are as follows: children, 5–15 ml every 1–2 hours; adults, 30–60 ml every 3–6 hours. In general, the aim is to provide enough antacid to neutralize a total of 1000 mEq of gastric acid every day (4). When ingested in the fasting state, antacids reduce the acidity for about 30 minutes. However, when an antacid is administered about 1 hour following meal ingestion, its effect lasts for approximately 3 hours. Longer duration of action by the antacids during the postprandial period is related to slower gastric emptying as compared with the fasting state (5). Several studies with antacids indicate that total acid neutralization up to 180–400 mEq is effective in healing inflammation and ulceration of gastroduodenal mucosa in most clinical settings. In Zollinger-Ellison syndrome, a much higher dose of antacids is often needed in conjunction with H_2 antagonists or omeprazol (6).

Drug Interactions. (*a*) Antacids increase the intraluminal gastric pH and can alter the solubility, ionization, and gastric emptying of various drugs and their metabolites. As a result of antacid ingestion, absorption of acidic drugs (digitalis, phenytoin, chlorpromazine) may be reduced. (*b*) Adsorption or binding of drugs to the surface of antacids can result in decreased bioavailability of some drugs (i.e., tetracycline, ranitidine, isoniazid, ethambutol, etc.). (*c*) Antacids can affect the rate of elimination of many drugs by increasing urinary pH. Antacid ingestion potentially can increase the rate of urinary excretion of salicylates and phenobarbital and decrease the elimination of amphetamine, quinidine, and pseudoephedrine.

Most commercially available antacids contain sodium bicarbonate, aluminum hydroxide, magnesium hydroxide, or calcium carbonate. A comparison of contents and neutralizing capacity of the commercially available antacids is summarized in Table 10.1 (7).

Aluminum Compounds. Aluminum hydroxide gel is actually a mixture of aluminum hydroxide and other oxide hydrates. Aluminum hydroxide usually is marketed in combination with magnesium hydroxide to offset its constipating effect. Aluminum compounds are used alone or in combination with H_2 blockers for prevention of bleeding from stress gastritis.

Adverse Effects. (*a*) Administration of aluminum-containing antacids except aluminum phosphate over a period of time can cause clinically significant hypophosphatemia resulting from acid binding of aluminum to indigenous phosphates (8, 9). This binding property of aluminum hydroxide frequently is used in patients with renal failure to lower plasma phosphate levels. (*b*) Aluminum antacids can also cause an increase in calcium absorption, with resultant hypercalcemia and bone resorption. (*c*) In addition, administration of aluminum-containing antacids

TABLE 10.1. Composition and Neutralizing Capacity of Commercially Available Antacids[a]

Antacids	*Composition (mg/5 ml)*				*Acid Neutralizing Capacity (per 5 ml)*
	$Al(OH)_3$	*$Mg(OH)_2$*	*$CaCO_3$*	*Other*	
Maalox	225	200	0	Na (1.4)	13
Mylanta	200	200	0	Simeth[b] (20) Na (0.7)	13
Gelusil	200	200	0	Simeth[b] (25) Na (0.7)	12
Amphojel	320	0	0	Na (2.0)	10
Milk of Magnesia	0	390	0	Na (0.1)	14
Gaviscon	32	0	0	$MgCO_3$ (137) Na alginate	4
Riopan	0	0	0	Magaldrate (540) Simeth[b] (40)	15

[a] Adapted from Brunton LL: Agents for control of gastric acidity and peptic ulcer. In Gilman AG, Rall TW, Nies AS, Taylor P (eds): *The Pharmacological Basis of Therapeutics*, ed 8. McGraw-Hill, New York, 1990, pp 897–913.
[b] Simeth, simethicone.

can result in an increase of aluminum levels in renal failure patients (10).

Special Considerations. Aluminum-containing antacids can be used to reduce hyperphosphatemia in patients with chronic renal failure. However, this approach should be done with caution, as aluminum-containing antacids can induce disequilibrium syndrome.

Magnesium Compounds. Magnesium-containing antacids generally include magnesium hydroxides and magnesium oxide. Magnesium salts are also used for treatment of hypomagnesemia resulting from starvation, alcoholism, and malnutrition. About 5% of orally administered magnesium-containing antacids is absorbed systemically (11). Cathartic action of magnesium salts results from an increase in the osmotic load and stimulation of intestinal secretions and motility.

Adverse Effects. In renal failure, administration of magnesium-containing antacids can result in fatal hypermagnesemia. All magnesium compounds have also been implicated in causing the milk alkali syndrome. This is an acute illness characterized by headaches, nausea, irritability, weakness, and azotemia with hypercalcemia.

Calcium Compounds. Calcium carbonate was the first antacid used and still remains popular. Calcium-containing antacids are highly soluble and interact avidly with gastric acid, resulting in production of calcium chloride. In the small intestine, 90% of calcium chloride is converted by pancreatic bicarbonate to insoluble calcium salts. Approximately 9–16% of calcium is absorbed from normal human intestines, and up to 34% in patients with peptic ulcer disease (12). The main route of absorbed calcium excretion is through the kidney, the amount of which varies with creatinine clearance. It has been estimated that the amount of calcium absorbed from the intestine increases with a higher dose. Transient hypercalcemia has been observed with a single 4-g dose of calcium carbonate. Furthermore, of all the antacids, calcium carbonate has been shown to produce acid rebound, which is defined as sustained hypersecretion of gastric acid after calcium-containing antacid has been emptied from the stomach (13).

Adverse Effects. Long-term use of calcium-containing antacids is associated with a positive phosphate balance, decreased magnesium absorption, and development of milk alkali syndrome (14–17).

SUCRALFATE

Sucralfate is a complex compound of aluminum hydroxide and sucrose sulfate. It is approved for treatment of acute duodenal ulcers and prevention of their recurrence (18–21). Several studies have examined the healing rates of duodenal ulcers in patients treated with sucralfate and cimetidine, an H_2 blocker antagonist. These healing rates have been reported to be 57, 88, and 96% at weeks 4, 8, and 12, respectively, and compare favorably with those rates of cimetidine (22–24). Sucralfate is not approved for either acute or maintenance therapy of gastric ulcers.

Similar to antacids and H_2 blockers, the benefit of sucralfate therapy in patients with bleeding ulcers lies in healing the ulcers and not in stopping the bleeding (25, 26). There is no significant difference in the mortality rates of patients treated with sucralfate or H_2 antagonists or antacid-treated patients with stress-induced erosive gastritis and bleeding. However, sucralfate has been demonstrated to be just as effective in preventing stress gastritis-related bleeding in critically ill patients receiving mechanical ventilation. In treatment of patients with nonsteroidal antiinflammatory drug (NSAID)-induced duodenal ulcers, sucralfate is just as efficacious as ranitidine (27–29). Sucralfate, however, does not prevent NSAID associated gastric or duodenal ulcers. Furthermore, in patients with gastroesophageal reflux, sucralfate seems to be only modestly effective in nonerosive esophageal disease (30, 31). Controlled trials of its efficacy in healing esophageal ulcers after sclerotherapy as well as other esophageal ulcers have not shown clinically important benefit (32, 33).

Mechanism of Action. Sucralfate forms a viscous suspension that binds with high affinity to both injured and normal mucosa.

At a pH less than 4.0 there is extensive polymerization and cross-linking of sucralfate. The condensed polymer is a very sticky, viscid, yellowish white gel. Even though the pH in the duodenum is well above 4.0, the gel retains its viscid demulcent properties in the duodenal bulb. Endoscopic studies have demonstrated that the gel remains adherent to the ulcerated epithelium for more than 6 hours. The binding of sucralfate to the ulcer crater probably represents its main therapeutic action. In addition, sucralfate releases the aluminum moiety in the presence of gastric acid and binds positively charged molecules, such as peptides, proteins, glycoproteins, drugs, and metals. It seems that various physical, mechanical, absorbent, ion exchange, and buffering properties of sucralfate may all contribute to its actions to protect gastric mucosa. It has also been suggested that sucralfate stimulates formation of prostaglandins by the gastric mucosa, thus exerting a cytoprotective effect by a mechanism similar to that of misoprostol (34). This effect is particularly relevant because sucralfate has only minimal acid neutralizing capability. It is noteworthy that in vitro studies indicate that sucralfate absorbs bile acids (35).

Pharmacokinetics. Sucralfate is poorly soluble in water, and little is absorbed from the GI tract. It is a very safe medication, and studies in animals using oral doses up to 1 g/kg have failed to establish a lethal dose (36). Aluminum absorption during sucralfate therapy is comparable to antacid therapy with aluminum hydroxide (37). Most of the aluminum (98%) is excreted in feces, and some in the urine. Sucralfate lowers the plasma phosphate level in uremic patients. However, sucralfate also results in increased plasma concentration of aluminum in these patients. Like aluminum-containing antacids, sucralfate can cause severe hypophosphatemia (38). Aluminum retention associated with sucralfate may be a problem in patients with renal insufficiency.

Drug Interactions. Sucralfate reduces the bioavailability and absorption of certain drugs when given simultaneously with them. Important drugs involved in this interaction include ciprofloxacin (39), norfloxacin (40, 41), theophylline (42), tetracycline (43), phenytoin (44), digoxin (45), and amitriptyline (46). The effect of combined therapy of sucralfate with antacids or H_2 blockers has not been evaluated in humans. However, since sucralfate is activated by acids, antacids should not be administered 30 minutes before or after sucralfate in the treatment of duodenal ulcer. Sucralfate does not seem to affect the bioavailability of acetaminophen, aspirin, diazepam, erythromycin, ethinyl estradiol, ibuprofen, imipramine, indomethacin, naprosyn, prednisone, propranolol, quinidine, and warfarin.

Dosage and Route of Administration. In the treatment of duodenal ulcer the recommended adult dosage of sucralfate is 1 g four times a day, administered orally. Interestingly, a dose of 2 g of sucralfate twice a day also appears to be equally effective in short-term treatments of duodenal ulcer (47). Sucralfate tablets can be dissolved in 15–30 ml of water and administered orally to patients with esophageal stricture or mucosal inflammation.

Side Effects. Because of minimal systemic absorption, side effects of sucralfate are rare (48, 49). In placebo-controlled clinical studies designed to evaluate the efficacy of sucralfate in duodenal ulcer healing, the most common side effect was constipation, which occurred in 0–15% of patients. Other side effects included dry mouth (0.7%), dizziness (0.4%), nausea, vomiting, headache, urticaria, and rashes. Rare side effects of sucralfate include gastric bezoar formation (50), aluminum intoxication (51), and hypophosphatemia (38). There have been no prospective safety studies of sucralfate in pregnant women, lactating women, children, and the elderly.

Special Considerations. Although sucralfate has no effect on gastric acid secretion, it is as effective as antacids or H_2 receptor antagonists in prevention of acute stress gastritis and bleeding in critically ill patients. It is interesting to note that, contrary to earlier claims, the frequency of nosocomial pneumonia is not significantly lower with sucralfate therapy than with antacid therapy in critically ill patients (52, 53).

OMEPRAZOLE

Chemically, omeprazole is a substituted benzimidazole (5-methoxy-2-(4-methoxy)-3-5-dimethyl-2-pyridinyl-sulfinyl-14-benzimidazole). It is a prototype of H^+K^+ ATPase (proton pump) inhibitor, which is being used pharmacologically as a potent inhibitor of gastric acid secretion. At present, omeprazole is the treatment of choice for patients with Zollinger-Ellison syndrome and severe gastroesophageal (GE) reflux disease.

The secretion of HCl by gastric parietal cells ultimately depends on the function of the hydrogen ion pump, which transports H^+ ions across the cell membrane in exchange for K^+ ions (54, 55). On activation of parietal cells by appropriate hormonal stimuli (i.e., histamine, gastrin, or acetylcholine), the proton pump, located in the apical portion of the parietal cell, is translocated to the plasma membrane of the acid-secreting canaliculi of the cell (56, 57). Within the acidic milieu of the parietal cells ($pH \leq 3$) it is converted to its active form, sulfenic acid and sulfonamide (58, 59). The end products react with the sulfhydryl group in the enzyme H^+K^+ ATPase, forming an irreversible enzyme-inhibitor complex. Omeprazole is a weak base and is absorbed at an alkaline pH in the small intestine. After intestinal absorption, it is carried to the parietal cells in the stomach through the bloodstream. Thus, the resumption of acid secretion after the administration of omeprazole requires synthesis of new H^+K^+ ATPase protein (60), which takes about 72 hours. Since omeprazole is a weak base, its exposure to acid in the stomach decreases its bioavailability (61). Consequently, it is administered in a pH-sensitive enteric coated form that releases omeprazole in the small intestine. Peak plasma concentration of omeprazole occurs within 2–3 hours, and its duration of action exceeds 24 hours. Plasma levels tend to increase during the first few days of treatment as increasing inhibition of gastric acid results in less degradation of omeprazole and more absorption from the small intestine (62). No significant correlation is seen between the absolute plasma level of the drug and decreased acid secretion, but it correlates well with the area under the curve (63).

Dosage and Route of Administration. Omeprazole inhibits acid secretion in a dose range of 5–30 mg/day by the oral route. Although omeprazole may have only little effect on acid secretion on the first day of oral ingestion, it significantly inhibits gastric HCl secretion by day 5. In human studies, oral administration after 7 days of 10, 20, or 30 mg of omeprazole caused reduction in acid secretion by 27, 90, and 97%, respectively (64). Inhibition of gastric acid secretion with 10 mg of omeprazole ranges between 10 and 90% (64, 65). A standard 20-mg dose of omeprazole given orally causes steady-state inhibition of acid secretion between 35 and 65% within 24 hours after drug administration. Larger doses of omeprazole reduce variations in acid inhibition among patients and inhibit acid secretion more profoundly (63, 64, 66). It takes at least 3 days for acid secretion to return to pretreatment levels on cessation of omeprazole therapy. Omeprazole is metabolized extensively by the hepatic cytochrome P-450 system and is secreted in bile. About 20% of an orally administered dose of omeprazole is excreted in the feces, and 80% in urine.

Adverse Effects. The main side effect of omeprazole is related to development of hypergastrinemia and carcinoid tumors in rats. Several studies have shown that plasma gastrin levels do not increase in humans as much as in rats (67). Additional clinical trials must be performed to examine more carefully the long-term side effects of omeprazole. Oral administration of omeprazole reversibly increases the bacterial cell counts and nitrosamine levels in the stomach (68), which potentially can lead to GI infections (69) and cancers (70).

Drug Interactions. As a result of its interaction with cytochrome P-450, competitive inhibition of hepatic metabolism of certain drugs by omeprazole has been reported. Hepatic clearance of diazepam is reduced by about 50%, necessitating administration of smaller doses of the drug. Similarly, omeprazole also reduces elimination of phenytoin and Coumadin.

H_2 BLOCKERS (HISTAMINE$_2$ RECEPTOR ANTAGONISTS)

The H_2 blockers act by competitively and selectively blocking the histamine receptors on the basolateral membrane of the acid-secreting parietal cells in the stomach. These histamine receptors are called H_2 type because they are not blocked by conventional H_1-type antihistamines such as diphenhydramine (71). The blockade of H_2 receptors, in turn, inhibits a cascade of reactions involving activation of adenyl cyclase, which decreases cyclic adenosine monophosphate (cAMP) concentration. In the parietal cell, cAMP is essential for optimal functioning of the hydrogen potassium ATPase pump and acid secretion. H_2 receptors are found at many other sites, including the atrium, ilium, uterus, adipocytes, T-suppressor cells, and mesenteric and percutaneous vascular beds. Structurally, all clinically approved H_2 blockers (i.e., cimetidine, ranitidine, nizatidine, and famotidine) are analogues of histamine with a bulky side chain in place of the ethylamine moiety. The relative potency of H_2 blockers varies 20- to 50-fold, with cimetidine being the least potent and famotidine the most. A comparison of the potency of various H_2 blockers is shown in Table 10.2 (182). It is noteworthy that magnesium- and aluminum-containing antacids reduce the bioavailability of all H_2 blockers (cimetidine, ranitidine, and famotidine) by 30–50% and should be administered about 2 hours after the dose of the H_2 blocker (72, 73).

Cimetidine. Cimetidine shares the imidazole ring structure of histamine and inhibits all phases of gastric acid secretion. Both basal and nocturnal acid secretions are reduced by 60–70% with a 300-mg dose of cimetidine (74). Fasting serum gastrin levels are unaffected by cimetidine, but postprandial levels are raised because of the reduction in acid feedback and inhibition of gastrin release (75). Pepsin secretion by chief cells of gastric glands also decreases in parallel with the reduction in volume of gastric juice.

Pharmacokinetics. The bioavailability of an orally ingested cimetidine dose ranges between 30 and 80% and has a plasma half-life of 2 hours. About 50% of the ingested dose is excreted unchanged by the kidneys, and the remainder is metabolized to sulfoxide prior to renal excretion. Only a very small amount of the ingested dose of cimetidine is excreted in the bile. Cimetidine easily crosses the placental barrier and blood-brain barrier and is excreted in breast milk. It is widely distributed in all organs

TABLE 10.2. Comparison of H_2 Receptor Antagonists[a]

Variable	Cimetidine	Ranitidine	Nizatidine	Famotidine
1. Absorption				
Bioavailability (%)	30–80 (60)	30–88 (50)	75–100 (98)	37–45 (43)
Time to peak plasma concentration (h)	1–2	1–3	1–3	1–3.5
2. Distribution				
Volume (liters/kg of body weight)	0.8–1.2	1.2–1.9	1.2–1.6	1.1–1.4
Protein binding in plasma (%)	13–26	15	25–35	16
3. Elimination				
Total systemic clearance (ml/min)	450–650	568–709	667–850	417–483
Half-life in plasma (h)	1.5–2.3	1.6–2.4	1.1–1.6	2.5–4
Hepatic clearance (%)				
Oral	60	73	22	50–80
Intravenous	25–40	30	25	25–30
Renal clearance (%)				
Oral	40	27	57–65	25–30
Intravenous	50–80	50	75	65–80
4. Relative potency	1	4–10	4–10	20–50
Dose to heal duodenal ulcer (mg)	300 qid 400 bid 800 hs	150 bid 300 hs	150 bid 300 hs	40 hs
Dose to prevent recurrence (mg)	400 hs	150 hs	150 hs	20 hs

[a] Adapted from information appearing in *The New England Journal of Medicine*, in Feldman M, Burton ME: Comparison of H_2-receptor antagonists. *N Engl J Med* 323:1672–1680, 1990.

of the body, and 70% of the total body content of cimetidine is found in the skeletal muscles. In the presence of renal failure, the dose of cimetidine is calculated by using the creatinine clearance formula. Hemodialysis decreases the level of circulating drug by at least 50%, and the dosage schedule should be adjusted to coincide with the hemodialysis (76, 77). With increasing age, a decline in volume of distribution resulting from a decrease in body mass has also been observed (78). Consequently, a one-third reduction of the cimetidine dose is justified in patients older than 65 years of age. Cimetidine can be given parenterally, and parenteral administration achieves higher peak levels than does an oral dose. After administration of a high dose of cimetidine parenterally, a clinically effective drug level is observed for approximately 4 hours (79).

Adverse Effects and Contraindications. The reported incidence of adverse effects of cimetidine is approximately 5%. Most commonly, headaches, dizziness, skin rash, and myalgia are observed. Cimetidine crosses the blood-brain barrier and can cause mental confusion. This effect may result from blockage of the H_2 receptors in the brain tissue and consequent partial inhibition of the neurotransmitters. Blockage of histamine receptors in the brain has been shown to interfere with endogenous enkephalins (80). Symptomatic adverse effects of cimetidine tend to be more frequent in the elderly and in those patients with hepatic and renal failure.

Cimetidine increases the serum concentration of prolactin and causes galactorrhea in women and gynecomastia in men. In addition, cimetidine binds to androgen receptors and reduces sperm counts in young males. Cimetidine also inhibits cytochrome P-450 and catalyzes hydroxylation of estradiol. It is also shown to inhibit release of aldosterone in vivo (81, 82).

Adverse hematologic reactions of cimetidine are uncommon (0.01–0.07%) and include leukopenia, thrombocytopenia, anemia, and pancytopenia (83). Reversible increases of serum aminotransferase are also seen in patients taking i.v. cimetidine (84, 85). Rarely, bradycardia has been reported with cimetidine as a result of the effect on cardiac H_2 receptors (86, 87).

Drug Interactions. Impairment of the hepatic metabolism of several drugs by cimetidine is caused by its inhibition of the P-450 enzyme system. Most importantly, hepatic metabolism of warfarin, theophylline, phenytoin, phenobarbital, and the benzodiazepines is prolonged. Consequently, smaller doses of these drugs may be required when they are administered with an oral dose of cimetidine. Other drugs such as digoxin, mexiletine, nifedipine, propranolol, and tricyclic antidepressants also are shown to have prolonged actions as a result of cimetidine.

Dosage. For oral use, cimetidine is available in tablet form in 200-, 300-, 400-, or 800-mg doses. Cimetidine is also available in liquid form as 60 mg/ml. For duodenal ulcers or benign gastric ulcers, the usual dose of cimetidine is 800 mg qhs or 300 mg qid to 400 mg bid to be administered for 4–8 weeks. A much higher dose of cimetidine is required in patients with Zollinger-Ellison syndrome. For parenteral administration, the drug is given as 300 mg i.v. every 6 hours or as a continuous i.v. infusion of 40–50 mg every hour.

Special Considerations. Cimetidine is shown to augment cell-mediated immunity in vitro because of H_2 receptor blockade of T-lymphocytes (88). In uncontrolled studies, cimetidine has been reported to accelerate healing of herpetic skin lesions in immunocompromised patients (89). The dose of cimetidine may need to be reduced in patients with renal function impairment. Furthermore, very small amounts of cimetidine are removed from plasma by peritoneal dialysis as a result of tight binding to plasma proteins (90).

Overdosage. Physostigmine has been reported to arouse obtunded patients, with evidence of cimetidine-induced central nervous system toxicity. Assisted renal excretion over a period of time reduces cimetidine toxicity.

Ranitidine. Structurally, ranitidine contains a furan ring instead of the imidazole ring of histamine. Ranitidine is considered effective in the treatment of both duodenal and gastric ulcers. Ranitidine is preferred over cimetidine because it binds minimally to other sites such as androgen receptors, the hepatic P-450 system, and peripheral lymphocytes (91). Furthermore, ranitidine is five to 12 times more potent than cimetidine on a molar basis in inhibiting stimulated gastric acid secretion in humans (92).

Pharmacokinetics. Ranitidine is absorbed rapidly from the small intestine and its absorption is not influenced by food ingestion. A single oral dose (150 mg) achieves a peak plasma concentration within 1–3 hours. In most cases, 50% inhibition of gastric acid output can be achieved with a plasma ranitidine concentration of 100–200 ng/ml (93). Bioavailability is influenced by hepatic function, since the drug is taken up and metabolized by the liver by first-pass kinetics. Up to 30% of ranitidine is metabolized by the liver to sulfuric oxide, nitrogen oxide, and desmethyl derivatives (94). About 50% or more of absorbed ranitidine is excreted unchanged by the kidney. In patients with liver disease, bioavailability of ranitidine is increased and serum half-life prolonged as a result of reduced hepatic metabolism. Ranitidine, however, is essentially free of dose-related adverse effects (95).

Dosage and Route of Administration. Ranitidine is available in tablet form (150 or 300 mg) and in liquid form (15 mg/ml). The usual dose for treatment of active duodenal ulcer is 150 mg bid or 300 mg qhs. Ranitidine can be given intravenously at a dose of 50 mg q8h or as a continuous infusion (6 mg/h). The dose of i.v. ranitidine should be adjusted to intragastric pH, which should be maintained at 5.0 or higher. With ranitidine, ulcer healing has been documented endoscopically in 70% of patients by the end of 4 weeks and in 85–90% by the end of 8 weeks (96, 97). In patients with Zollinger-Ellison syndrome in whom cimetidine produced ineffective control of symptoms, suppression of gastric acid secretion was achieved with high doses (600–1200 mg) of ranitidine daily (98).

Side Effects. Side effects of ranitidine are quite infrequent and include minor events such as rash, malaise, or constipation. Sinus bradycardia has been reported with rapid i.v. infusion of ranitidine (99–101). Ranitidine does not increase basal levels of testosterone and is devoid of antiandrogenic activity, as it does not bind to androgen receptors (102). In patients with cimetidine-induced impotence, complete remission of impotence was observed with ranitidine after discontinuation of cimetidine

(103). Furthermore, unlike cimetidine, ranitidine does not inhibit metabolism of estradiol (104). Anicteric hepatitis and mild increase of transaminase have been observed rarely with ranitidine administration. Mental confusion and other CNS symptoms have also been reported rarely with ranitidine, as it minimally crosses the blood-brain barrier and binds minimally to brain receptors. Ranitidine does not bind to the cells of the hemopoietic system, and thus anemia, thrombocytopenia, and other hematologic abnormalities are not observed with ranitidine, which is another advantage over cimetidine (105). It minimally alters hepatic metabolism of diazepam, warfarin, and propranolol. It predisposes to bezoar formation (106) and achlorhydria, which can lead to breakdown of the gastric barrier with proliferation of enteric and nitrate-producing bacteria. The proliferation of enteric bacteria is a common side effect of all H_2 blockers and is a matter of concern on a long-term basis (107–109).

Famotidine. Famotidine is a chemically distinct H_2 blocker with a thiazole ring structure. It is 50–80 times more potent than cimetidine and 5–8 times more potent than ranitidine. It is indicated for short-term treatment (4–8 weeks) of acute duodenal ulcer and maintenance of healed duodenal ulcer. It has also been used for hypersecretory states such as Zollinger-Ellison syndrome.

Pharmacokinetics. Famotidine is rapidly but incompletely absorbed on oral administration, with bioavailability of 35–45%. Seventy percent of the drug is eliminated intact in the urine (110). With renal failure (CrCl <10 ml/min), the daily dose of famotidine should be reduced from 40 to 20 mg. Famotidine dosage adjustment is not required with hepatic failure. Peak antisecretory activity is reached within 1–3 hours after oral administration and persists for 10–12 hours.

Dosage and Route of Administration. Famotidine can be given intravenously, with a similar time for onset of antisecretory effects but twice the potency of the oral dose. Famotidine is available in tablet (20 or 40 mg) or liquid (40 mg/5 ml) form.

Drug Interactions and Side Effects. No drug interaction has been reported so far, but experience with this medication is limited at the present time. Famotidine does not interfere with compounds that are metabolized by hepatic microsomal enzyme processes, including diazepam, phenytoin, theophylline, and warfarin. Furthermore, no adverse effects on the central nervous, endocrine, or renal systems have been reported (111). Several minor side effects have been documented with famotidine and include headaches, dizziness, constipation, and diarrhea (112, 113). However, the frequency of these side effects is exceedingly low (1–4%) and the drug is very well-tolerated.

Overdosage. Doses up to 640 mg/day have been given with no reported untoward effects. Symptomatic treatment and gastric lavage within the first few hours are warranted.

Nizatidine. Nizatidine has a substituted imidazole ring compared with the other H_2 blockers. It is available in 150- and 300-mg capsules for oral use. Because it has little first-pass hepatic metabolism, the bioavailability of the oral dose is close to 100% (114, 115). In patients with renal failure its effect is prolonged, as renal excretion is the principal pathway for its elimination. It is the only H_2 blocker whose active metabolite (N_2-monodesmethyl nizatidine) has about 60% of the activity of the parent drug. Nizatidine does not bind notably to the cytochrome P-450 enzyme system and thus has no drug interactions with drugs that are metabolized by the hepatic route.

Adverse Reactions. Sweating (1%), hyperuricemia unassociated with gout or nephrolithiasis, and asymptomatic ventricular tachycardia can be seen.

Overdosage. If overdosage of nizatidine is encountered, renal dialysis should be initiated within the first 4–6 hours. This increases plasma clearance of the drug by 84%.

Misoprostol. Misoprostol is a synthetic prostaglandin E_1 analogue that has antisecretory (gastric acid inhibition) and mucosal protection properties (116, 117).

Mechanisms of Action. Misoprostol produces a definite decrease in gastric acid secretion and a moderate decrease in pepsin secretion. It does not seem to affect fasting or postprandial gastrin levels. Furthermore, misoprostol does not interfere with the antiinflammatory and analgesic actions of the NSAIDs.

NSAIDs act by inhibiting prostaglandin synthesis, and a deficiency of prostaglandins in the gastric mucosa leads to diminished mucus and bicarbonate secretion. These diminished defense barriers are presumed to be responsible for NSAID-induced peptic ulcerations.

Indications for Use. Prevention of NSAID- and aspirin-induced gastric ulcerations is an indication for use of misoprostol. People on high doses of NSAID have a high risk of GI bleeding (118).

Pharmacokinetics. Misoprostol is absorbed extensively and undergoes rapid change to its free acid, misoprostic acid. Misoprostic acid is responsible for the clinical activity of misoprostol and can be measured in the plasma. Peak concentration of the drug on oral administration is achieved in 12 minutes, and it has a plasma half-life of 20–35 minutes. Mean plasma levels of misoprostol are linearly correlated in the dose range of 200–400 μg. Eighty percent of the drug is excreted in the urine. The serum protein binding of misoprostol is about 80–90%, and the binding is concentration independent in the therapeutic range. It is noteworthy that misoprostol and its active metabolite have no effect on the cytochrome P-450 system.

Dosage and Route of Administration. Misoprostol is generally recommended for the full duration of the NSAID intake. The usual dose is 200 μg four times a day with food (119). It is advisable to start with a much smaller dose and increase it gradually over a period of time.

Contraindications. (*a*) The most important and definite contraindication is pregnancy. Misoprostol has abortifacient properties. Misoprostol is relatively contraindicated in all women of child-bearing age unless the risk:benefit ratio truly warrants its use. All patients who are sexually active should be warned of this risk and be advised to use adequate contraception. (*b*) A history of severe allergic reaction to misoprostol and other synthetic prostaglandins is a contraindication.

Adverse Reactions. (*a*) Development of diarrhea is seen in 13–40% of all patients who are started on misoprostol therapy. Diarrhea is dose-related and usually appears within the first 6 weeks after initiation of misoprostol therapy. Diarrhea usually is self-limiting and resolves in 1–2 weeks. Because of abdominal cramps and diarrhea, misoprostol therapy is discontinued in a small percentage of patients. Development of diarrhea can be minimized by administration of the drug after meals and at bedtime, and by starting with a small dosage of the medication. Concomitant use of magnesium-containing antacids should be avoided to minimize the problem of diarrhea (120). (*b*) Other adverse effects include headaches (2–3%), vaginal spotting (1%), abdominal cramps, and dysmenorrhea. Postmenopausal vaginal bleeding has also been reported in about 5.5% of female patients.

Overdosage. The toxic dose of misoprostol has yet to be determined. A cumulative total oral dose of 1600 μg has been tolerated, with some GI symptoms. Higher doses may cause cardiac arrhythmias, hepatic and renal tubular necrosis, and testicular atrophy. Treatment of misoprostol overdose is mainly supportive.

ANTIDIARRHEAL AGENTS

Management of diarrhea should be directed mainly at treating the underlying cause. Most commonly, the underlying causes of diarrhea in the ICU setting include infection, malabsorption, drugs, endocrine disorders, or enterocolitis. In the critical care setting, symptomatic relief of diarrhea with prevention of fluid losses and electrolyte imbalance assumes prime importance. Apart from the nonspecific antidiarrheal drugs, oral or parenteral replacement of fluid and electrolytes is essential and life-saving. Salient pharmacologic compounds that reduce diarrhea promptly include the drugs discussed below.

OPIATES

Hydroalcoholic solutions of opium (opium tincture and paregoric) and synthetic opiates (diphenoxylates and loperamide) are the principal drugs in this class. Opioid agonists act at the μ- and possibly δ-receptors on enteric neurons and disrupt aboral peristaltic movements, which results in prolonged transit time of intestinal contents. These agents also reduce interstitial fluid secretion and enhance mucosal absorption, ameliorating abdominal cramps and diarrhea.

Loperamide. Loperamide is a piperidine opioid that is slowly and partially absorbed from the gastrointestinal tract after oral ingestion.

Mechanism of Action. Loperamide slows intestinal motility via its direct effects on the circular and longitudinal muscles of the intestinal wall. It also slows the intestinal transit of water and electrolytes (121).

Pharmacokinetics. After oral administration, 40% of loperamide is absorbed from the GI tract. Peak plasma levels occur 5 hours after oral administration of the capsular form and 2.5 hours after intake of the liquid form. Elimination half-life of loperamide is 9–12 hours.

Dosage and Route of Administration. Loperamide is administered orally and is available as a 2-mg capsule or a liquid preparation (1 mg/ml). Because the drug is long-acting, it is given initially as a 4-mg dose followed by a 2-mg dose after each unformed stool, up to a maximum of 16 mg/day.

Contraindications. (*a*) Loperamide should not be used if infectious (i.e., *Salmonella, Campylobacter, Shigella,* etc.) enterocolitis is suspected (122). (*b*) Pseudomembranous colitis contraindicates its use. (*c*) Hypersensitivity to opioids is a third contraindication.

Adverse Reactions. Reactions include dry mouth, nausea, vomiting, abdominal pain, and distension. All adverse reactions are self-limiting and are seen only after months of chronic use.

Special Considerations. Loperamide is relatively devoid of central nervous system effects, as it does not cross the blood-brain barrier. It can be given to the elderly with negligible neurologic effects. Safety and efficacy of opioid analogues has not been established clearly for pregnant patients and lactating mothers.

Overdosage. Up to 60 mg of the drug has been tolerated, with minimal side effects such as constipation and CNS depression. These side effects can be reversed by naloxone. In addition, activated charcoal and gastric lavage are recommended to reduce intestinal absorption of loperamide.

Diphenoxylate HCl with Atropine Sulfate. Diphenoxylate is a piperidine opioid related to meperidine but lacking analgesic activity. To discourage abuse of this preparation, atropine is added.

Mechanism of Action and Pharmacokinetics. Diphenoxylate is metabolized rapidly and extensively to diphenoxylic acid, which is the biologically active metabolite. Fifty percent of a single orally ingested dose is excreted in the feces and 14% in the urine over a 4-day period. Elimination half-life of diphenoxylate is 12–14 hours.

Dosage and Route of Administration. Orally, the dose is 2.5–5 mg every 3–4 hours. In combination with atropine, the drug is called lomotil, which has 25 μg of atropine for every 2.5 mg of diphenoxylate.

Adverse Reactions. Adverse reactions occur mainly because of the anticholinergic actions of atropine, which include dry skin, dry mouth, dry eyes, hyperesthesia, and urinary retention. Anorexia, nausea, vomiting, and paralytic ileus are the other common GI side effects. Allergic reactions ranging from mild pruritus to angioneurotic edema can also be seen. CNS side effects include dizziness, headaches, malaise, and lethargy (120).

Contraindications. (*a*) Pregnant and lactating mothers should not take the drug. (*b*) Neonates should not be given diphenoxylate, as it has been shown to cause cholestatic jaundice in them.

Drug Interactions. When administered with monoamine oxidase inhibitors, diphenoxylate may precipitate hypertensive crisis. Furthermore, diphenoxylate can potentiate the depressant actions of alcohol, barbiturates, and tranquilizers.

Overdosage. Anticholinergic overactivity and respiratory depression are the main toxic effects of diphenoxylate overdosage. GI lavage, naloxone, and physostigmine may be considered to reduce and reverse its toxic effect.

BISMUTH SALICYLATES

Bismuth salicylates are a mixture of trivalent bismuth and salicylates that frequently are used to treat mild to moderate diarrhea.

Mechanism of Action. Local antiinflammatory action of salicylates is thought to be the primary mode of action, as a result of inhibition of prostaglandins, which have been implicated as the cause of various forms of diarrhea (123). Bismuth has antimicrobial activity, which contributes to its antidiarrheal action in cases of infectious diarrhea.

Dosage and Route of Administration. Orally, 2 tablets (15 mg each) or 30 ml (1 mg/ml) generally are given every 30 minutes to 1 hour as needed, for a maximum of 8 doses in 24 hours.

Side Effects. Salicylism may be observed and is characterized by tinnitus. Caution should be exercised in administering this drug simultaneously with anticoagulants, oral hypoglycemic agents, and colchicine.

Drug Interactions. Bismuth salicylate may decrease GI absorption and bioavailability of tetracycline, thus reducing its antimicrobial activity. Concomitant use of aspirin can further increase the likelihood of developing salicylism.

Special Considerations. Along with ampicillin and metronidazole, bismuth subsalicylate is used as adjunctive treatment for *Helicobacter pylori*-associated gastritis and ulcer disease.

MISCELLANEOUS

In the past, a variety of starches, talcs, and chalks have been used to treat diarrhea. Kaolin or pectin, alone and in combination, have been used extensively for the treatment of diarrhea. Presumably, these compounds absorb water from the intestine and produce a more formed stool. There is little evidence that Kaopectate diminishes the number of evacuations or decreases intestinal fluid losses (124–126). In addition, α_2 central agonists such as clonidine have also been used to treat diarrhea in patients with diabetes mellitus (127). The dose of clonidine is 0.5 mg every 12 hours orally.

SOMATOSTATIN

Somatostatin is a neuropeptide that has a potent growth hormone inhibitory action. It has been demonstrated to have strong antisecretory and antimotility effects. The long-acting somatostatin analogue octreotide is considered to be the new drug of choice in the treatment of secretory diarrhea, carcinoid syndrome, and vasointestinal peptide-secreting tumors (128). The commercially used preparation octreotide is effective in the treatment of endocrine tumors of the gastroenteropancreatic axis. These tumors are well known to cause accumulation of fluid in the intestinal lumen and produce voluminous diarrhea by secreting vasoactive intestinal polypeptide, serotonin, and/or prostaglandins.

Mechanism of Action. Somatostatin exerts its effects by binding to specific receptors on the surface of target cells, which then mediate a number of intracellular events. The most important intracellular event is the inhibition of adenylate cyclase activity and accumulation of cyclic AMP. Another effect is enhanced potassium conduction, causing cell membrane hyperpolarization. Either of these events could lead to reduction in the intracellular concentration of calcium necessary for cell secretion.

Pharmacokinetics. Somatostatin has a short half-life of about 2 minutes. Octreotide, the specific analogue of somatostatin, has a longer half-life in plasma (90–115 minutes). Octreotide has a smaller ring and contains a *d*-amino acid side chain, which decreases the rate of degradation. Octreotide currently is available only for parenteral administration. Octreotide attains peak plasma concentration within 1 hour, and the height of plasma concentration is proportional to the dose administered. Injection of 50–100 μg results in a plasma concentration of 2 to 4 μg/liter. Clinical effects are seen within 2 hours of administering the dose (129, 130).

Dosage and Route of Administration. Octreotide is available in ampules containing 0.05, 0.10, or 0.5 mg/ml. It is administered subcutaneously two to four times a day for a total dose of 50–1500 μg/day. A starting dose is generally 50 μg twice a day and can be increased gradually to 600–1000 μg/day or as tolerated by the patient.

Side Effects. The major effect of somatostatin analogue is minor pain at the injection site and abdominal cramping on initiation of therapy. Glucose intolerance, diabetes, gallstone development as a result of decreased contraction of the gallbladder, and malabsorption resulting from decreased pancreatic secretions have all been shown to be clinically significant side effects in patients on long-term (>4–6 months) use of this medication. None of these side effects has resulted in cessation of Sandostatin when indicated.

Special Consideration. Somatostatin has been shown to decrease basal and stimulated gastric acid secretion. In addition, somatostatin decreases plasma gastrin levels and pepsin secretion. It also stimulates mucus production in the stomach and thus may act as a cytoprotective agent (131, 132). Somatostatin has been used in clinical trials for control of variceal hemorrhage because of its effect on decreasing splanchnic circulation. Somatostatin has also been advocated as a treatment for acromegaly, thyrotropinomas, carcinoid syndrome, VIPoma, and glucagonomas (133).

DRUGS FOR GASTROPARESIS AND COLONIC INERTIA

METOCLOPRAMIDE

Metoclopramide is a procainamide analogue (methoxy-2-chlor-5-procainamide) that was developed as an antiemetic agent for the treatment of nausea and vomiting during pregnancy (134). Although structurally related to procainamide, it has no local anesthetic or antiarrhythmic effects.

Mechanism of Action. Metoclopramide is a dopamine antagonist that causes dopamine receptor blockade. Its antiemetic effect against drugs such as apomorphine and ergotamine is achieved by this mechanism. In addition to being an antiemetic agent, metoclopramide is also a prokinetic agent that promotes motility of the GI tract by stimulating the smooth muscle. Dopaminergic blockade by metoclopramide improves gastric emptying by decreasing relaxation in the upper part of the stomach and increasing antral contractions. In addition, pylorus and duodenum are relaxed while the lower esophageal sphincter tone is enhanced. It also increases peristalsis of the jejunum and accelerates intestinal transit time from duodenum to ileocecal valve (135).

These pharmacologic actions of metoclopramide accelerate gastric emptying and reduce gastroesophageal reflux. Metoclopramide has minimal effect on gastric secretion or colonic motility. Apart from its antidopaminergic effect on gut smooth muscle, metoclopramide is also intrinsically cholinergic for the intramural neurons and augments acetylcholine release from postganglionic nerve terminals.

Dosage. The oral dosage is 10–15 mg 30 minutes before each meal and at bedtime for 2–8 weeks. The parenteral dose for antiemetic effect in cancer chemotherapy patients is 1 mg/kg diluted with normal saline or 5% dextrose solution administered intravenously over 15 minutes.

Pharmacokinetics. Onset of action is within 1–3 minutes following an i.v. dose, 10–15 minutes after an i.m. dose, and 30 to 60 minutes after an oral dose. The clinical effect of metoclopramide persists for 1–2 hours. It is well-absorbed from the GI tract but is subject to first-pass metabolism, with a total bioavailability of 50–70%. After oral ingestion on an empty stomach, intestinal absorption of metoclopramide is rapid. It is weakly protein bound (13–22%) and rapidly distributed in all tissues.

Adverse Reactions. Mild and transient side effects of the drug are observed in 20–30% of cases. Principal CNS effects include fatigue, restlessness, extrapyramidal reactions, and dystonia. Common GI side effects include nausea and diarrhea. Transient hypertension may also be seen at times. Metoclopramide is known to increase serum prolactin levels, causing gynecomastia in males and amenorrhea in females.

Special Considerations. Caution should be applied when metoclopramide is given to a patient with previously detected breast cancer. Chronic administration raises prolactin levels, and one-third of breast cancers are prolactin dependent in vitro. Metoclopramide readily enters breast milk and thus should be used cautiously in nursing mothers. In infants, methemoglobinemia has been reported with the use of metoclopramide.

BETHANECHOL

Bethanechol is a cholinomimetic drug that seems to augment the prokinetic effects of metoclopramide. This observation supports the idea that enhanced responsiveness to acetylcholine

(ACh) may also be a mechanism of action by which metoclopramide acts on target tissues. Bethanechol is not usually used as a single agent in the treatment of gastroparesis.

Pharmacokinetics. Bethanechol is rapidly and completely absorbed after oral administration. Sulfate conjugation during the first pass through the liver is the principal determinant of bioavailability of the oral form (136). Thirty percent of the drug is excreted unchanged in the urine, and the rest after conjugation with sulfate or glucuronic acid, also in the urine. Bethanechol is distributed rapidly into most tissues and readily crosses the blood-brain barrier. It also crosses the placental barrier and is secreted in breast milk in high concentrations.

Onset of action of bethanechol takes 1–15 minutes after i.v. administration, 10–30 minutes after i.m. injection, and 30–60 minutes after an oral dose. Plasma half-life of bethanechol is about 4–6 hours.

Dosage. Bethanechol is available in tablet (5 and 10 mg) and syrup (5 mg/ml) form and as an injectable solution (5–10 mg/ml). The usual dose of bethanechol is 10 mg qid orally, taken 15–30 minutes prior to meals and at bedtime. It has also been shown to be effective subcutaneously with sustained plasma levels.

Side Effects. The frequency of various side effects ranges between 15 and 20%. Most frequently, drowsiness, restlessness, and anxiety are observed with bethanechol therapy. Extrapyramidal reactions such as opisthotonus, torticollis, and oculogyric crisis are seen infrequently (1%). Extrapyramidal reactions secondary to bethanechol can be treated with diphenhydramine or benzotropine administration. Hyperprolactinemia with breast tenderness and menstrual irregularities has also been reported in patients treated with bethanechol.

Contraindications. Bethanechol is contraindicated in patients with suspected intestinal obstruction or perforation. In patients with pheochromocytoma, bethanechol can exacerbate a hypertensive crisis, necessitating reversal by phentolamine (137). Similarly, bethanechol should not be used in patients with Parkinson's disease. Simultaneous use of anticholinergic and dopamine agonist drugs must be monitored very closely for potentiation of action and side effects.

DOMPERIDONE

Domperidone is a benzimidazole derivative that possesses both prokinetic and antiemetic properties. It is a specific dopamine antagonist that stimulates the GI tract smooth muscle. It does not cross the blood-brain barrier and acts on the chemoreceptor trigger zone to provide antiemetic properties. Its mode of action on the chemoreceptor trigger zone may account for the absence of extrapyramidal and other CNS side effects. Domperidone's action is not blocked by atropine, suggesting that it may have no intrinsic cholinergic activity.

Pharmacokinetics. Domperidone is absorbed rapidly after oral intake, and its bioavailability is about 10–15% of a single oral dose. Bioavailability of domperidone increases to 90% on intravascular administration. About 70% of the drug and its metabolites are excreted in the feces, while the rest passes through the urine. Plasma half-life of domperidone is about 7–8 hours. This drug is shown to have a high affinity for the tissue in the GI tract, and high concentrations of the drug have been reported in the esophagus, stomach, and small intestine of humans and animals.

Dosage. The optimal dose of domperidone is 20–30 mg orally four times daily. This dose has been shown to improve gastric motility in patients with idiopathic gastric stasis (138).

Side Effects. Breast enlargement, nipple tenderness, galactorrhea, and amenorrhea secondary to hyperprolactinemia are observed more commonly with domperidone than with metoclopramide. Fatal cardiac arrhythmias have been reported from Japan after intravenous administration of domperidone. In the United States, domperidone has not been released for routine clinical use. Phase IV clinical trials are currently in progress to evaluate and establish clinical efficacy of the drug in the United States.

CISAPRIDE

Cisapride is a benzamide derivative that is currently undergoing clinical trials in the United States. Animal data suggest a prokinetic effect of cisapride on esophagus, stomach, and small bowel. In addition, unlike other prokinetic agents, cisapride has a stimulating effect on the colonic smooth muscle as well. It is devoid of any antidopaminergic actions but acts by facilitating acetylcholine release in the myenteric plexus. Cisapride is also demonstrated to be an effective serotonin antagonist in guinea pig intestinal mucosa (139). Because of its prokinetic action on the colon, cisapride promises to be an effective drug in patients with colonic inertia. Cisapride has also been used in patients with idiopathic gastric stasis, diabetic gastroparesis, and intestinal pseudoobstruction.

Pharmacokinetics. On oral administration, cisapride has a bioavailability of 30–40%. Peak plasma levels were observed after a standard oral dose at 1.5–2 hours. After intravenous administration, cisapride has been shown to disappear exponentially, with a half-life of approximately 19 hours.

Dosage. Clinical trials of cisapride are currently in progress. No consensus has been reached about its precise dose in various disorders. Cisapride is available in 4- and 16-mg tablets and in 2-, 4-, and 8-mg vials for intravenous administration. All of these doses have been shown to increase gastric emptying and intestinal peristalsis. The drug has no effect on plasma prolactin levels and is shown to have fewer side effects than domperidone.

ERYTHROMYCIN

Erythromycin is a macrolide antibiotic that can be both bacteriostatic or bactericidal, depending on the microorganism and the concentration of the drug. Erythromycin is most effective against Gram-positive cocci, and it is used frequently in patients who are allergic to penicillin. It is the drug of choice against *Legionella* and *Mycoplasma* infections. More recently, erythromycin in small doses has been shown to be an effective agent in promoting motility in patients with diabetic gastroparesis.

Mechanism of Action. (*a*) Erythromycin acts as an antibiotic by inhibiting protein synthesis. It does so by binding reversibly to the 50S ribosomal subunits of sensitive microorganisms (140).

(*b*) Erythromycin mimics the effect of the gastrointestinal polypeptide motilin by binding to motilin receptors and acts as an agonist to enhance gastrointestinal motility.

Dosage and Route of Administration. As an antibiotic, doses of erythromycin vary from 250–500 mg every 6 hours orally or intravenously. The dose of erythromycin for patients with gastroparesis has not been clearly established. In a study from Belgium that demonstrated the efficacy of erythromycin in the treatment of diabetic gastroparesis, 250-mg tablets of erythromycin were administered twice a day (141). There is a general consensus that the dose of erythromycin needed for promoting motility is much less than its dose as an antibiotic.

Pharmacokinetics. When given orally, erythromycin base is incompletely but adequately absorbed from the upper part of the small intestine. It is inactivated by gastric juice and thus has to be taken as enteric coated tablets. A dose of 250 mg in estolate form produces peak plasma concentration after 2 hours of administration. Only 2–5% of orally administered erythromycin is excreted in the active form in the urine, whereas 12–15% is excreted in the urine after i.v. infusion. Most of the drug is concentrated in the liver and excreted in an active form in the bile.

Plasma half-life of erythromycin is approximately 1–6 hours. The drug diffuses rapidly into intercellular fluids but does not cross the blood-brain barrier.

Side Effects. Allergic reactions include fever, eosinophilia, and skin eruptions, which disappear in a few days after cessation of therapy. (*b*) Cholestatic hepatitis is caused primarily by the estolate salt of erythromycin. (*c*) GI side effects are commonly seen if the drug is administered on an empty stomach. These commonly include epigastric distress, cramping, nausea, vomiting, and diarrhea.

Drug Interactions. Erythromycin is reported to potentiate the effect of carbamazepine and cyclosporine.

DRUGS FOR TREATMENT OF VARICEAL HEMORRHAGE

In the ICU setting, variceal hemorrhage is encountered frequently and presents a potentially life-threatening condition. Variceal hemorrhage usually results from portal hypertension from chronic liver disease and frequently is associated with concomitant encephalopathy, coagulopathy, and / or renal insufficiency. Bleeding from esophageal varices usually occurs from the lower 5 cm of the esophagus as a result of disruption of a varix (142, 143). Because of accompanying coagulopathy, encephalopathy, and ascites, the management of these patients presents a special challenge. The diagnosis of variceal hemorrhage generally is established by endoscopic evaluation of the esophagus following the diagnosis. Several pharmacologic agents are used to control variceal bleeding.

VASOPRESSORS

Vasopressin (Table 10.3). Vasopressin is a neurohypophyseal peptide that has a potent vasoconstrictor action on mesenteric circulation. Because of its effect on mesenteric blood flow, vasopressin is commonly used as an adjunctive therapy not only in control of variceal bleeding but also in hemorrhagic gastritis and in patients with portal hypertension undergoing abdominal surgery (144).

Mechanism of Action. The principal clinical effect of vasopressin is caused by marked splanchnic vasoconstriction when the drug is administered by the intravenous or intraarterial route. A single bolus of vasopressin administered intravenously causes a marked reduction in portal blood flow and portal pressure, lasting for about 30 minutes. In patients with suspected coronary artery disease, vasopressin should be administered with caution and, if necessary, in combination with nitrates to decrease the incidence of serious myocardial ischemia (145, 146).

Dosage and Route of Administration. Vasopressin is administered initially at a dose of 0.2–0.4 U/min intravenously, but higher doses up to 1–3 U/min have been used in cases with unmanageable bleeding. Close hemodynamic monitoring is essential during intravenous infusion of vasopressin. Although vasopressin can acutely slow down or stop bleeding, it does not prevent recurrence of bleeding from varices.

Side Effects. The most important limiting factor for the use of vasopressin is reduced coronary blood flow in patients with

TABLE 10.3. Vasopressin Analogues[a]

Agent	*Dose*	*Duration*	*Formulation*
Desmopressin (dDAVP)	10 μg i.n.[a]	12–24 h	2.5 and 5.0 ml for i.n. (100 μg/ml)
	or 1–2 μg i.v. or s.c. q12 h	12–24 h	1- and 10-ml vials for i.v. or s.c. (4 μg/ml)
Aqueous vasopressin	1.6–2 mIU/kg/h i.v. or 5–10 U s.c. q4–6h; (children 3–5 U s.c.)	3–6 h 4–8 h	Pitressin 0.5- and 1.0-ml ampules; (20 U/ml)
Lysine vasopressin (lypressin)	2–4 U i.n. q4–6h	3–6 h	5-ml bottle (50 U/ml)

[a] i.n., intranasal.

coronary artery disease. Vasopressin also causes some peripheral vasoconstriction, with increased systemic afterload. In addition, cardiac arrhythmias and direct impairment of cardiac contractility have also been reported. Nausea, belching, and abdominal cramps frequently are observed as a result of increased gut motility secondary to smooth muscle stimulation. Furthermore, allergic reactions ranging from a mild rash to severe anaphylaxis have also been reported (147).

Glypressin. More recently, a synthetic analogueue of vasopressin, glypressin, has become available (148). Glypressin has a much longer duration of action after administration of a single bolus (2 mg) intravenously. The pharmacologic effect of glypressin lasts for 6 hours, and consequently a continuous infusion is not necessary. Availability of glypressin may reduce the duration of ICU stay for patients with variceal hemorrhage.

SCLEROSING AGENTS

Injection sclerotherapy of esophageal varices commonly is used for control of acute variceal bleeding. Injection sclerotherapy of esophageal varices is effective in controlling variceal hemorrhage in 90–95% of all patients and seems to be superior to balloon tamponade or pharmacologic therapy alone (149–151). In one study, definitive control of variceal bleeding was achieved in 95% of patients with a single sclerotherapy session (152). A large number of pharmacologic compounds have been used as sclerosing agents.

Sodium Morrhuate. Sodium morrhuate is a mixture of sodium salts of the saturated and unsaturated fatty acids present in cod liver oil. On venous injection, sodium morrhuate causes inflammation of the intima layer of the blood vessels, leading to the formation of a thrombus. Intimal inflammation leads to the occlusion of the vein followed by fibrosis around it. In most cases of variceal hemorrhage, 1–2 ml of a solution of sodium morrhuate (5%) is injected locally, with an average total volume of 15–25 ml per endoscopic sclerotherapy session. The principal side effects of sodium morrhuate include hypersensitivity reaction, fever, chest pain, and mucosal ulceration. There have been concerns about sodium morrhuate's role in causing acute respiratory distress syndrome (ARDS) in patients with variceal hemorrhage. However, it has now become evident that the pulmonary endothelium is relatively safe, as only 20% of injected sodium morrhuate reaches the lungs and causes no change in diffusing capacity of the lungs (153).

Sodium Tetradecyl Sulfate. Sodium tetradecyl sulfate is a synthetic anionic surfactant that causes variceal thrombosis when injected locally. Sodium tetradecyl sulfate is available as a 1–5% solution containing 10–30 mg of drug in benzyl alcohol along with diabasic sodium phosphate. This compound has been used extensively in the management of variceal hemorrhage and is considered from a clinical viewpoint to be relatively safe . Impairment of pulmonary function has not been observed with this agent (154).

Ethanolamine Oleate. The oleic acid component of the ethanolamine oleate molecule is responsible for the inflammatory response in the intima varices and activation of coagulation cascade by release of tissue factor and activation of Hageman factor. It has been suspected that the ethanolamine component of the compound may act by inhibiting fibrin clot formation as a result of chelation of calcium ions. Generally, 1.5–2 ml of a solution of ethanolamine oleate is injected at one site. The pharmacologic preparation is available in 2-ml vials as a 5% solution. More than 20 ml of ethanolamine oleate should not be used at one sclerotherapy session.

Several adverse effects have been reported with the use of ethanolamine in clinical trials. These side effects include pleural effusion, pulmonary edema, and pneumonia. Case reports of anaphylactic reactions, acute renal failure, pyrexia, and retrosternal discomfort have also been recorded.

LAXATIVES

Constipation is a common clinical condition in the ICU setting. It is related primarily to lack of oral intake and impaired intestinal motility resulting from associated physical and emotional stress. Consequently, a large number of patients need laxatives to initiate defecation during their recovery from critical illness. A large variety of laxatives currently is available, ranging from stimulant laxatives to saline and bulk laxatives (Table 10.4). Stimulant or saline laxatives are used at cathartic doses prior to radiologic exam of the GI tract, kidneys, and other abdominal organs and prior to bowel surgery. Saline laxatives are also used for emptying the large bowel prior to colonoscopy and a variety of surgical procedures.

BULK LAXATIVES

Dietary fiber is plant cell wall that escapes digestion by enzymatic secretions of the human GI tract. It can bind water in the colonic lumen, thus softening feces and increasing its bulk. In addition, some components of dietary fiber are digested by colonic bacteria to metabolites that contribute to the laxative action by increasing the osmotic activity of the luminal fluid. Dietary fiber and bulk-forming laxatives are also used for symptomatic relief of acute diarrhea in patients with ileostomy or colostomy.

Adverse Effects. Bulk laxatives generally are safe, and few side effects have been reported with their use. However, abdominal fullness, flatulence, and borborygmi are observed frequently. These agents can bind and reduce intestinal absorption of cardiac glycosides, salicylates, nitrofurantoin, and a variety of other drugs. Bulk laxatives should be taken with caution when taking other medications that affect GI motility (155).

Preparations and Dosages. (*a*) Psyllium husk is rich in mycelioid, which, on reaction with water, forms a sticky gelatinous mass. The usual dose is 2.5–4 g orally two to three times a day in 250 ml of fruit juice, water, or other liquid. (*b*) Methylcellulose and carbomethylcellulose sodium are also available as capsules and oral solution. The usual dose is 2–6 g/day in two or three divided doses. (*c*) Polycarbophil and calcium polycarbophil are polyacrylic resins with maximal water-binding capacity. As calcium polycarbophil contains calcium, its use should be avoided in patients with disorders of hypercalcemia. The dose is 1 g once a day, to four times a day. Each dose should be taken with 250 ml of water.

TABLE 10.4. Classification and Comparison of Representative Laxatives[a]

	Onset of Action (h)	*Site of Action*	*Mechanism of Action*	*Comments*
1. Bulk producing				
Methylcellulose Psyllium Polycarbophil	12–24 (up to 72)	Small and large intestine	Holds water in stool; mechanical distension reduces fecal pH	Safest and most physiologic
2. Saline and osmotic				
Magnesium sulfate Magnesium hydroxide Magnesium citrate	0.5–3	Small and large intestine	Retains water in intestinal lumen, increasing intraluminal pressure; cholecystokinin release	May alter fluid and electrolyte balance; sulfate salts are considered potent
Sodium phosphate/biphosphate enema	0.03–0.25	Colon		
Glycerin suppository	0.25–0.5	Colon	Local irritation; hyperosmotic action	
Lactulose	24–48	Colon	Delivers osmotically active molecules to colon	Also indicated in portal systemic encephalopathy
3. Irritant/stimulant				
Phenolphthalein Bisacodyl tablets	6–10	Colon	Direct action on intestinal mucosa; stimulates myenteric plexus; alters water and electrolyte secretion	Bile must be present for phenolphthalein to produce its effect
Bisacodyl suppository	0.25–1			
Senna				
Castor oil	2–6	Small intestine	Converted to ricinoleic acid (active component) in the gut	
Docusate	24–72	Small and large intestine	Detergent activity; facilitates admixture of fat and water to soften stool	Beneficial when feces is hard or dry

[a] Adapted from Olin BR: Gastrointestinal drugs. In *Drug Facts and Comparisons*. JB Lippincott, St Louis, 1990, pp 1355–1462.

SALINE AND OSMOTIC LAXATIVES

The saline and osmotic laxatives include various magnesium salts, lactulose, glycerine, and sorbitol. These laxatives act via their osmotic properties in the luminal fluids, as they are poorly absorbed. In addition, the magnesium salt can stimulate cholecystokinin, which, in turn, stimulates fluid secretion and mobility (156). Lactulose is metabolized by bacteria in the colon to lactate, which is partially absorbed and augments lactulose's osmotic effects. Lactulose also causes reduction in the intestinal absorption of ammonia as a result of its decreased production and increased utilization by intestinal bacteria. Furthermore, fecal secretion of ammonia is enhanced because lactulose traps ammonia as ammonium ions and helps to lower ammonia concentration in patients with hepatic encephalopathy associated with chronic liver disease.

Adverse Effects. Administration of magnesium salts should be avoided in patients with impaired renal function because there is a greater likelihood of accumulation and toxicity. Similarly, sodium salts should be avoided in patients with congestive heart failure. Furthermore, hypertonic solutions of saline laxatives can lead to dehydration and should be administered with a sufficient quantity of water. Lactulose can cause abdominal discomfort, flatulence, cramps, and, occasionally, nausea and vomiting. Since lactulose contains glucose and fructose, it should also be used with caution in patients with diabetes mellitus.

Preparation and Dosages. (*a*) *Magnesium sulfate:* The usual dose is 10–15 g (5 g contains 40 mEq of magnesium). This compound has a bitter taste and should be taken with citrus fruit juice. (*b*) *Milk of Magnesia* (*aqueous suspension of magnesium hydroxide*): The usual dose for adults is 15–40 ml and contains 40–110 mEq of magnesium. Magnesium hydroxide in tablet form has a dose of 1.8–3.6 g, which contains 62–124 mEq of magnesium. (*c*) *Sodium phosphate:* This is a pleasant-tasting bulk laxative. The usual dose is 1.8 g in 20–30 ml, to be taken with plenty of water. (*d*) *Polyethylene glycol (solution):* This laxative provides 67 g of polyethylene glycol per liter and contains a mixture of sodium sulfate, sodium bicarbonate, sodium chloride, and potassium chloride in an isotonic solution. The patient drinks 4 liters of this solution over a 4-hour period to clean the bowel. Dehydration does not occur, as the fluid administered is isotonic. (*e*) *Lactulose:* This preparation is available as lactulose syrup. Each 15 ml of lactulose syrup contains 10 g of lactulose, 2.2 g of galactose, 1.2 g of lactose, and 1.2 g of other sugars. Doses vary from 7–10 g to 40 g / day. For chronic hepatic encephalopathy, the maintenance dose is 20–30 g (i.e., 30–45 ml) given three or four times a day and adjusted to provide a fecal pH of 5–5.5. (*f*) *Glycerin:* This agent acts as an osmotic to soften and lubricate the passage of inspissated feces. It may also stimulate rectal contraction. Rectal suppositories of glycerin promote colonic motility within 30 minutes and are available in strengths of 4–10 ml per suppository. (*g*) *Sorbitol:* This agent acts as an osmotic when administered rectally as an enema (120 ml of a 25–30% solution for adults and 30–60 ml for children). Sorbitol can also be administered as a 70% solution (60 ml every 2 hours to induce osmotic diarrhea) and can counteract the constipating effects of sodium polystyrene sulfonate used in the treatment of hyperkalemia.

STIMULANT LAXATIVES

These compounds stimulate accumulation of water and electrolytes in the colonic lumen and enhance intestinal motility. These pharmacologic agents also increase the permeability of the intestinal mucosa by making tight junctions leaky. Stimulant laxatives also increase the synthesis of prostaglandins and cAMP and thus contribute to increased secretion of water and electrolytes. Diphenylmethane derivatives (i.e., phenolphthalein and bisacodyl) act primarily on the colon.

Phenolphthalein. The onset of laxative action takes at least 6 hours. Fifteen percent of the dose is absorbed and eliminated by the kidney, mostly in a conjugated form. The urine becomes pink if sufficiently alkaline. Phenolphthalein needs bile to produce its laxative effect. It is available in tablet form for adults in doses of 30–200 mg, and 15–60 mg for children.

Bisacodyl. Five percent of the orally administered dose of bisacodyl is absorbed and excreted in urine as glucuronidase. Bisacodyl commonly is marketed in 5-mg enteric coated tablets, 10-mg suppositories, and suspension (10 mg/30 ml). The recommended oral dose of bisacodyl is 10–15 mg for adults and 5–10 mg for children. Adverse effects of both derivatives of diphenylmethane include fluid and electrolyte deficits resulting from excessive and chronic laxative abuse. Allergic reactions include fixed drug eruption, Steven Johnson syndrome, lupus-like syndrome, osteomalacia, and protein-losing gastroenteropathy.

ANTHRAQUINONE DERIVATIVES

The anthraquinone derivatives are glycoside derivatives of 1,8-dihydroxyanthraquinone and are poorly absorbed from the small intestine. Their adverse effects include excessive laxative effect and abdominal pain. As the anthraquinone is secreted in breast milk, nursing mothers should be warned against its usage. In high doses, these pharmacologic agents can cause nephritis. Senna produces bowel evacuation within 6 hours, with considerable griping abdominal pain. The adult dose is 30 mg, which is available in both tablet and liquid form.

Castor Oil. In the intestine, pancreatic lipase hydrolyzes castor oil to glycerol and ricinoleic acid. Ricinoleic acid and its salts reduce net absorption of fluid and electrolytes in the colon and stimulate intestinal peristalsis. Castor oil stimulates uterine contractions and can cause abortions in pregnancy. The adult dose is 15–60 ml orally at bedtime.

Docusates. Docusates are used primarily as stool softeners. These compounds hydrate and soften the stool by emulsifying the feces and also facilitate admixture of water and fat. Occasionally, these compounds can cause nausea. Available as capsules, the daily dose is 50–500 mg, with a usual dose of 100 mg twice daily.

ANTIEMETICS

Symptomatic relief of nausea and vomiting is frequently a very important issue with critically ill patients. Proper control of nausea and vomiting is essential to prevent fluid and electrolyte imbalances in the presence of other illnesses. Although the underlying causes of vomiting should be treated primarily, antiemetic agents prove invaluable to tide over the acute illness. Available antiemetic agents can be divided into four classes: (*a*) phenothiazines, (*b*) benzamides, (*c*) cannabinoids, and (*d*) antihistaminics. The important role of dopamine in the function of the chemoreceptor trigger zone and as a mediator of motor reflexes in the stomach presumably is the basis for the antiemetic effect of dopamine antagonists.

PHENOTHIAZINE

Representative drugs of this group are prochlorperazine (compazine) and chlorpromazine (thorazine). These drugs constitute an important group of antiemetic agents that are commonly used to counteract vomiting secondary to radiation exposure, gastroenteritis, cancer chemotherapy, exposure to anesthetic agents, and ingestion of drugs such as estrogens and tetracycline (157). Phenothiazines also have antihistaminic and anticholinergic properties. These compounds reduce the dopamine transmission in the chemoreceptor trigger zone (CTZ) area and decrease afferent signals to the vomiting center. Prochloperazine has a high incidence of dystonia, especially when given intramuscularly. Administration of phenothiazine can mask diagnostic symptoms in acute surgical conditions. Sedation, dysphagia, and jaundice have been described as side effects of these drugs.

ANTIHISTAMINICS

These drugs have H_1 receptor antagonistic activity and occasionally are used in the treatment of nausea associated with pregnancy (morning sickness). Antihistaminics have also been shown to be very useful in motion sickness or vomiting resulting from other vestibular disorders. Scopolamine, another H_1 antihistamine, is widely used for motion sickness and is available as a transdermal patch.

CANNABINOLS

Tetrahydrocannabinoid is the active ingredient in marijuana and is quite effective in preventing nausea and vomiting after cancer chemotherapy. It has also been shown to be more effective than phenothiazine in such instances (158, 159). Side effects of these drugs include drowsiness, orthostatic hypotension, tachycardia, and dry mouth. Less common side effects include anxiety, depression, visual hallucinations, and manic psychosis. These symptoms have been seen more in elderly patients.

BENZAMIDE

The primary agent of the benzamide class is metoclopramide, which was discussed in detail in the section on Drugs for Gastroparesis and Colonic Inertia.

MISCELLANEOUS AGENTS

High-dose dexamethasone and adrenocorticotropic hormone (ACTH) have also been shown to be effective in counteracting emesis in chemotherapy patients (160). Furthermore, neither ACTH nor dexamethasone is particularly effective as a single agent, but each is very effective in combination with any of the agents described previously (161).

DRUGS FOR INFLAMMATORY BOWEL DISEASE

SULFASALAZINE AND AMINOSALICYLATES

Indications. Sulfasalazine is indicated for the treatment of ulcerative colitis and Crohn's colitis. In patients with ulcerative colitis, sulfasalazine is also used to maintain remission (162–164).

Pharmacokinetics and Mechanism of Action. Sulfasalazine is partially absorbed in the proximal jejunum, and a small fraction of the absorbed drug is excreted unchanged in the urine. The remaining portion of the absorbed drug is returned to the intestine unchanged in the bile, while a portion of the drug traverses the intestine intact until it encounters bacterial flora in the distal ileum and colon (165, 166). The intestinal bacteria initiate the first step in the metabolism of sulfasalazine, cleaving the azo bond that joins the sulfapyridine and the 5-aminosalicylic acid (5-ASA) moieties (167, 168). The sulfa portion is largely absorbed and, after achieving high blood levels, is metabolized by the liver and excreted in the urine. Most of the intolerance associated with sulfasalazine can be attributed to the serum sulfapyridine level. The 5-ASA portion remains largely intact and acts on the colonic mucosa until excreted in the stool. If either sulfapyridine or 5-ASA is orally ingested separately, each is absorbed in the proximal small bowel, metabolized by the liver, and excreted in the urine, thus never achieving substantial levels in the distal intestine (169). Therefore, the parent drug sulfasalazine may be merely a vehicle for the delivery of the active component, 5-ASA, to the distal ileum and colon. Both 5-ASA and sulfasalazine act as inhibitors of the initial enzyme lipoxygenase in arachidonic acid metabolism, and this results in the lowering of leukotriene levels in patients with inflammatory bowel disease (170, 171). 5-ASA may also act as a scavenger of oxygen-derived free radicals that are known to be toxic to the cell. As a possible inhibitor of antibodies, its action may be directed at colonic antigens that promote intestinal cell destruction (172).

Dosage and Route of Administration. A comparison of 5-ASA enemas with sulfapyridine and sulfasalazine enemas has shown that significant clinical and sigmoidoscopic improvement occurred in 5-ASA and sulfasalazine groups as compared with response in the sulfapyridine group. Some additional trials have documented the efficacy of 5-ASA enemas (dose 1–4 g/day) in patients with distal ulcerative colitis. In addition, 5-ASA suppositories (dose 200 mg to 1 g two or three times daily) in patients with active proctitis and/or distal colitis provide high doses to the most distal bowel and are effective.

Sulfasalazine is available in 500-mg tablets and a suspension of 250 mg/5 ml. The initial therapy begins with a total dose of 1 or 2 g and then is slowly brought up to the dose of 3–4 g (173, 174). Oral forms of 5-ASA have been developed (i.e., olsalazine) (175) and currently are available in the United States (dose 500 mg twice daily, orally). 5-ASA enemas are also commercially available.

Adverse Reactions. The sulfapyridine moiety is considered to be responsible for most of the adverse effects of sulfasalazine. Adverse effects of sulfasalazine include Heinz body anemia, acute hemolysis in patients with glucose-6-phosphatase deficiency (G, PD), and agranulocytosis. Nausea, fever, arthralgia, and rash occur in up to 20% of patients treated with sulfasalazine. More recently, several patients have been reported to have an exacerbation of colitis with 5-ASA enemas that presumably may be related to sulfides used as preservatives in them. Furthermore, several side effects have been reported with oral 5-ASA, which include perimyocarditis and pancreatitis (176, 177). Ten to twenty percent of patients will experience a reaction to 5-ASA identical to that to sulfasalazine, which clearly implicates 5-ASA, rather than sulfur, as the offending agent. Therefore, care must be taken when placing any patient who is allergic to sulfasalazine on 5-ASA.

Special Considerations. The disappointment in drug therapy for inflammatory bowel disease has been the inability of sulfasalazine to show efficacy in maintaining remission in patients with Crohn's disease. Although topical steroids have proved to be effective for patients with distal colitis, oral prednisone continues to be the principal medication against moderate or severely active ulcerative colitis and Crohn's disease. Neither sulfasalazine nor steroids are effective in maintaining remission in patients with Crohn's disease. Both azathioprine and 6-mercaptopurine appear to be effective agents in patients with Crohn's disease and ulcerative colitis that is in remission (175, 178, 179). However, the use of these two drugs is limited by adverse side effects such as development of lymphoma and occurrence of life-threatening neutropenia in patients with hematologic malignancy and rheumatoid arthritis (180, 181). At present, azathioprine or 6-mercaptopurine should be considered only in patients with Crohn's disease that is refractory to treatment with other agents such as sulfasalazine and corticosteroids. In recent years, metronidazole has been demonstrated to be effective in patients with Crohn's disease involving the perineal area and colon. Furthermore, metronidazole is also currently recommended for patients with Crohn's colitis or ileocolitis of mild to moderate severity who do not respond to or tolerate sulfasalazine therapy.

REFERENCES

1. Lucas CE, Sugawa C, Ridelle J, et al: Natural history and surgical dilemma of "stress" gastritis bleeding. *Arch Surg* 102:266–273, 1971.
2. Skillimann JJ, Bushnell LS, Silen W, et al: Respiratory failure, hypotension, sepsis and jaundice: a clinical syndrome associated with lethal hemorrhage from acute stress ulceration of the stomach. *Am J Surg* 117(4):523–530, 1969.
3. Fiddian-Green RG, McGough E, Pittenger G, et al: Predictive value of intramural pH and other risk factors for massive bleeding from stress ulceration. *Gastroenterology* 85:613–620, 1983.
4. Peterson WL, Sturdervant R, McCallum RW, et al: Healing of a duodenal ulcer with antacid regimen. *N Engl J Med* 227:341–347, 1977.
5. Lam SK: Antacids: the past, the present, the future. In Bayless TM (ed): *Current Therapy in Gastroenterology and Liver Disease,* Vol 2. BC Decker, Philadelphia, pp 641–654, 1988.
6. Kumar N, Vij J, Kamal A, et al: Controlled therapeutic trial to determine the optimum dose of antacids in duodenal ulcer. *Gut* 25:1199–1202, 1984.
7. Brunton LL: Agents for control of gastric acidity and peptic ulcer. In Gilman AG, Rall TW, Nies AS, Taylor P (eds): The Pharmacological Basis of Therapeutics, ed 8. McGraw-Hill, New York, pp 897–913, 1990.
8. Ansari A: Antacid induced phosphorous depletion and repletion. *Minn Med* 53:837–838, 1970.
9. Harvey SC: Gastric antacids and digestants. In Gilman AG, Goodman LS (eds): *A Pharmacologic Basis of Therapeutics,* ed 6. MacMillan New York, pp 988–1001, 1980.
10. Berlyne GM, Ben Air J, Pist D, et al: Hyperaluminemia from aluminum resins in renal failure. *Lancet* 2:494–496, 1970.
11. Drake D, Hollander D: Neutralizing capacity and cost effectiveness of antacids. *Ann Intern Med* 94:215–217, 1981.
12. Ivanovich P, Fellows H, Ruth C: The absorption of calcium carbonate. *Ann Intern Med* 60:917–923, 1967.
13. Fordtran JS: Acid rebound. *N Engl J Med* 279:900–905, 1968.
14. Clarkson EM, McDonald SJ, DeWardner HW: The effect of high intake of calcium carbonate in normal subjects and patients with chronic renal failure. *Clin Sci* 30:425–438, 1966.
15. Makoff DZ, Gordon A, Franklin AS, et al: Chronic calcium carbonate therapy in uremia. *Arch Intern Med* 123:15–21, 1969.
16. McMillan DE, Freeman RB: The milk alkali syndrome: a study of the acute disorder with comments on development of the chronic condition. *Medicine (Baltimore)* 44:485–501, 1965.
17. Orwell ES: The milk alkali syndrome: current concepts. *Ann Intern Med* 97:242–248, 1982.
18. Elsborg L, Boysen K, Bruusgaard A, et al: Sucralfate versus placebo treatment in duodenal and prepyloric ulcer: a clinical endoscopic double-blind controlled investigation. *Hepatogastroenterology* 31:269–271, 1984.
19. Hollander D: Efficacy of sucralfate for duodenal ulcers: a multicenter double-blind trial. *J Clin Gastroenterol* 3(suppl 2):153–157, 1981.
20. McHardy GG: A multicenter double-blind trial of sucralfate and placebo in duodenal ulcer. *J Clin Gastroenterol* 3(suppl 2):147–152, 1981.

21. Lam SK, Hui WM, Lau WY, et al: Sucralfate overcomes adverse effect of cigarette smoking on duodenal ulcer healing and prolongs subsequent remission. *Gastroenterology* 92:1193–1201, 1987.
22. Martin F, Farley A, Gagnon M, et al: Short-term treatment with sucralfate or cimetidine in gastric ulcer: preliminary results of a controlled randomized trial. *Scand J Gastroenterol Suppl* 83:37–41, 1983.
23. Hallerback H, Anker-Hansen O, Carling I, et al: Short-term treatment of gastric ulcer: a comparison of sucralfate and cimetidine. *Gut* 27:778–783, 1986.
24. Hjortrup A, Svendsen LB, Beck H, et al: Two daily doses of sucralfate or cimetidine in the healing of gastric ulcer: a comparative randomized study. *Am J Med* 86(suppl 6A):113–115, 1989.
25. Peterson WL: Pharmacotherapy of bleeding peptic ulcer—is it time to give up the search? *Gastroenterology* 97:796–797, 1989.
26. Jensen DM, Osterhaus J, You S, et al: Health and economic impact of ranitidine in a randomized controlled study of patients with a recent severe duodenal ulcer hemorrhage (abstract). *Gastroenterology* 98(suppl):A5, 1990.
27. Barrier CH, Hirshowitz BI: Controversies in the detection and management of nonsteroidal and antiinflammatory drug-induced side effects of the upper gastrointestinal tract. *Arthritis Rheum* 32:926–932, 1989.
28. Caldwell JR, Roth SH, Wu WC, et al: Sucralfate treatment of nonsteroidal antiinflammatory drug-induced gastrointestinal symptoms and mucosal damage. *Am J Med* 83(suppl 3B):74–82, 1987.
29. Wu WC, Semble EL, Castell DO, et al: Sucralfate therapy of nonsteroidal antiinflammatory drug-induced gastritis (abstract). *Gastroenterology* 88:1636, 1985.
30. Carling L, Cronstedt J, Engqvist A, et al: Sucralfate versus placebo in reflux esophagitis: a double-blind multicenter study. *Scand J Gastroenterol* 23:1117–1124, 1988.
31. Weiss W, Brunner H, Buttner GR, et al: Treatment of reflux esophagitis with sucralfate. *Dtsch Med Wochenschr* 108:1706–1711, 1983.
32. Singal AK, Sarin SK, Misra SP, et al: Ulceration after esophageal and gastric variceal sclerotherapy—influence of sucralfate and other factors on healing. *Endoscopy* 20:238–240, 1988.
33. Tabibian N, Smith JL, Graham DY: Sclerotherapy associated esophageal ulcers: lessons from a double-blind, randomized comparison of sucralfate suspension versus placebo. *Gastrointest Endosc* 35:312–315, 1989.
34. Lingusky M, Karmski F, Ruchmilewitz D: Sucralfate stimulation of gastric PGE synthesis: possible mechanism to explain its effective cytoprotective mechanism. *Gastroenterology* 86:1164, 1984.
35. Nagishumo R: Mechanisms of action of sucralfate. *J Clin Gastroenterol* 3(suppl 2):117–127, 1981.
36. Carafate (sucralfate): package insert. Marion Laboratories, Kansas City, MO, 1985.
37. Leung ACT, Henderson IS, Halls DJ, et al: Aluminum hydroxide versus sucralfate as a phosphate binder in uremia. *Br Med J* 286:1379–1381, 1983.
38. Sherman RA, Hwang ER, Walker JA, et al: Reduction in serum phosphorus due to sucralfate. *Am J Gastroenterol* 78:210–211, 1983.
39. The effect of sucralfate pretreatment on the pharmacokinetics of ciprofloxacin. *Pharmacotherapy* 9:377–380, 1989.
40. Nix DE, Wilton JH, Schentag JJ, et al: Inhibition of norfloxacin absorption by antacids and sucralfate (abstract). *Rev Infect Dis* 11(suppl 5):S1096, 1989.
41. Parpia SH, Nix DE, Hejmanowski LG, et al: Sucralfate reduces the gastrointestinal absorption of norfloxacin. *Antimicrob Agents Chemother* 33:99–102, 1989.
42. Cantral KA, Schaaf LJ, Jungnickel PW, et al: Effect of sucralfate on theophylline absorption in healthy volunteers. *Clin Pharm* 7:58–61, 1988.

43. Lacz JP, Groschang AG, Giesing DH, et al: The effect of sucralfate on drug absorption in dogs (abstract). *Gastroenterology* 82:1108, 1982.
44. Hall TG, Cuddy PG, Glass CJ, et al: Effect of sucralfate on phenytoin bioavailability. *Drug Intell Clin Pharm* 20:607–611, 1986.
45. Giesing DH, Lanman RC, Dimmit DC, et al: Lack of effect of sucralfate on digoxin pharmacokinetics (abstract). *Gastroenterology* 84:1165, 1983.
46. Ryan R, Carlson J, Farris F: Effect of sucralfate on the absorption and disposition of amitriptyline in humans (abstract). *Fed Proc* 45:205, 1986.
47. Brandstaetter G, Kratochvil P: Comparison of two sucralfate dose (2 gm bid vs 1 gm bid) in duodenal ulcer healing. *Am J Med* 79(suppl 2C):18–20, 1985.
48. Ishimori A: Safety experience with sucralfate in Japan. *J Clin Gastroenterol* 3(suppl 2):169–173, 1981.
49. Konturek SJ, Bizozowski T, Bielanski W, et al: Epidermal growth factor in the gastroprotective and ulcer-healing actions of sucralfate in rats. *Am J Med* 86(suppl 6A):32–37, 1989.
50. Algozzine GJ, Hill G, Scoggins WG, et al: Sucralfate bezoar. *N Engl J Med* 309:1387, 1983.
51. Campistol JM Cases A, Botey A, et al: Acute aluminum encephalopathy in an uremic patient. *Nephron* 51:103–106, 1989.
52. Driks MR, Craven DE, Celi BR, et al: Nosocomial pneumonia in intubated patients given sucralfate as compared with antacids or histamine type 2 blockers: the role of gastric colonization. *N Engl J Med* 317:1376–1382, 1987.
53. Tryba M: Risk of acute stress bleeding and nosocomial pneumonia in ventilated intensive care unit patients: sucralfate versus antacids. *Am J Med* 83(suppl 3B):117–124, 1987.
54. Sachs G: The parietal cell as a therapeutic target. *Scand J Gastroenterol Suppl* 118:1–10, 1986.
55. Sachs G, Carllson E: H^+K^+ ATPase as therapeutic target. *Annu Rev Pharmacol* 28:269–284, 1988.
56. Helander NF, Herschowitz BI: Quantitative ultrastructural studies on inhibited and on partly stimulated gastric paretial cells. *Gastroenterology* 67:447–452, 1974.
57. Smotke A, Helander NF, Sachs G: Monoclonal antibodies against gastric H^+K^+ ATPase. *Am J Physiol* 245:6589–6596, 1983.
58. Lundberg P, Nordberg P, Almenger T, et al: The mechanism of action of the gastric acid secretion inhibitor—omeprazole. *J Med Chem* 24:1327–1329, 1986.
59. Lorentizen P, Jackson R: Inhibition of H^+K^+ ATPase by omeprazole in isolated gastric vesicles requires proton transport. *Biochem Biophys Acta* 897:41–51, 1987.
60. Im WB, Blakeman D, Davis JP: Irreversible inactivation of the rate of gastric acid secretion in vivo by omeprazole. *Biochem Biophys Res Commun* 126:78–82, 1985.
61. Reganth CB: Pharmacokinetics and metabolism of omeprazole in man. *Scand J Gastroenterol Suppl* 118:99–104, 1986.
62. Pichard PJ, Yeomans NK, Mihly GW: Omeprazole: a study of its inhibition of gastric pH and oral pharmacokinetics after morning or evening doses. *Gastroenterology* 88:64–69, 1985.
63. Lind T, Cederburg C, Ebenved G, et al: Effect of omeprazole—a gastric proton pump inhibitor—on pentagastrin stimulated acid secretion in man. *Gut* 24:2470–2476, 1983.
64. Sharma BK, Walt RP, Pounder RE, et al: Optimal dose of oral omeprazole for maximal 24 hr decrease of intragastric acidity. *Gut* 25:957, 1984.
65. Gowden CW, Derodra JK, Burget DW, Hunt RN: Effects of low dose omeprazole on gastric secretion and plasma gastrin in patients with healed duodenal ulcer. *Hepatogastroenterology* 33:267, 1986.

66. Festen HPM, Tuynman NA, Defizi T, et al: Effect of single and repeated doses of oral omeprazole on gastric acid and pepsin secretion and fasting serum gastrin and serum pepsinogen I levels. *Dig Dis Sci* 23:1259–1266, 1986.
67. Carlsson E, Larsson H, Mattsson N, et al: Pharmacology and toxicology of omeprazole with special reference to effects on the gastric mucosa. *Scand J Gastroenterol Suppl* 118:31–38, 1986.
68. Sharma BK, Santana IA, Wood EC: Intragastric bacterial activity and nitrosation before, during and after treatment with omeprazole. *Br Med J* 289:717–719, 1984.
69. Howden CW, Hurt RH: Relationship between gastric secretion and infection. *Gut* 28:96–107, 1987.
70. Wormsley KG: Assessing the safety of drugs for long term treatment of peptic ulcers. *Gut* 25:1416–1423, 1984.
71. Wolfe MM, Soll AH: The physiology of gastric acid secretion. *N Engl J Med* 319:1707–1715, 1988.
72. Steinberg HM, Lewis JH, Katz DM: Antacids inhibit absorption of cimetidine. *N Engl J Med* 98; 307(2):400–404.
73. Gugler R, Brand M, Somogyi A: Impaired cimetidine absorption due to antacids and metoclopramide. *Eur J Clin Pharmacol* 20:225–228, 1981.
74. Binder HJ, Donaldson Jr RM: Effect of cimetidine on intrinsic factor and pepsin secretion in man. *Gastroenterology* 74:371–375, 1978.
75. Longstreth AF, Go CLW, Malagelada JR: Postprandial gastric, pancreatic and biliary response to histamine H_2 receptor antagonists in active duodenal ulcer. *Gastroenterology* 72:9–13, 1977.
76. Ma KW, Brown D, Masler DS, et al: Effects of renal failure on blood levels of cimetidine. *Gastroenterology* 74(2):473–477, 1978.
77. Vaziri ND, Ness RL, Barton CH: Peritoneal dialysis clearance of cimetidine. *Am J Gastroenterol* 71(6):572–576, 1979.
78. Somogyi A, Gugler R: Clinical pharmacokinetics of cimetidine. *Clin Pharmacokinet* 8:463–495, 1983.
79. Festen HPM, Diemel J, Lamers CBH: Is the measurement of blood cimetidine levels useful? *Br J Clin Pharmacol* 12:417–421, 1981.
80. Bulkard WP: Histamine H_2 receptor binding with ^{3}H-cimetidine in brain. *Eur J Pharmacol* 50:449–450, 1978.
81. Sancho JM, Garcia-Robles R, Mancheno E, et al: Interference by ranitidine with aldosterone secretion in vivo. *Eur J Clin Pharmacol* 27:495–497, 1984.
82. Fujimura A, Ohashi K, Sudo T, et al: Effects of H_2 receptor antagonists on plasma aldosterone response to angiotensin II in healthy subjects. II. Comparison of cimetidine and ranitidine. *J Clin Pharmacol* 29:230–233, 1989.
83. Aymard J-P, Aymard B, Netter P, et al: Haematological adverse effects of histamine H_2 receptor antagonists. *Med Toxicol Adverse Drug Exp* 3:430–448, 1988.
84. Brogden RN, Heel RC, Speight TM, et al: Cimetidine: a review of its pharmacological properties and therapeutic efficacy in peptic ulcer disease. *Drugs* 15:93–131, 1978.
85. Lewis JH: Hepatic effects of drugs used in the treatment of peptic ulcer disease. *Am J Gastroenterol* 82:987–1003, 1987.
86. Matthews SJ, Michelson PA, Cersosimo RJ: Cimetidine-induced sinus bradycardia. *Clin Pharm* 11:556–558, 1982.
87. Hughes DG, Dowling EA, DeMeesman RE, et al: Cardiovascular effects of H_2 receptor antagonists. *J Clin Pharmacol* 29:472–477, 1989.
88. Mavligit GM: Immunologic effects of cimetidine: potential uses. *Pharmacotherapy* 7(suppl 2):120S–124S, 1987.
89. Kurzrock R, Auber M, Mavligit GM: Cimetidine therapy of herpes simplex virus infections in immunocompromised patients. *Clin Exp Dermatol* 12:326–331, 1987.

90. Kogan FJ, Sampliner RE, Mayersohn M, et al: Cimetidine disposition in patients undergoing continuous ambulatory peritoneal dialysis. *J Clin Pharmacol* 23:252–256, 1983.
91. Binder HJ, Cocco A, Crossley RJ, et al: Cimetidine in the treatment of duodenal ulcer: a multicenter double blind study. *Gastroenterology* 74:380–388, 1978.
92. Brogden RN, Carmine AA, Heel RC, et al: Ranitidine: a review of its pharmacology and therapeutic use in peptic ulcer disease and other allied diseases. *Drugs* 24:267–303, 1982.
93. Peden NR, Saunders JHB, Wormsley KG: Inhibition of pentagastrin-stimulated and nocturnal gastric secretion by ranitidine: a new H_2 receptor antagonist. *Lancet* 1:690–692, 1979.
94. Martin LE, Oxford J, Tanner RJN: Use of high-performance liquid chromatography-mass spectrometry for the study of the metabolism of ranitidine in man. *J Chromatogr* 251:215–224, 1982.
95. Young CJ, Daneshmend TK, Roberts CJC: Effects of cirrhosis and aging on the elimination and bioavailability of ranitidine. *Gut* 23:819–823, 1982.
96. Berner BD, Conner CS, Sawyer DR, et al: Ranitidine: a new H_2 receptor antagonist. *Clin Pharm* 1:499–509, 1982.
97. Langman MJS, Henry DA, Bell GD, et al: Cimetidine and ranitidine in duodenal ulcer. *Br Med J* 281:473–474, 1980.
98. Mignon M, Vallot T, Bonfils S: Use of ranitidine in the management of Zollinger-Ellison syndrome. In Misiewicz JT, Wormsley KG (eds): The Clinical Use of Ranitidine. Medicine Publishing Foundation, Oxford, pp 281–282, 1982.
99. Jack D, Richards DA, Granata F: Side effects of ranitidine. *Lancet* 2:264–265, 1982.
100. Jack D, Smith RN, Richards DA: Histamine H_2 antagonists and the heart. *Lancet* 2:1281, 1982.
101. Camarri E, Chirone E, Fanteria G, et al: Ranitidine induced bradycardia. *Lancet* 2:160, 1982.
102. Grant SM, Langtry ND, Brogden RN: Ranitidine: an updated review of its pharmacodynamic and pharmacokinetic properties and therapeutic use in peptic ulcer disease and other allied diseases. *Drugs* 38:551–590, 1989.
103. Jensen RT, Collen MJ, Pandol SJ, et al: Cimetidine-induced impotence and breast changes in patients with gastric hypersecretory states. *N Engl J Med* 308:883–887, 1983.
104. Galbraith RA, Michnovicz JJ: The effects of cimetidine on the oxidative metabolism of estradiol. *N Engl J Med* 321:269–274, 1989.
105. deGalocsy C, van Ypersele de Strihou C: Pancytopenia with cimetidine. *Ann Intern Med* 90:274, 1979.
106. Nichols TW Jr: Phytobezoar formation: a new complication of cimetidine therapy. *Ann Intern Med* 95:70, 1981.
107. Reed PI, Smith PLR, Haines K, et al: Effect of cimetidine on gastric juice *N*-nitrosamine concentration. *Lancet* 2:553–556, 1981.
108. Stockbrugger RW, Cotton PB, Eugenides N, et al: Intragastric nitrites, nitrosamines, and bacterial overgrowth during cimetidine treatment. *Gut* 23:1048–1054, 1982.
109. Milton-Thompson CGJ, Lightfoot NF, Ahmet Z, et al: Intragastric acidity, bacteria, nitrite, and *N*-nitroso compounds before, during, and after cimetidine treatment. *Lancet* 1:1091–1095, 1982.
110. Campoli S, Richards DM, Clissold SP: Famotidine: pharmacodynamic and pharmacokinetic properties and preliminary review of its therapeutic use in peptic ulcer disease and Zollinger-Ellison syndrome. *Drugs* 32:197–221, 1986.
111. Burck JD, Myka JA, Kokelman DK: Famotidine: summary of preclinical safety assessment. *Digestion* 32:7–14, 1985.
112. Drug Information File: Merck Sharp & Dohme, West Point, PA, 1988.
113. Smith J, Torey C: Clinical pharmacology of famotidine. *Digestion* 32:15–23, 1985.

114. Knadler MP, Bergstrom RF, Callaghan JT, et al: Absorption studies of the H_2 blocker nizatidine. *Clin Pharmacol Ther* 42:514–520, 1987.
115. Aronoff GR, Bergstom RF, Bopp RJ, et al: Nizatidine disposition in subjects with normal and impaired renal function. *Clin Pharmacol Ther* 43:688–695, 1988.
116. Konturek SJ: Gastric cytoprotection. *Scand J Gastroenterol* 20:543–553, 1985.
117. Robert A: Cytoprotection of the gastrointestinal mucosa. *Adv Intern Med* 28:325–337, 1983.
118. Stern WC: Summary of the 33rd meeting of the FDA's Gastrointestinal Drugs Advisory Committee, September 15–16, 1988. *Am J Gastroenterol* 84:351–354, 1989.
119. Graham DY, Agrawal NM, Roth SM: Prevention of NSAID induced gastric ulcer with misoprostol: multi-center double-blind, placebo-controlled trial. *Lancet* 2:1277-1280, 1988.
120. Olin BR: Gastrointestinal drugs. In *Drug Facts and Comparisons*. JB Lippincott, St Louis, MO, pp 1355–1462, 1990.
121. Binder HJ: Absorption and secretion of water and electrolytes by small and large intestine. In Sleisienger MH, Fordtran JS (eds): *Gastrointestinal Disease*, ed 4. WB Saunders, Philadelphia, pp 1022–1045, 1984.
122. DuPont NL: Nonfluid therapy and selected chemoprophylaxis of acute diarrhea. *Am J Med* 78(suppl 6B):81–90, 1985.
123. Gorbach SL (ed): Pathophysiology of gastrointestinal infections: the role of bismuth subsalicylate. *Rev Infectious Dis* 112:580–586, 1990.
124. Durrington PN, Manning AP, Bolton CH, et al: Effect of pectin on serum lipids and lipoproteins, whole gut transit time and stool weight. *Lancet* 2:394–396, 1976.
125. Cummings TN, Southgate DAT, Branch WJ, et al: The digestion of pectin in the human gut and its effect on calcium absorption and large bowel function. *Br J Nutr* 41:477–485, 1979.
126. Portnoy BL, Dupont HL, Pruitt D, et al: Antidiarrheal agents in the treatment of acute diarrhea in children. *JAMA* 236:844–846, 1976.
127. Fedorak RN, Field M, Chang EB: Treatment of diabetic diarrhea with clonidine. *Ann Intern Med* 102:197, 1985.
128. Bauer W, Briner U, Doepfrier W, et al: SMS 201-995. A very potent and selective octapeptide analogue of somatostatin with prolonged actions. *Life Sci* 31:1133–1140, 1982.
129. Davies RR, Miller M, Turner SJ, et al: Effects of somatostatin analogue SMS 201-995 in normal man. *Clin Endocrinol (Oxf)* 24:665–674, 1986.
130. Kutz K, Neusch E, Rosenthaler J: Pharmacokinetics of SMS 201-995 on healthy subjects. *Scand J Gastroenterol* 119(suppl 21):84–85, 1986.
131. Schrezenmier J, Plewe G, Sturmer W, et al: Treatment of APUDomas with the long acting somatostatin analogue (SMS 201–995). Investigation of therapeutic use and digestive side effects. *Scand J Gastroenterol* 21(suppl 119):223–227, 1986.
132. Buchanan KD, Johnston CV, O'Hare MM, et al: Neuroendocrine tumors. A European view. *Am J Med* 81(suppl B):14–22, 1986.
133. Ruskone A, Rene E, Chayville JA, et al: Effect of somatostatin on diarrhea and on small intestinal water and electrolyte transport in a patient with pancreatic cholera. *Dig Dis Sci* 27:459–466, 1982.
134. Justin-Besancon, Laville L: Le metoclopramide et ses homologues. *CR Acad Sci* (Paris) 258:4384, 1964.
135. Johnson AG: Gastroduodenal motility and synchronization. *Postgrad Med J* 4:649, 1968.
136. McCallum RW, Albibi R: Metoclopramide: pharmacology and clinical application. *Ann Intern Med* 98:86, 1983.
137. Maddern GT, Chatterton BE, Collins PT, et al: Solid and liquid gastric emptying in patients with gastroesophageal reflux. *Br J Surg* 72:344, 1985.

138. McCallum RW, Ricci D, Du Boric S, et al: Effect of domperidone on gastric emptying and symptoms in patients with idiopathic gastric stasis (abstract). *Gastroenterology* 66:1179, 1984.
139. Cooke HT, Carey HV: The effects of cisapride on serotonin-evoked mucosal responses in guinea pig ileum. *Eur J Pharmacol* 98:148, 1984.
140. Brisson-Noel A, Trieu Chot P, Courralis P: Mechanism of action of spiramycin and stress macrolides. *J Antimicrob Chemother* 22(suppl B):13–23, 1988.
141. Janssens J, Peeters TL, Vantrappen et al: Improvement of gastric emptying in diabetic gastroparesis by erythromycin. *N Engl J Med* 322(15):1028–1031, 1990.
142. Spence RAJ, Sloan JM, Johnston GW: Esophagitis in patients undergoing esophageal transection for varices: a histological study. *Br J Surg* 70:332–334, 1983.
143. Garcia-Tsao G, Grozman RJ, Fisher RL, et al: Portal presence of gastroesophageal varices and variceal bleeding. *Hepatology* 5:419–424, 1985.
144. Hays MR: Agents affecting the renal conservation of water. In Goodman LS, Gilman AG, Rall TW, Nies AS, Taylor P (eds): *Goodman & Gilman's The Pharmacologic Basis of Therapeutics,* ed 6. Macmillan, New York, pp 732–790, 1985.
145. Tsia Y-T, Lay CS, Lai K-N, et al: Controlled trial of vasopressin plus NTG versus vasopressin alone in the treatment of bleeding esophageal varices. *Hepatology* 6:406–409, 1986.
146. Gimson AES, Westaby D, Hegarty J, et al: A randomized trial of vasopressin and vasopressin and nitroglycerin in the control of acute variceal hemorrhage. *Hepatology* 6:410–413, 1986.
147. Recter WG: Drug therapy for portal hypertension. *Ann Intern Med* 105:96–107, 1986.
148. Freeman TG, Cobden I, Leshman AN, et al: Controlled trial of Terlipressin (glypressin) versus vasopressin in the early treatment of esophageal varices. *Lancet* 2:202–204, 1982.
149. Barsoum MS, Bolous FI, El Rooby AA, et al: Tamponade and injection sclerotherapy in the treatment of bleeding esophageal varices. *Br J Surg* 69:76–78, 1982.
150. Paquet K-J, Feussner H: Endoscopic sclerosis and esophageal balloon tamponade in acute hemorrhage from esophagogastric varices: a prospective controlled randomized trial. *Hepatology* 5:580–583, 1985.
151. Lasson A, Cohen H, Zweiban B, et al: Acute esophageal variceal sclerotherapy. Results of prospective randomized controlled trial. *JAMA* 255:497–500, 1986.
152. Tarblanche J, Yakoob HJ, Bornman PC, et al: Acute bleeding varices. A 5 year prospective evaluation of tamponade and sclerotherapy. *Ann Surg* 194:521–530, 1981.
153. Connors AF, Bacon BR, Miron SD: Sodium morrhuate delivery to the lung during endoscopic variceal sclerotherapy. *Arch Intern Med* 105:539–542, 1986.
154. Korula J, Baydur A, Sasoon C, et al: Effect of esophageal variceal sclerotherapy on lung function: a prospective controlled study. *Arch Intern Med* 14:1517–1520, 1986.
155. Brunton LL: Agents effecting water flux and motility, digestants and bile acids. *Goodman and Gilman's The Pharmacological Basis of Therapeutics,* ed 8. Macmillan, New York, pp 918–923, 1990.
156. Harvey RF, Read AE: Mode of action of the saline purgatives. *Am Med J* 89:810–812, 1975.
157. Wapler G: The pharmacology and clinical effectiveness of phenothiazines and related drugs for managing chemotherapy induced emesis. *Drugs* 25(suppl 1):35, 1983.
158. Synthetic marijuana for nausea and vomiting due to cancer chemotherapy. *Med Lett Drug Ther* 27:97, 1985.
159. Ott LE, McKernan JF, Bloome B: Antiemetic effect of tetrahydrocannabinol. *Arch Intern Med* 140:1431, 1980.

160. Markman L, Sheidler V, Ettinger DS, et al: Antiemetic efficacy of dexamethasone in a randomised double blinded crossover study with prochlorperazine in patients receiving cancer chemotherapy. *N Engl J Med* 311:549, 1984.

161. Eyre HJ, Ward JH: Control of cancer chemotherapy induced nausea and vomiting. *Cancer* 54:2642, 1984.

162. Baron JH, Connell PM, Lennard-Jones JE, et al: Sulphasalazine and salicylazosulphadimidine in ulcerative colitis. *Lancet* 1:1094–1096, 1962.

163. Dissanayake AS, Truelove SC: A controlled therapeutic trial of long term maintenance treatment of ulcerative colitis with sulphasalazine (salazophyrin). *Gut* 14:923–926, 1973.

164. Goldstein F, Murdock MG: Clinical and radiologic improvement of regional enteritis and enterocolitis after treatment with salicylazosulfapyridine. *Am J Dig Dis* 16:421–431, 1981.

165. Schroder H, Campbell DE: Absorption, metabolism, and excretion of salicylazosulfapyridine in man. *Clin Pharmacol Ther* 13:539–551, 1972.

166. Das KM, Chowdhury JR, Zapp B, et al: Small bowel absorption of sulfasalazine and its hepatic metabolism in human beings, cats, and rats. *Gastroenterology* 77:280–284, 1979.

167. Peppercorn MA, Goldman P: The role of intestinal bacteria in the metabolism of salicylazosulfapyridine. *J Pharmacol Exp Ther* 181:555–562, 1972.

168. Das KM, Eastwood MA, McManus JP, et al: The role of the colon in the metabolism of salicylazosulfapyridine. *Scand J Gastroenterol* 9:137–141, 1974.

169. Peppercorn MA, Goldman P: Distribution studies of salicylazosulfapyridine and its metabolites. *Gastroenterology* 64:240–245, 1973.

170. Stenson WF, Lobos E: Sulfasalazine inhibits the synthesis of chemotactic lipids by neutrophils. *J Clin Invest* 69:494–497, 1982.

171. Nielsen OH, Bukhave K, Elmgreen J, et al: Inhibition of 5-lipoxygenase pathway of arachidonic acid metabolism in human neutrophils by sulfasalazine and 5-aminosalicylic acid. *Dig Dis Sci* 6:577–582, 1987.

172. MacDermott RP, Schloemann SR, Bertovich MJ, et al: Inhibition of antibody secretion by 5-aminosalicylic acid. *Gastroenterology* 96:442–448, 1989.

173. Willoughby CP, Campieri M, Lanfranchi G, et al: 5-Aminosalicylic acid (Pentasa) in enema form for the treatment of active ulcerative colitis. *Ital J Gastroenterol* 18:15–17, 1986.

174. Danish 5-ASA Group: Topical 5-aminosalicylic acid versus prednisolone in ulcerative proctosigmoiditis. A randomized, double-blind multicenter trial. *Dig Dis Sci* 32:598–602, 1987.

175. O'Donoghue DP, Dawson AM, Powell-Tuck J, et al: Double-blind withdrawal trial of azathioprine as maintenance treatment for Crohn's disease. *Lancet* 2:955–957, 1987.

176. Bernstein LH, Frank MS, Brandt LJ, et al: Healing of perineal Crohn's disease with metronidazole. *Gastroenterology* 79:357–365, 1980.

177. Brandt LJ, Bernstein LH, Boley SJ, et al: Metronidazole therapy for perineal Crohn's disease: a follow-up study. *Gastroenterology* 83:383–387, 1982.

178. Nyman M, Hansson I, Eriksson S: Long-term immunosuppressive treatment in Crohn's disease. *Scand J Gastroenterol* 20:1197–1203, 1985.

179. Korelitz BI: The treatment of ulcerative colitis with "immunosuppressive" drugs. *Am J Gastroenterol* 76:297–298, 1981.

180. Kinlen LF: Incidence of cancer in rheumatoid arthritis and other disorders after immunosuppressive treatment. *Am J Med* 78(suppl 1A):44–49, 1985.

181. Present DH, Meltzer SJ, Wolke A, et al: Short-and long-term toxicity to 6-mercaptopurine in the treatment of inflammatory bowel disease (abstract). *Gastroenterology* 88:1545, 1985.
182. Feldman M, Burton ME: Comparison of H_2 receptor antagonists. *N Engl J Med* 323:1672–1680, 1990.

CHAPTER

11

Infectious Disease Medications[a]

Infection is frequently suspected or documented in critically ill patients either as the primary process that brings the patient to an intensive care unit (ICU) or as a complication of diagnostic procedures, surgical intervention, drug therapy, or nosocomial exposure in patients who originally entered the ICU for other indications. Therapy of suspected infections in critically ill patients must often be more empiric than in other hospitalized patients, because the critically ill patient may be too sick to tolerate diagnostic procedures. Treatment must also be more encompassing since the critically ill patient may not survive if a causative organism is not treated immediately, whereas a less ill patient may be able to tolerate inadequately treated infection for a few days until the specific pathogens are identified.

Another major consideration for treating critically ill patients is the route of drug administration and the dose and interval that are required. Oral and intramuscular routes usually must be avoided because of uncertainty of absorption. Hepatic and renal dysfunction must be monitored carefully and the fluid and colloid status assessed so that drug levels are maintained in therapeutic but nontoxic ranges.

The focus of this chapter is the antimicrobial agents commonly employed for critically ill patients in the United States.

[a] Henry Masur, M.D., contributed this chapter to *The Pharmacologic Approach to the Critically Ill Patient*, Third Edition.

In the early 1990s a plethora of antimicrobial agents has become available, and a major issue is which of these agents really represent an advance in terms of improved efficacy, lower cost, or reduced toxicity, and which agents should no longer be used (57, 69, 80). These newer drugs vary greatly in antimicrobial spectrum, toxicity, doses, distribution, half-lives, and routes of elimination. It is probably preferable for intensivists to be very familiar with a limited number of antimicrobial drugs so that these drugs are used correctly rather than to attempt the use of numerous costly agents, many of which are quite similar to each other (3, 46, 58).

SPECIFIC ANTIMICROBIAL AGENTS

ANTIBACTERIAL AGENTS

Penicillins. The penicillins are a group of natural and semisynthetic compounds that share a basic structure that consists of a thiazolidine ring connected to a β-lactam ring with an attached side chain (83). The biologic activity of the penicillins is determined by the integrity of the thiazolidine and β-lactam structures. The antibacterial and pharmacologic properties of penicillin are modified by altering the side chain, resulting in a wide variety of available penicillin compounds (Table 11.1). These penicillins are most usefully classified according to their antibacterial spectrum. They all have similar, though not necessarily identical, mechanisms of action, the details of which are currently being elucidated. Penicillins kill bacteria by interfering with synthesis of the peptidoglycan component of the bacterial cell wall. Without effective cell walls the bacteria either fail to divide or swell and rupture.

Penicillins do not kill or inhibit all bacteria. Bacteria may be intrinsically resistant or may acquire resistance to the penicillins. Differential permeability to penicillins and differential binding of a specific penicillin to receptor proteins account for different activity of various penicillin compounds against specific bacteria. Other bacteria contain enzymes that inactivate the drugs. In Gram-positive bacteria, for instance, the peptidoglycan polymer is near the cell surface and is thus readily acted upon. In

Gram-negative bacteria, however, the cell wall is protected from the hydrophilic penicillins by a complex surface structure. Whereas some microorganisms are inherently resistant to the penicillins, other microorganisms produce enzymes that can inactivate various β-lactam drugs. Gram-positive organisms generally secrete extracellular enzymes, whereas Gram-negative organisms produce small quantities of enzymes that remain in the periplasmic space between the inner and outer cell membranes. Each bacterial species produces a somewhat different β-lactamase, and each specific penicillin, or cephalosporin, varies in its susceptibility to the particular enzyme produced. The information for penicillinase is encoded on a plasmid that can be transferred by phages to other organisms. Ability to produce the enzyme is often inducible by exposure to the appropriate substrate. Some of the β-lactamases secreted by Gram-negative bacteria are inducible, whereas others are constitutive (19). In recent years, β-lactam drugs have been combined with β-lactam inhibitors such as clavulanate acid and sulbactam to produce drug combinations that are stable in the presence of β-lactamase drugs. Ampicillin-sulbactam (Unasyn) and ticarcillin-clavulanate (Timentin) are examples that are finding increasing clinical utility.

Penicillins are most readily classified for clinical purposes on the basis of their antimicrobial spectrum. Table 11.1 lists the most commonly used penicillins and their major routes of excretion. Table 11.2 indicates organisms for which penicillin drugs are effective therapy.

Distribution and Elimination. Most penicillins are widely distributed throughout the body, though local concentrations may vary substantially. In cerebrospinal fluid (CSF), levels generally are well below serum concentrations, though the presence of fever or meningeal inflammation usually augments penetration such that subarachnoid concentrations are therapeutic for the most common community-acquired organisms that cause meningitis. Concentrations in obstructed bile and in prostatic tissue are often subtherapeutic for the most likely pathogens.

Adverse Reactions. The most common adverse reactions to the penicillins are hypersensitivity reactions. All of the penicillin

TABLE 11.1. Antimicrobial Agents for Bacterial, Fungal, and Viral Infections in Critically Ill Patients

Drug	*Usual Adult Daily Dose (recommended dose interval)*	*Route of Administration*	*Peak Serum (μg/ml) Concentration (i.v. dose)*	*Hepatic Metabolism/ Excretion*	*Dose Alteration with Renal Dysfunction*	*Serum Concentration Altered by:*	
						Hemodialysis	*Peritoneal Dialysis*
Penicillins							
Aqueous crystalline penicillin G	0.6–20 million units/day (continuous q4h)	i.v.	18(1×10^8 U/h)	No	Major	No	No
Ampicillin	4–12 g/day (q4–6h)	i.v.	6 (0.5 g)	Yes	Major	Yes	No
Ampicillin-sulbactam	4–12 g/day[a] (q4–6h)	i.v.	6 (0.5 g)	Yes	Major	Yes	No
Carbenicillin	0.5 g/kg/day (q4h)	i.v.	150 (2 g)	Yes	Major	Yes	Yes
Ticarcillin	0.25 g/kg/day (q4h)	i.v.	140 (3 g)	Yes	Major	Yes	Yes
Ticarcillin-clavulanate	6–18.0 g/day (q4–6h)[b]	i.v.		Yes	Major	Yes	Yes
Piperacillin	0.2–0.5 g/kg/day (q4h)	i.v.	320 (4 g)	Yes	Minor	Yes	Yes
Oxacillin	4–8 g/day (q4–6h)	i.v.	50 (0.5 g)	No	Minor	No	No
Nafcillin	4–8 g/day (q4h)	i.v.	11 (0.5 g)	Yes	Minor	No	No
Methicillin	6–12 g/day q4–6h)	i.v.	72 (2.0 g)	No	Minor	No	No
Cephalosporins and cephamycins							
Cephalothin	4–12 g/day (q4–6h)	i.v.	100 (2 g)	Yes	Minor	Yes	Yes
Cefazolin	2–6 g/day (q4–6h)	i.v.	188 (1 g)	Yes	Major	Yes	No
Cefoxitin	4–12 g/day (q4–6h)	i.v.	110 (1 g)	Yes	Major	Yes	
Cefamandole	4–12 g/day (q4–6h)	i.v.	80 (1 g)	Yes	Major	No	No
Cefoperazone-sulbactam	4–16 g/day (q6–12h)			Yes	Minor	Yes	No
Cefotaxime	4–12 g/day (q6–8 h)	i.v.	214 (2 g)	Yes	Minor	No	No
Ceftazidime	4–6 g/day (q6–8 h)	i.v.	130 (2 g)	No	Major	Yes	Yes
Ceftriaxone	2–4 g/day (q12h)	i.v.	250 (2 g)	Yes	Minor	No	No
Other β-lactams							
Imipenem/cilastatin	3 g/day (q6–8 h)	i.v.	70 (1 g)	No	Major	Yes	
Aztreonam	8 g/day (q8–12h)	i.v.	125 (1 g)	Yes	Major	Yes	Yes

Aminoglycosides							
Gentamicin	3–6 mg/kg/day (q6–8h)	i.v.	3–6 (1 mg/kg)	No	Major	No	Yes
Tobramycin	3–6 mg/kg/day (q6–8h)	i.v.	4–10 (1 mg/kg)	No	Major	No	Yes
Amikacin	15 mg/kg/day (q12h)	i.v.	20 (1.0 g)	No	Major	No	Yes
Antimycobacterial agents							
Isoniazid	300 mg/day (q24h)	p.o., i.m.	1.0 (10 mg/kg)	Yes	Minor	Yes	
Rifampin	600 mg/day (q24h)	p.o., i.v.	7 (600 mg)	Yes	Minor	No	No
Ethambutol	15 mg/kg/day (q24h)	p.o.		No	Major	Yes	
Pyrazinamide	25 mg/kg/day (q24h)	p.o.					
Ofloxacin	400–800 mg (q12h)	i.v., p.o.			Minor	Yes	Yes
Other antibacterial agents							
Trimethoprim/ sulfamethoxazole	320–960 mg trimethoprim/ day	i.v.	100–150 S[c] (25 mg/kg)	Yes	Major	Yes	Yes
Vancomycin	2 g/day (q6h or q12h)	i.v.	20–40 (0.5 g)	No	Major	Yes	No
Erythromycin lactobionate	2 g/day (q6h)	i.v.	9.9 (0.50 g)	Yes	No	No	No
Clindamycin	2–4 g/day (q6h)	i.v.	14 (0.6 g)	Yes	Minor	No	No
Chloramphenicol	2–6 g/day (q6h)	i.v.	11 (1.0 g)	Yes	Minor	No	No
Metronidazole	2.25 g/day (q6h)	i.v.	26 (0.5 g)	Yes	Major	Yes	
Tetracycline	2 g/day (q6h)	i.v.	8.5 (0.5 g)	Yes	Avoid	Yes	No
Antiprotozoal/antipneumocystis agents							
Pentamidine	4 mg/kg/day (q24h)	i.v.	0.612 (4 mg/kg)	?	No	No	No
Trimethoprim/ sulfamethoxazole	15–20 mg/kg/day (T) and 75–100 mg/kg/day (S) (q6h)	i.v., p.o.	100–150 S (25 mg/kg)	Yes	Major	Yes	Yes
Sulfadiazine	4–8 g/day (q6h)	i.v.		Yes	Yes	Yes	Yes
Pyrimethamine	25–100 mg/day (q24h)	p.o.		No			

TABLE 11.1. *(Continued)*

Drug	Usual Adult Daily Dose (recommended dose interval)	Route of Administration	Peak Serum (µg/ml) Concentration (i.v. dose)	Hepatic Metabolism/ Excretion	Dose Alteration with Renal Dysfunction	Serum Concentration Altered by:	
						Hemodialysis	Peritoneal Dialysis
Antifungal agents							
Amphotericin B	0.6–1.5 mg/kg/day (q24h)	i.v.		No	Minor	No	
Flucytosine	150 mg/kg/day (q6h)	p.o.	75 (2.0 g)	No	Yes	Yes	Yes
Fluconazole	100–800 mg/day	p.o., i.v.	1.0 (50 mg)	Yes	Major	Yes	Yes
Antiviral agents							
Acyclovir	15–30 mg/kg/day (q8h)	i.v.	20 (10 mg/kg)	No	Yes	Yes	
Amantadine	100–200 mg/day (q24h)	p.o.	0.3 (100 mg)	No	Yes		
Dideoxyinosine	Variable by weight	p.o.					
Azidothymidine	600 mg/day (q8h)	p.o.		Yes			
Ribavirin	1.1 g/day	aerosol					
Ganciclovir	10 mg/kg/day (q12h)	i.v.		No	Major		
Foscarnet	180 mg/kg/day (q8h)	i.v.			Major		

[a] Ampicillin component with 2 to 6 g sulbactam.
[b] Ticarcillin component.
[c] *S*, sulfamethoxazole; *T*, trimethoprim.

compounds have potential to cause allergic phenomena (61, 77). In order of decreasing frequency, these reactions include maculopapular rash, urticaria, fever, bronchospasm, vasculitis, serum sickness, exfoliative dermatitis, and anaphylaxis. The true incidence of such reactions is probably between 0.5 and 10%, although some hypersensitivity reactions may occur particularly frequently with one penicillin compound. A hypersensitivity response after one administration of a drug does not guarantee a similar response for each of its subsequent administrations. It is not safe clinical practice to give a patient a penicillin compound if the patient has a reliable history of immediate hypersensitivity response to any drug in the β-lactam group, with the exception of aztreonam, a monobactam that does not appear to cross-react. Whether or not desensitization of the patient to the penicillin compound decreases the likelihood of a subsequent allergic response is uncertain, but desensitization in a controlled medical setting, such as an ICU, is a standard practice for patients who have no therapeutic alternative to penicillin. Skin testing with both major and minor determinants of penicillin is useful for predicting which patients are most likely to have a hypersensitivity response. Reliable preparations of antigens should be used for skin testing. Both major and minor determinants must be employed.

Serious toxic reactions to the penicillins are unusual events. The drugs provoke an inflammatory response that appears to be concentration dependent: inflammation at injection sites and thrombophlebitis occasionally occur. Very high serum concentrations, which may occur if doses are not adjusted appropriately for severe renal dysfunction, are associated with confusion, lethargy, and seizures, especially in those patients with preexisting cerebral disorders. Intrathecal administration of penicillins can cause arachnoiditis, and such administration is almost never warranted. Other toxic reactions reported include nephritis (especially with methicillin), bone marrow depression (especially with methicillin or nafcillin), hepatitis (especially with oxacillin), and impaired platelet aggregation (especially with carbenicillin and ticarcillin).

TABLE 11.2. Antimicrobial Drugs of Choice for the Treatment of Specific Infectious Agents in Critically Ill Patients

Organism	*Antimicrobial Agent of Choice*	*Alternative Agents*
BACTERIA		
Gram-positive cocci (aerobic)		
Staphylococcus aureus		
Non-penicillinase-producing	Penicillin	Vancomycin, cephalosporin
Penicillinase producing	Nafcillin, oxacillin	Vancomycin, cephalosporin
α-Streptococci (*S. viridans*)	Penicillin	Erythromycin, clindamycin, cephalosporin
β-Streptococci (A, B, C, G)	Penicillin	Cephalosporin, erythromycin
Streptococcus faecalis		
Serious infection	Ampicillin + aminoglycoside	Vancomycin + aminoglycoside
Uncomplicated urinary infection	Ampicillin	Vancomycin
Streptococcus bovis	Penicillin	Cephalosporin, vancomycin
Streptococcus pneumoniae	Penicillin	Erythromycin, vancomycin cephalosporin
Gram-negative cocci (aerobic)		
Neisseria meningitidis	Penicillin	Cefotaxime
Neisseria gonorrhoeae	Penicillin	Ceftriaxone
Gram-positive bacilli (aerobic)		
Corynebacterium JK	Vancomycin	
Gram-negative bacilli (aerobic)		
Acinetobacter sp.	Aminoglycoside + carbenicillin	Trimethoprim-sulfamethoxazole
Campylobacter sp.	Erythromycin	Tetracycline
Enterobacter sp.	Aminoglycoside	Third-generation cephalosporin
Escherichia coli	Ampicillin	Cephalosporin, aminoglycoside
Haemophilus influenzae	Second- or third-generation cephalosporin	Trimethoprim-sulfamethoxazole

Klebsiella pneumoniae	Aminoglycoside	Cephalosporin, aztreonam
Legionella sp.	Erythromycin + rifampin	Quinolone
Proteus mirabilis	Ampicillin	Aminoglycoside, cephalosporin
Other *Proteus* species	Aminoglycoside	Cephalosporin, aztreonam
Providencia sp.	Aminoglycoside (amikacin)	Cephalosporin, aztreonam
Pseudomonas aeruginosa	Aminoglycoside + piperacillin	Third-generation cephalosporin, aztreonam
Salmonella sp.	Trimethoprim-sulfamethoxazole	Ampicillin, quinolone, third-generation cephalosporins
Serratia marcescens	Aminoglycoside	Third-generation cephalosporin
Shigella sp.	Ampicillin	Third-generation cephalosporin, quinolone
Anaerobes		
Anaerobic streptococci	Penicillin	Clindamycin, metronidazole
Bacteroides sp.		
Oropharyngeal strains	Penicillin	Clindamycin
Gastrointestinal strains	Clindamycin	Metronidazole, cefoxitin
Clostridium sp. (except *C. difficile*)	Penicillin	Clindamycin, metronidazole
Clostridium difficile	Vancomycin	Metronidazole
Other bacteria		
Actinomyces and *Arachnia*	Penicillin G	Tetracycline
Nocardia sp.	Trimethoprim-sulfamethoxazole	Minocycline
Mycobacterium tuberculosis	Isoniazid + rifampin + pyrizinamide + ethambutol	Streptomycin
FUNGI		
Aspergillus sp.	Amphotericin B	
Blastomyces dermatitidis	Amphotericin B	
Candida sp.	Amphotericin B	Fluconazole
Coccidioides immitis	Amphotericin B	

TABLE 11.2. *(Continued)*

Organism	*Antimicrobial Agent of Choice*	*Alternative Agents*
Cryptococcus neoformans	Amphotericin B + flucytosine	Fluconazole
Histoplasma capsulatum	Amphotericin B	
Mucor-Absidia-Rhizopus	Amphotericin B	
PROTOZOA		
Pneumocystis carinii	Trimethoprim-sulfamethoxazole	Pentamidine, trimetrexate
Toxoplasma gondii	Sulfadiazine + pyrimethamine	Clindamycin-pyrimethamine
VIRUSES		
Herpes simplex	Acyclovir	Foscarnet
Influenza A	Amantadine	
Herpes zoster	Acyclovir	Foscarnet
OTHER ORGANISMS		
Mycoplasma pneumoniae	Erythromycin	Tetracycline, quinolone
Chlamydia psittaci	Tetracycline	Quinolone
Chlamydia trachomatis	Erythromycin	Tetracycline
Leptospira sp.	Penicillin G	Tetracycline
Rickettsia sp.	Tetracycline	

Clinical Use. Because of their proven clinical efficacy and their safety, penicillins are commonly used in critically ill patients. Table 11.1 indicates the recommended doses for the commonly used penicillin drugs.

Numerous new penicillin compounds have appeared in recent years. The acylamino penicillins, for example (azlocillin, mezlocillin, piperacillin), are broad-spectrum penicillins with activity against many enterobacteriaceae and *Pseudomonas aeruginosa.* Piperacillin is widely used because of its excellent in vitro activity against *P. aeruginosa,* but the major determinant of the drug of choice among these acylamino penicillins is probably cost rather than efficacy or safety, because the efficacy and safety profiles of these drugs are so similar. Ticarcillin has been marketed as a combination with potassium clavulanate, a noncompetitive inhibitor of many β-lactamases. The combination is available as Timentin and has increased in vitro activity against a variety of organisms. Similarly, ampicillin has been marketed as a combination with clavulanate (Unasyn). This drug combination may be useful against certain aerobic Gram-negative bacilli, anerobes, and *Staphylococcus aureus* that produce β-lactamase.

Cephalosporins. Cephalosporins are a group of natural and semisynthetic compounds with broad antibacterial activity (20, 29). They are structurally similar to penicillins and inhibit bacterial cell wall synthesis in much the same manner as the penicillins. Cephamycins are structurally similar to cephalosporins and act in a similar manner and thus are also considered in this section.

A large and expanding number of cephalosporin and cephamycin compounds are available, which vary considerably in antibacterial spectrum, pharmacokinetics, and cost (20, 29). For most clinicians it is necessary to be knowledgeable about only a few of these many compounds but to be aware that, if the cephalosporin they are accustomed to using does not have the desired antimicrobial spectrum or tissue penetration, other cephalosporin compounds should be considered. The availability of new, extended-spectrum cephalosporins may make it possible to use a relatively nontoxic cephalosporin drug as a single agent rather than a multiple-drug regimen that includes an aminoglycoside. The relative role of newer cephalosporins compared with imipenem, Timentin, aztreonam, or the quinolones and the role of monotherapy vs. combination therapy for life-threatening infection are currently matters of great debate (16, 38, 51).

Cephalothin and cefazolin are the prototype compounds against which subsequent cephalosporins should be judged. They have wide activity against almost all aerobic cocci, including *S. aureus* (but not *Streptococcus faecalis*), and against many enteric Gram-negative bacilli (but not against *P. aeruginosa*). Cefazolin is less phlebogenic than cephalothin and can be given either intramuscularly or intravenously, unlike cephalothin, which should not be given intramuscularly.

Cefoxitin offers the advantage, compared with cephalothin or cefazolin, of outstanding activity against almost all anaerobic organisms, including *Bacteroides fragilis*, and more activity for indole-positive *Proteus* and *Serratia*. Thus, it can be of particular use for purulent pulmonary infections such as empyemas and abscesses and for mixed abdominal infections. Cefotetan and cefmetazole are newer agents with similar spectra (28). The choice of which agent among cefoxitin, cefotetan, and cefmetazole to use often is determined by cost. The former has a longer half-life. Cefamandole has excellent activity against *Haemophilus influenzae* as well as aerobic Gram-positive cocci and an extended spectrum of enteric bacilli. Cefuroxime, however, probably has more activity than cefamandole and is preferred over cefamandole by some experts. Its usefulness is primarily for mixed upper and lower respiratory infections that are likely to involve Gram-positive cocci and *H. influenzae*.

The extended-spectrum cephalosporins (the so-called third generation) offer improved in vitro activity compared with second-generation cephalosporins for aerobic Gram-negative bacilli. As a group these drugs are active against most aerobic Gram-positive cocci (but not *S. faecalis*, methicillin-resistant *S. aureus*, or many *Staphylococcus epidermidis*), *Neisseria meningitidis*, *Neisseria gonorrhoeae*, and many anaerobic Gram-negative bacilli including, for a few cephalosporins, *P. aeruginosa*. Cefotaxime, ceftizoxime, and ceftriaxone are the most commonly used third-generation cephalosporins that have broad-spectrum activity, which includes good activity against most aerobic Gram-positive cocci (except enterococci), but which does not include *P. aeruginosa.* Ceftriaxone has the advantage of a longer half-life (10). Ceftazidime has a similar (but not identical) spectrum of activity to these latter drugs. Ceftazidime is also active against *P. aeruginosa* but has weak activity against aerobic streptococci. Cefoperazone has been combined with sulbactam to extend its spectra: it may have a role for broad-spectrum therapy that needs to include *P. aeruginosa.* All the third-generation cephalosporins mentioned above cross-inflamed meninges. The emergence of resistance during therapy has been reported for third-generation cephalosporins. The major advantage of this group of cephalosporins is their low toxicity compared with aminoglycosides, activity against certain unusual multiple-drug-resistant bacilli, and the opportunity in many situations to administer a single drug rather than multiple agents. These drugs clearly are effective clinically, but their relative efficacy compared with older antibiotic combinations has not been clearly established, particularly when these agents are used as monotherapy for immunologically abnormal patients (e.g., the efficacy of ceftazidime compared with combination regimens for therapy of sepsis and neutropenia has not been established unequivocally).

Distribution and Elimination. Therapeutic cephalosporin levels can be found in most body sites, including bile, synovial fluid, and pericardial fluid. Cephalothin, cefazolin, cefoxitin, and cefamandole penetrate the subarachnoid space poorly, but several of the third-generation cephalosporins appear to penetrate sufficiently to have therapeutic potential. These include cefotaxime, ceftriaxone, ceftizoxime, and ceftazidime. The elimination of cephalosporins varies with the specific agent (Table 11.1).

Adverse Effects. Hypersensitivity reactions are the most common adverse effects for the cephalosporins and cephamycins (77). No single cephalosporin or cephamycin seems to cause dramatically more hypersensitivity responses than the others. Clinical manifestations of hypersensitivity are similar to those described with the penicillins. Clinically, about 5–10% of patients with a penicillin allergy demonstrate an allergic response when challenged with a cephalosporin. Skin test antigen is not available to assess cephalosporin hypersensitivity. It is imprudent to administer a cephalosporin to any patient with a history of immediate hypersensitivity reactions to a penicillin drug.

Other serious adverse effects are uncommon. They include positive Coombs' test, hemolytic anemia, nephrotoxicity (especially when cephalosporins are used in combination with aminoglycosides), thrombocytopenia, and granulocytopenia (59).

Carbapenems. Imipenem is a β-lactam antibiotic that is sold in a fixed combination with cilastatin (33). Cilastatin inhibits the renal metabolism of imipenem and is included to decrease the production of potentially nephrotoxic compounds. Imipenem has the broadest activity of any β-lactam drug, including extended-spectrum cephalosporins: its spectrum includes Gram-positive cocci (except some *Enterococcus faecium,* a few *E. fecalis, S. epidermidis,* and methicillin-resistant staphylococci), most aerobic Gram-negative bacilli, including *P. aeruginosa* (but excluding *Pseudomonas capacia* and *Pseudomonas maltophilia*), and many anaerobic bacteria, including *B. fragilis;* it does not cover *Corynebacterium JK.* Emergence of resistance during therapy, particularly for *P. aeruginosa,* is a concern, as is superinfection and the induction of β-lactamases, which would make Gram-negative bacilli more resistant to other β-lactam drugs. The role for imipenem is similar to that for extended-spectrum cephalosporins, but imipenem should not be used as a single agent for *P. aeruginosa* infections because of the possible emergence of resistance (7). Patients who are allergic to other β-lactam drugs are likely to be allergic to imipenem. Imipenem should be avoided in patients with seizures or high seizure potential.

Monobactams. Aztreonam is a synthetic β-lactam antibiotic that is structurally different from cephalosporins and penicillins (9, 47). It is the first monobactam approved for clinical use. Aztreonam has broad activity against aerobic Gram-negative organisms, including *N. gonorrhoeae,* most enteric Gram-negative rods, and *P. aeruginosa.* It has no activity against Gram-positive organisms or anaerobes. Aztreonam is clinically effective against a broad range of Gram-negative organisms (64). It crosses the blood-brain barrier adequately. Adverse effects are similar to those of other β-lactam drugs. There appears to be little cross-allergenicity with penicillins and cephalosporins (62). The major advantage of aztreonam is that it has potent activity against Gram-negative bacilli without the toxicity of aminoglycosides.

Aminoglycosides. The aminoglycosides are a group of natural and semisynthetic compounds that have broad activity against Gram-negative bacilli (21, 42). The clinically useful drugs are gentamicin, tobramycin, amikacin, and netilmicin. The group also includes streptomycin, neomycin, and kanamycin, which are used infrequently in the 1990s. Because aminoglycosides have broad activity against Gram-negative bacilli and because they are proved to be clinically efficacious, they are a major component of the antimicrobial armamentarium for the critically ill. They are widely used as part of multiple-drug empiric therapy and as specific therapy for infections caused by organisms not susceptible to less toxic drugs.

Gentamicin, tobramycin, netilmicin, and amikacin have excellent activity against aerobic Gram-negative bacilli including most *Pseudomonas* species. These drugs have no activity against anaerobic organisms and limited activity against aerobic Gram-positive cocci. *S. faecalis* are susceptible to aminoglycosides in the presence of penicillins. Aminoglycosides have excellent activity against most *P. aeruginosa;* they act synergistically against these organisms and against some *Enterobacteriaceae* when used in combination with ticarcillin or piperacillin. Aminoglycosides are active in vitro against most *S. aureus* and *S. epidermidis,* but clinical efficacy against staphylococci has never been proved, and staphylococci rapidly become resistant when treated with aminoglycosides alone. The aminoglycosides act at the 30S bacterial ribosomal unit, where they inhibit protein synthesis and interfere with the translation of mRNA. These mechanisms do not, however, explain the bactericidal effects of these drugs.

Bacterial resistance to aminoglycosides is usually caused by elaboration of enzymes that inactivate the drugs, though failure to penetrate into the bacteria and low affinity of the drug for ribosomes are also factors. These enzymes are located in the bacterial membrane. They adenylate, acetylate, and phosphorylate the aminoglycosides at numerous sites. Aminoglycosides that are poor substrates for these enzymes are active against more organisms. Thus, amikacin, a compound that is a substrate for only one of the common enzymes, an acetylase, is active against more Gram-negative bacilli than are the other aminoglycosides. However, it is not clear whether clinicians should use this semisynthetic compound in preference to the other aminoglycosides, since resistance to amikacin could spread if this drug were used more commonly. Many consultants prefer to withhold amikacin for the treatment of microorganisms that are suspected or documented to be resistant to other aminoglycosides (66).

Distribution and Elimination. Aminoglycoside concentrations are high in the renal cortex. Levels are low in other tissues, and aminoglycosides do not reliably penetrate into the subarachnoid space. Concentrations in bile are about 30% of serum levels unless the biliary system is obstructed, in which case levels are even lower. Aminoglycosides are eliminated by glomerular filtration. Some tubular reabsorption of these agents probably occurs.

Adverse Effects. Aminoglycosides are toxic to renal, auditory, and cochlear function (44, 45, 67, 68). Toxicity is concentration dependent, and the predilection for site of toxicity varies with each specific drug. Ototoxicity occurs as a result of progressive destruction of vestibular or cochlear sensory cells when the aminoglycoside is concentrated in the perilymph of the inner ear. Ototoxicity can occur abruptly or gradually. Gentamicin and streptomycin primarily affect auditory function, and tobramycin affects both equally. All the aminoglycosides are nephrotoxic. The frequency of clinical nephrotoxicity is influenced by the frequency and severity of concurrent nephrotoxic insults and by preexisting renal pathology. Nephrotoxicity characteristically occurs after 5–7 days of therapy: proteinuria and tubular casts initially occur, followed by a reduction in glomerular filtration. The process is usually reversible. Tobramycin is slightly less nephrotoxic than gentamicin; the difference is probably not clinically important. In patients who are seriously ill it is important to measure serum levels of aminoglycosides in order to avoid drug accumulation and toxicity, and, conversely, to avoid inappropriately low levels and ineffectiveness. Peak serum levels of 2–3 μg/ml usually are needed to produce concentrations greater than the minimum inhibitory concentration of most *Pseudomonas* and many *Enterobacteriaceae.* Gentamicin or tobramycin levels greater than 12 mg/ml are associated with toxicity. There is controversy concerning the optimal peak and trough levels to maximize efficacy but avoid toxicity. It seems reasonable to try to maintain peak gentamicin or tobramycin levels of 6–12 μg/ml, and trough levels of 1–2 μg/ml. Peak amikacin levels should be maintained at 25–30 μg/ml. Serum aminoglycoside levels (peak and trough) should be measured at least two or three times weekly in seriously ill patients regardless of renal function. Many factors affect serum level, including the underlying disease and fever. Although nomograms and formulas are available, measurement of serum levels is the only accurate method of ensuring the desired range. Either the total daily dose or the interval between doses can be altered. A useful method of estimating the appropriate interval between 1 mg/kg doses of gentamicin or tobramycin while awaiting laboratory results is to estimate the interval in hours to be equal to the product of eight times the serum creatinine. Thus, if the serum creatinine is 3 mg/dl, 1 mg/kg of gentamicin should be given every 24 hours (8 × 3). Peak and trough levels should then be measured and the dose readjusted as indicated by the levels. Recent interest has focused on once daily dosing regimens; while these are promising, they cannot yet be recommended for critically ill patients.

Quinolones. *Fluoroquinolones.* Fluoroquinolones have become recent additions to the antibiotic armamentarium of intensivists with the introduction of intravenous preparations of ciprofloxacin and ofloxacin (34, 76). These agents inhibit the enzyme deoxyribonucleic acid (DNA) gyrase, and members of this class may have broad activity against many aerobic Gram-positive cocci, aerobic Gram-negative bacilli including *P. aeruginosa,* and some mycobacteria. These drugs have found wide application in outpatient settings, but their role in seriously ill patients is still being defined.

Ciprofloxacin has broad activity against Gram-negative bacilli, including most *Enterobacteriaceae, P. aeruginosa,* and *H. influenzae.* For Gram-negative bacilli, it is the most active of the fluoroquinolones and is generally more active than ofloxacin. Ciprofloxacin is active against many aerobic Gram-positive cocci, including *S. aureus,* and some enterococci, but has poor activity against *Streptococcus pyogenes* and some pneumococci, and no activity against anaerobes. There is increasing resistance among Gram-positive cocci against fluoroquinolones so that this class is not a first- or second-line drug for Gram-positive cocci, especially in the respiratory tract. Ofloxacin has better activity than ciprofloxacin against Gram-positive cocci. Both ciprofloxacin and ofloxacin have excellent activity against *Legionella* species.

The development of resistance to fluoroquinolones by Gram-negative bacilli as well as Gram-positive cocci is a major problem. Their major role in the intensive care unit is in the therapy of Gram-negative bacilli that are resistant to other drugs, in patients with cystic fibrosis, and perhaps in the therapy of legionellosis (48). These agents probably should not be used in prepubertal children, since evidence in some animal models indicates that they cause arthropathies. In adults, the major toxicity of fluoroquinolones is nausea.

Macrolide Antibiotics. The macrolide antibiotics are a group of compounds that contain a lactone ring to which are attached one or more deoxy sugars. Because of their excellent gastrointestinal absorption, erythromycin and clindamycin are widely used antibiotics in ambulatory medicine. In critically ill patients, their use as intravenous preparations relates primarily to their excellent activity against agents that cause atypical pneumonia and anaerobic infections, respectively.

Erythromycin. Erythromycin is either bacteriostatic or bactericidal, depending on the microorganism and the serum concentration. The drug is effective in vitro for almost all *S. pyogenes, S. pneumoniae,* and *Streptococcus viridans,* though a few strains of these organisms may be resistant, particularly if the patient has been exposed recently to a macrolide antibiotic. The antibiotic is also useful against all *Mycoplasma pneumoniae, Legionella pneumophila,* and *N. gonorrhoeae.* Erythromycin is active against only some *S. aureus* and *H. influenzae,* and thus is not recommended as first-line therapy for infections involving these organisms. Erythromycin has little activity against most Gram-negative bacilli, with the exception of *Campylobacter* species. In critically ill patients the major role for erythromycin is to treat suspected *Legionella* or *Mycoplasma* pneumonias.

Erythromycin binds to the 50S subunit of bacterial ribosomes and thus interferes with protein synthesis.

Newer macrolides with more extended spectra (azithromycin and clarithromycin) are available as oral agents, but they are not available in parenteral form and thus are seldom used in intensive care units.

Distribution and Elimination. Erythromycin diffuses into intracellular fluids, and adequate concentration is attained in almost all tissues except the brain and CSF. It penetrates the prostate well, though its antimicrobial spectrum renders it of little utility in prostatic infections.

Erythromycin is concentrated in the liver and excreted in the bile. About 15% of the intravenous form is excreted in the urine.

Adverse Effects. Serious adverse effects caused by erythromycin are rare. The drug is irritating in its intravenous form and frequently causes phlebitis. Fever, eosinophilia, and rashes occasionally occur. Cholestatic hepatitis rarely occurs with the intravenous preparations. This complication is more often observed with the oral estolate. Erythromycin causes reversible hearing loss, a complication that intensivists using high doses must be aware of (36).

Clindamycin. Clindamycin is a macrolide antibiotic that, like erythromycin, has excellent activity against *S. pyogenes, S. pneumoniae,* and *S. viridans* (65). It is active against many but not all

S. aureus. Because clindamycin is bacteriostatic only against *S. aureus,* and because resistance develops during experimental infection, clindamycin is not first-line antistaphylococcal therapy. Clindamycin differs from erythromycin in that it has excellent activity against almost all anaerobic bacteria except for a few peptococci, a few *Clostridium perfringens,* a few *B. fragilis,* and many nonperfringens clostridia. The major role for clindamycin in the treatment of critically ill patients is to provide therapy for anaerobic infections.

Clindamycin inhibits protein synthesis by binding to the 50S subunit of bacterial ribosome.

Distribution and Elimination. Clindamycin penetrates most body sites well, particularly bone. It does not reliably enter the CSF. Only about 10% of clindamycin is excreted unchanged in the urine. The rest of the drug is metabolized in the liver and excreted in the bile and urine.

Adverse Effects. The most prominently described adverse effect of clindamycin is pseudomembranous colitis, which is a serious inflammatory process caused by the toxin of *Clostridium difficile,* a normal bowel organism. The frequency of its occurrence differs sharply in various series, from 0.2–20% of patients. It must be recognized, however, that pseudomembranous colitis has been reported with almost every currently used antibiotic, not just clindamycin, and concern about this potential complication should not be an important factor in deciding whether or not to include clindamycin in an antibiotic regimen.

Skin rashes, transaminasemia, and bone marrow suppression occasionally have been associated with clindamycin administration. Diarrhea without pseudomembrane formations is quite common. This form of diarrhea probably results from alteration of bowel flora. It usually resolves when antimicrobial therapy is stopped.

Vancomycin and Teicoplanin. Vancomycin is a natural compound that is structurally unlike the other antimicrobial compounds (79). It is bactericidal against essentially all staphylococci (both *S. aureus* and *S. epidermidis*), all *S. pneumoniae, S. pyogenes,* and *S. viridans.* It is bacteriostatic against most *faecalis* and most *Corynebacterium* species. A few anaerobes are susceptible, but virtually no Gram-negative organisms are susceptible to vancomycin. Vancomycin has a prominent role in therapy of critically ill patients. To an increasing extent, critically ill patients have temporary or permanent foreign bodies implanted as pacemakers, vascular access, valves, or shunts. These devices are especially predisposed to infection by staphylococci, including *S. aureus* and *S. epidermidis,* an increasing fraction of which are methicillin resistant (1, 50). In addition, the importance of *S. epidermidis* and diphtheroid species in patients with prosthetic valves or malignant tumors and the emergence of drug-resistant *S. pneumoniae* have made vancomycin a particularly useful bactericidal antibiotic. Vancomycin is also useful for patients with Gram-positive infection and a history of serious penicillin allergy (24). Enterococci and staphylococci resistant to vancomycin are being reported in increasing numbers in Europe and occasionally in North America (32, 35). Teicoplanin and daptomycin may have a role in treating some vancomycin-resistant strains (35, 39, 43, 63).

Distribution and Elimination. Vancomycin penetrates most body tissues well, including the brain and inflamed meninges. It is excreted almost unchanged by the kidneys.

Adverse Effects. Nephrotoxicity and ototoxicity are uncommon with the modern drug preparation if peak serum levels are maintained below 50 μg/ml (25, 82). Phlebitis is common with intravenous vancomycin. Flushing, tingling, and erythema are usually associated with rapid infusion, especially if 1-g doses are used (18, 49). Leukopenia occasionally occurs.

Sulfonamides, Trimethoprim, and Pyrimethamine. Sulfonamides are a large group of compounds that were the first chemotherapeutic agents employed systematically for the prevention and treatment of bacterial infection in humans. They have a wide antibacterial spectrum that includes Gram-positive cocci, Gram-negative rods, *Chlamydia, Nocardia, Neisseria,* and Protozoa (*Toxoplasma, Pneumocystis,* malaria). More effective drugs have taken the place of sulfonamides for the treatment of most bacterial processes. They have an important role for treating uncomplicated urinary tract infections. They are also first-line therapy for *Nocardia, Pneumocystis,* and *Toxoplasma* infections, particularly when combined with trimethoprim and pyrimethamine.

The sulfonamides are structural analogues and competitive antagonists of *para*-aminobenzoic acid and thus interfere with the production of folic acid. Sulfonamides exert a synergistic effect when they are combined with agents such as trimethoprim or pyrimethamine that act at sequential steps in folic acid synthesis. For this reason a fixed combination preparation of two of these sequential blockers, trimethoprim-sulfamethoxazole (in a ratio of 1:5), has proved to be an effective and widely used therapeutic product (13). It is the drug of choice for pneumocystosis. Sulfadiazine or sulfisoxazole are still preferred for nocardiosis. Pyrimethamine is the preferred choice in combination with sulfadiazine for toxoplasmosis, although both of these drugs must be given orally.

Distribution and Elimination. Sulfonamides are widely distributed throughout the body, including the CSF. They are metabolized in the liver to varying degrees depending on the compound involved. The parent drug and the metabolites are excreted in the urine.

Adverse Effects. For most patient groups, about 5% of recipients have adverse reactions to sulfonamides. Hypersensitivity reactions, especially those of the skin and mucous membranes, and vasculitic lesions can be life-threatening. Acute hemolytic anemia, often associated with glucose-6-phosphate dehydrogenase deficiency, and agranulocytosis, thrombocytopenia, aplastic anemia, crystalluria, and hepatic necrosis are also seen. For human immunodeficiency virus (HIV)-infected adults, up to 70% can have fever, leukopenia, hepatitis, nephritis, or rash when treated with trimethoprim-sulfamethoxazole; these reactions appear to be related to the sulfamethoxazole rather than to the trimethoprim and may necessitate cessation of therapy. Clinicians are becoming more familiar with completing courses of therapy despite the presence of non-life-threatening reactions.

Metronidazole. Metronidazole is a synthetic nitroimidazole that has an increasingly important role in the treatment of serious anaerobic infections as well as in the treatment of certain protozoal infections (65). Metronidazole is active against almost all anaerobes; some cocci and a few non-spore-forming Gram-positive bacilli are resistant. *Amoeba, Giardia,* and *Trichomonas* generally are susceptible. Because metronidazole is the only bactericidal drug available for most anaerobic organisms, it has a potentially important role for critically ill patients with anaerobic infections. Its role compared with that of clindamycin or chloramphenicol is currently being defined. With regard to mechanism of action, the nitro group of metronidazole is reduced by electron transport proteins with low redox potentials. The cell is thus deprived of reducing equivalents, and the reduced form of metronidazole is able to alter the helical structure of DNA.

Although metronidazole is well-absorbed after oral administration, it should be given intravenously to seriously ill patients.

Distribution and Elimination. Good drug levels are attained in most tissues; particularly high levels are found in the CSF. Both metabolized and unmetabolized metronidazole are excreted in the urine.

Adverse Effects. Metronidazole causes considerable headache and gastrointestinal symptoms, including anorexia, nausea, vomiting, diarrhea, epigastric pain, and cramps. Neurotoxic effects such as dizziness, vertigo, and ataxia and peripheral neuropathy may occur. Reversible neutropenia may be noted during therapy.

ANTIMYCOBACTERIAL THERAPY

Although many antituberculosis drugs are available, the most important drugs for therapy of critically ill patients are isoniazid, rifampin, streptomycin, and ethambutol (73). The first three are available for intramuscular administration. As the tuberculosis epidemic spreads in the United States, intensivists are likely to use these drugs with increasing frequency.

Isoniazid (INH) is the hydrazide of isonicotinic acid. It is bactericidal against dividing typical mycobacteria (*Mycobacterium tuberculosis*) and some atypical mycobacteria. It appears to work by inhibiting synthesis of the cell wall. About one in 10^5 *M. tuberculosis* are genetically impermeable to INH.

Isoniazid is readily absorbed orally. The drug penetrates all body tissues, including the CSF. The drug is acetylated and hydrolyzed and then excreted in the urine. The rate of acetylation is racially dependent. The serum INH concentration of rapid acetylators is 50–80% less than that of slow acetylators.

About 5% of patients develop INH-induced untoward reactions, including rash, jaundice, peripheral neuritis, fever, seizures, bone marrow depression, hypersensitivity reactions, and arthritis. The peripheral neuritis is quite common if pyridoxine is not given concurrently. The most common concern with isoniazid therapy is hepatic injury. Mild transaminasemia (SGOT and SGPT two to three times normal) is a common occurrence that does not predict more serious injury. Bridging necrosis can be caused by isoniazid. The drug should be stopped immediately in patients with symptoms of hepatitis (anorexia, nausea, malaise, and jaundice) and in those whose transaminases are more than three times normal. Older patients are more likely to have substantial hepatic damage than are younger patients.

Rifampin is a zwitterion that inhibits many Gram-positive and Gram-negative organisms by inhibiting DNA-dependent RNA polymerase, leading to suppression of the initiation of RNA chain synthesis. In vitro and in vivo resistance develops rapidly.

The drug is well-absorbed orally; the parenteral form is available only as an investigational drug. Rifampin is metabolized in the liver via an active deacetylation and ultimately excreted via bile in the gastrointestinal tract. Rifampin is widely distributed in body tissue, including the CSF.

Less than 4% of patients suffer fever, rash, jaundice, various gastrointestinal complaints, and hypersensitivity reactions.

Ethambutol is an oral compound with excellent tuberculostatic activity. The drug is widely distributed. About 50% is excreted unchanged in the urine. Optic retinitis occurs only rarely in patients who are receiving 15 mg/kg or less of the drug. Other adverse effects are rare.

Pyrizinamide is an oral agent that is bactericidal for intracellular organisms. This drug can cause hepatitis, arthralgias, and nausea.

Streptomycin is tuberculocidal. Vestibular toxicity, auditory toxicity, and nephrotoxicity are not uncommon.

A variety of other antimycobacterial drugs are available for the therapy of multiple-drug-resistant *M. tuberculosis* or atypical mycobacteria such as *M. avium intracellulare.* Clofazimine and rifabutin (investigational agents) and azithromycin, clarithromycin, and amikacin have been used in HIV infected patients to treat *M. avium intracellulare,* but their efficacy or the efficacy of any other agents for the treatment of this organism is not entirely clear.

ANTIFUNGAL AGENTS

Amphotericin B. Amphotericin B is a polyene antibiotic that is fungistatic or fungicidal for a wide variety of fungi but has no activity against bacteria or viruses (4, 71). Amphotericin B is active against most *Candida* species, *Cryptococcus neoformans,* and *Torulopsis glabrata* as well as some *Aspergillus* and *Rhizopus* species, and most *Histoplasma capsulatum, Coccidioides immitis, Blastomyces dermatiditis,* and *Sporotrichum schenkii.* Amphotericin B binds to the sterol component of fungal membranes, creating channels that increase the permeability of the membrane. Amphotericin B does not bind to the membranes of resistant organisms. Fungi do not become resistant to amphotericin B in vivo.

Amphotericin B must be administered by slow intravenous infusion after the amphotericin B has been dissolved in 5% dextrose in water. The drug precipitates in solutions containing acids, preservatives, or electrolytes. Because of the serious adverse effects, a 1-mg test dose is usually given in 20 ml of 5% dextrose solution over 1 hour. The next dose can be given immediately if there are no adverse effects. Although some experts suggest a gradual increase in dosage by 5-mg steps, it is prudent in critically ill patients to proceed directly to 0.6 mg/kg/day administered in 500 ml of 5% dextrose solution over 2–8 hours (4 hours is commonly used). Few patients tolerate higher daily doses, although for life-threatening infections, especially those caused by *Aspergillus* or *Mucor,* doses as high as 1.0–1.5 mg/kg/day have been used. Alternate-day therapy may be useful for some critically ill patients, especially after their fungal disease is clearly controlled. Hypersensitivity effects can be diminished by premedication with meperidine (50 mg i.v.) and diphenhydramine HCl (50 mg i.v.), and heparin (1000 units) added to the infusion (11). Premedication with hydrocortisone (10–100 mg i.v.) may be necessary to reduce the adverse effects, but this immunosuppressive agent should not be given automatically unless the other premedications are not effective. Amphotericin B can be administered intrathecally, although there are few cases where this is warranted. Coccidioidomycosis meningitis may be one such indication.

Amphotericin B is a highly tissue-bound drug that penetrates most body compartments, though concentrations in CSF and vitreous humor are low. Its metabolic pathways are incompletely understood. Very little of the drug is excreted in the urine, though the drug can be detected in the urine for 6–8 weeks after the last dose is given. Altered renal function or hemodialysis do not necessitate changes in drug dosage.

Adverse Effects. Amphotericin B is associated with a substantial number of adverse reactions such as flushing, chills, fever, anorexia, and headache. When severe, these untoward effects can be associated with tachypnea, hypoxemia, and hypotension. Slowing the infusion and premedicating the patient can diminish or eliminate these untoward effects.

Renal function is impaired by long courses of amphotericin B in more than half of patients. Renal dysfunction can be reduced in severity and frequency by maintaining good hydration for the patient, and perhaps by using concomitant pentoxifylline (8). Often the patient's serum creatinine, initially normal, will plateau in the 2–3 mg/dl range. In most cases, the renal dysfunction is largely (but not completely) reversible. If the serum creatinine rises beyond 3.0 mg/dl, the amphotericin B should be discontinued or the dose should be reduced if the danger of uremia outweighs the acute danger of the fungal process. Renal tubular function is often impaired by amphotericin B, resulting in hypokalemia, hypomagnesemia, and renal tubular acidosis that may be permanent. Anemia is also reported as a consequence of amphotericin B therapy, but leukopenia and thrombocytopenia are rare.

Flucytosine. Flucytosine, or 5-fluorocytosine, is a fluorinated pyrimidine that has activity against *C. neoformans,* some *Candida* species, and occasional isolates of other fungal species. Because 30% of cryptococci develop resistance during therapy, and resistance has also been observed to develop during therapy of *Candida* infection, flucytosine has no role as a single agent except perhaps in the treatment of chronic blastomycosis. Its primary use is in combination with amphotericin B for cryptococcal infections and some *Candida* infections (5).

Flucytosine is converted to fluorouracil by fungal cells, but not by host cells. The fluorouracil ultimately inhibits thymidylate synthetase.

Flucytosine is well-absorbed orally and is widely distributed in body tissues, penetrating CSF and aqueous humor quite well. About 80% of the drug is excreted unchanged in the urine.

Adverse Effects. Bone marrow depression is a common occurrence in patients receiving flucytosine, especially those whose marrows have been compromised previously by malignancy, radiation, or myelosuppressive drugs. Bone marrow suppression can be minimized by maintaining peak serum levels below 100–125 μg/ml. Hepatomegaly, transaminasemia, nausea, rash, emesis, diarrhea, and enterocolitis are also seen occasionally.

Fluconazole. There are an expanding number of imidazoles and triazoles with excellent antifungal activity. Fluconazole is the only member of the group that is currently available as an intravenous drug (27). Fluconazole has excellent activity against *C. neoformans* and many *Candida* species, but not *Candida krusei.* Fluconazole does not have activity against molds such as *Aspergillus* or *Mucor.* Some drugs in this class are active against these fungi (e.g., itraconazole), but these agents are not approved or readily available as parenteral products. Fluconazole is very well-tolerated, although nausea, rash, and hepatotoxicity can occur. Fluconazole penetrates the cerebrospinal fluid well (72).

Fluconazole is an excellent drug for treating mucosal candidiasis, including esophageal disease. At the doses tested for treating cryptococcal meningitis, fluconazole is not as effective as optimal doses of amphotericin B (70). Fluconazole has not yet been shown to be as effective as amphotericin B for the therapy of disseminated candidiasis. Thus, its role in treating serious, life-threatening disease has not yet been established.

Itraconazole has been used to treat some cases of aspergillosis, often in conjunction with amphotericin B. The utility of this oral investigational drug for treating serious infections needs further documentation.

Ketoconazole. Ketoconazole is an oral agent that is effective against mucosal candidiasis as well as less common fungal diseases such as histoplasmosis, coccidiomycosis, and blastomycosis. For patients with life-threatening fungal disease, ketoconazole has no role as a single agent. Nausea is the major adverse effect; numerous endocrinologic effects have also been described, although their clinical importance when conventional doses are used is unclear. Ketoconazole is not absorbed unless there is gastric acidity.

Miconazole. The indications to use miconazole in an intensive care setting are extremely rare, although this imidazole does have activity against yeasts and filamentous fungi.

ANTIVIRAL AGENTS

Ribavirin. Aerosolized ribavirin is effective therapy for severe respiratory syncytial virus (RSV) infections in children (17, 31, 37, 40, 55). Precipitation of the aerosolized drug on the valves and tubing of mechanical ventilators can lead to potentially hazardous malfunctions, especially if prefilters are not used. Other adverse effects associated with its use include anemia. There is no clear role for ribavirin in adults.

Acyclovir. Acyclovir is a purine nucleoside analogue that has excellent activity against herpes simplex and herpes zoster but not against cytomegalovirus or Epstein-Barr virus (2, 37, 78). The drug acts by inhibiting viral DNA synthesis. An increasing number of herpesviruses are resistant by virtue of thymidine kinase deficiency as well as other mechanisms. Resistance developing during therapy has been described. Intravenous acyclovir is the drug of choice for life-threatening herpes simplex or herpes zoster infections such as disseminated disease or herpes simplex encephalitis. Because herpes zoster is less sensitive to acyclovir than is herpes simplex, serious herpes zoster disease requires higher doses of acyclovir than does serious herpes simplex. Acyclovir is excreted largely unchanged by the kidney, so dose adjustments must be made in the presence of renal dysfunction. Acyclovir-resistant strains of herpes simplex and herpes zoster are being reported with increasing frequency.

Adverse Effects. Intravenous acyclovir is well-tolerated; phlebitis, rash, hypotension, nausea, headache, and encephalopathic changes can occur, as can reversible renal dysfunction (60). The dosage must be adjusted in the presence of severe renal dysfunction (6, 60).

Ganciclovir. Ganciclovir (9-1,3-dihydroxy-2-propoxymethylguanine, or DHPG) inhibits the replication of all herpes viruses in vitro, including cytomegalovirus (CMV), herpes zoster, and herpes simplex. Ganciclovir is highly bone marrow suppressive in the doses employed clinically, so it is less desirable than acyclovir for therapy of herpes simplex and herpes zoster infections. Its major clinical role is for therapy of cytomegalovirus disease. In acquired immune deficiency syndrome (AIDS) patients it has been used successfully to treat cases of cytomegalovirus retinitis, pneumonia, esophagitis, and colitis (15). It is also being used with increasing frequency in other populations of immunosuppressed patients, often in conjunction with immune globulin (22, 23, 53). Granulocyte colony-stimulating factor (G-CSF) may be needed in some patients to reduce neutropenia. CMV, herpesvirus (HSV), and varicella-zoster virus (VZV) isolates resistant to ganciclovir are being reported with increasing frequency.

Foscarnet. Trisodium phosphonoformate, or foscarnet, is a pyrophosphate analogue that inhibits viral DNA polymerases. It has activity against HIV, but its major current clinical use derives from its virustatic activity against the herpesviruses, especially cytomegalovirus and acyclovir-resistant herpes simplex or herpes zoster (12, 24).

Foscarnet is widely distributed and penetrates the central nervous system well. It is eliminated by the kidneys. Its major toxicities are renal failure, seizures, and chelation of ions, especially calcium. Nausea and vomiting also occur. Toxicity can probably be reduced by vigorous hydration. Foscarnet is not bone marrow toxic, although anemia can be caused by the drug.

Foscarnet is effective for treating CMV retinitis in AIDS patients and likely has good efficacy for treating CMV disease in other patient populations as well. Its role in intensive care units is to be an alternative to ganciclovir, probably with comparable efficacy but with a very different toxicity profile.

Azidothymidine/Dideoxyinosine/Dideoxycytidine. Azidothymidine (AZT, zidovudine) is a synthetic nucleoside that has activity against HIV. It was the first drug shown clearly to prolong the lives of patients with AIDS (26, 75). It is currently available commercially only in oral form. There is no evidence that therapy during life-threatening illness improves short-term survival. Major adverse effects include neutropenia, anemia, and headache. Few data are available about its interaction with other marrow suppressive drugs. Dideoxyinosine (DDI) and dideoxycytidine are newer nucleosides with antiviral efficacy. Their role in the ICU is uncertain. Both can cause life-threatening pancreatitis.

Vidarabine. Vidarabine (adenosine arabinoside) is a derivative of adenosine. It is effective for herpes simplex encephalitis and keratoconjunctivitis, but there is almost no occasion to use it since intravenous acyclovir has become available. Acyclovir is at least as effective and considerably less toxic. The vidarabine must be administered intravenously in large volumes of fluid (15 mg/kg dissolved in 25 liters) given over 12–24 hours. This fluid bolus presents a management problem for patients with increased intracranial pressure or renal failure.

ANTI-PNEUMOCYSTIS AGENTS

PENTAMIDINE

Pentamidine is a diamidine compound that is effective for the therapy of *Pneumocystis* pneumonia (56). For protozoa the mechanism of action of pentamidine is unclear; it may inhibit replication of protozoan kinetoplast DNA.

Pentamidine isethionate should be reconstituted in sterile water and administered by slow intravenous infusion (30–60 minutes). Clinically important hypotension is not frequently associated with slow intravenous infusion, despite older reports to the contrary. Intramuscular administration often causes painful sterile abscesses and is no longer recommended. Aerosolized pentamidine is well-tolerated and effective as prophylaxis for *Pneumocystis* pneumonia, but the drug should rarely, if ever, be delivered by this route for the therapy of acute *Pneumocystis* pneumonia.

Distribution and Elimination. Concentrations of drug are detectable for at least 24 hours after a 4 mg/kg intravenous dose. The half-life after intravenous administration is about 6.5 hours. The routes of metabolism and elimination are not well-worked out.

Adverse Effects. Parenteral pentamidine is associated with renal failure in a high percentage of patients, as well as dysglycemia (hypoglycemia followed by hyperglycemia, both of which can be clinically severe) and pancreatitis. HIV-infected patients appear to be particularly predisposed to leukopenia, which is usually reversed quickly when the drug is discontinued. Because trimetrexate is better tolerated than pentamide, there may be a role for this newer agent for treating patients who need parenteral therapy and cannot tolerate trimethoprim-sulfamethoxazole.

CLINICAL USE OF ANTIMICROBIAL AGENTS IN CRITICALLY ILL PATIENTS

GENERAL CONSIDERATIONS

The successful use of antimicrobial therapy in the critically ill depends on an understanding of the pharmacology of the agents employed (54, 57, 74, 80). For optimal therapy of an infectious process, the drug must have good activity against the suspected or documented pathogen, it must be administered in such a way that active forms of the drug reach the site of infection at concentrations greater than the minimum inhibitory concentration (MIC) of the organism, and adverse effects must be avoided. The activity of the drug against the presumed pathogens must be based on both in vitro susceptibility testing and clinical trials. Certain antibiotics have excellent in vitro activity but poor clinical efficacy. For example, polymyxins may be quite active against Gram-negative bacilli, yet clinical response is unimpressive. *Salmonella* species may be susceptible to cephalothin, and *S. aureus* may be susceptible to chloramphenicol, yet patients do not have dramatic clinical response to these drugs compared with ampicillin and methicillin, respectively. Similarly, drugs may fail because organisms quickly develop resistance, as with *S. aureus* and rifampin or *P. aeruginosa* and carbenicillin.

The mechanism of antimicrobial action is frequently considered in the choice of an antimicrobial agent. Common sense deems it preferable to use an agent that is bactericidal rather than bacteriostatic, especially if the patient's immune function is abnormal. In bacterial endocarditis, bactericidal agents are much more efficacious than bacteriostatic compounds (14, 30, 81). For the treatment of other infections, the importance of microbicidal as opposed to microbistatic drugs is unconvincing. Thus, the optimal antibiotic is probably best chosen on the basis of activity against the pathogen, distribution, and toxicity rather than mechanism of action.

Additive or synergistic drug combinations are popular approaches to the treatment of infectious processes (41, 52). For bacterial endocarditis the addition of an aminoglycoside to a penicillin enhances serum bactericidal activity and the likelihood of clinical cure. These observations have been applied to other clinical situations where in vitro testing shows synergy for the offending microbe. In fact, there are few data, except for endocarditis, that document the clinical usefulness of these drug combinations, and in many situations, toxicity of the second drug can outweigh its usefulness. In some situations, however, the addition of a second drug may provide sufficient synergy that the dose of the first drug can be reduced, thus decreasing the toxicity. This is the case when flucytosine is added to amphotericin B for the treatment of cryptococcal meningitis.

Antagonism between bactericidal and bacteriostatic drugs is another in vitro phenomenon that frequently is applied to clinical situations. With the exception of a trial of penicillin plus tetracycline for the treatment of pneumococcal meningitis, however, there is little documentation that antibiotic antagonism should be an important consideration in the choice of antibiotics. To ascertain that adequate antibiotic concentration reaches the site of infection is an essential consideration. An antibiotic must be present at a concentration equal to or greater than the MIC of the organism. Measuring antibiotic levels or measuring bacteriostatic activity in joint fluid, CSF, or bone may help determine the adequacy of drug dose. For anesthetic agents or for pressors, augmented clinical responses can be obtained by augmenting drug concentrations. With antibiotics, however, drug concentrations increased over the MIC for the pathogen do not correlate with enhanced clinical response in any predictable manner. The clinician often takes solace in attaining serum or body fluid drug levels that are much higher than the MIC of the causative organism. Attaining very high serum levels at peak and trough periods may, in fact, be useful—they assure the clinician that sufficient antibiotic will be available if renal or hepatic drug excretion suddenly increases or if the infection occurs at a site where drug diffusion is poor. Only in bacterial endocarditis, however, does a specific measurement of serum killing activity correlate with clinical efficacy.

Measuring serum levels of antibiotics is important for ensuring adequate dosing and for preventing toxicity. In critically ill patients, renal and hepatic function may be difficult to assess and may fluctuate rapidly. Formulas and nomograms may help to estimate proper drug dose. Drug levels should be measured on a regular basis, particularly if the drug is potentially toxic, such as an aminoglycoside or vancomycin. Measuring drug levels several times weekly may be expensive on an absolute basis, yet such measurements represent a small fraction of total patient cost and prevent distressing and expensive complications.

EMPIRIC THERAPY

When patients are critically ill their survival is often dependent on the prompt initiation of appropriate antimicrobial therapy. If the identity of the etiologic microorganism(s) is uncertain, empiric therapy must be initiated to cover the full range of likely pathogens pending the outcome of diagnostic procedures.

For many critically ill patients, however, the optimal diagnostic procedure cannot be performed because the patient is too hypoxic for a bronchoscopy, too thrombocytopenic for a biopsy, or too hemodynamically unstable to be transported to radiology or the operating suite. This scenario is especially common when dealing with immunosuppressed patients.

Traditionally, empiric antimicrobial regimens were likely to include multiple drugs, since no one agent has broad coverage that includes aerobic and anaerobic organisms, Gram-positive and Gram-negative bacteria, rods, and cocci. The past few years have been characterized by the appearance of third-generation cephalosporins, thienamycin, quinolones, and β-lactam/β-lactamase inhibitor combinations that can provide broad coverage. Single agents have the advantage of being less time-consuming to administer. Moreover, several of these drugs are considerably less toxic than the aminoglycosides that were previously included in most multiple-drug empiric regimens, particularly those used for neutropenic patients. In the middle 1980s a major unresolved issue was whether single agents such as ceftazidine, imipenem, or Timentin would be as effective as multiple-drug regimens, thus allowing clinicians the ease of monotherapy and the diminution in direct toxicity. Whether these benefits will outweigh the high absolute cost of many of these newer drugs remains to be determined.

EPIDEMIOLOGIC AND OTHER FACTORS

The epidemiology of highly pathogenic multiple-antibiotic-resistant organisms is an important consideration in the choice of antimicrobial agents in critically ill patients. Many patients who are critically ill have been exposed to hospital flora during previous hospitalization. Many critically ill patients are hospitalized in an ICU, where they can acquire resistant organisms and become superinfected. Substantial antibiotic pressure on these patients can also select out endogenous flora that are multiply antibiotic resistant. These organisms can cause serious disease in the infected patient, and they can be transmitted to other patients. A physician caring for a critically ill patient is obligated to use the most efficacious antimicrobial therapy available. The physician must also, however, introduce antibiotics appropriately so that resistance to newer antibiotics is delayed, thus saving these drugs for unusual situations in which they are uniquely useful. For instance, amikacin has decided advantages over gentamicin and tobramycin because it is often more active against more Gram-negative bacilli. Gram-negative bacilli that are resistant to gentamicin and tobramycin will sometimes be susceptible to amikacin, yet the more frequently this latter drug is used, the more amikacin-resistant organisms will likely appear. Thus, amikacin should probably be used only if the organism is known to be resistant to other therapeutic agents, or if there is some reason to suspect strongly such resistance. Similarly, some third-generation cephalosporins appear to be useful nontoxic agents for the treatment of organisms that previously required toxic agents such as the aminoglycosides. If they are used indiscriminately to treat organisms that are susceptible to more conventional agents, however, resistance may develop rapidly, thus decreasing their usefulness and the usefulness of other β-lactam drugs.

The cost of newer antibiotics should also influence the drug selected. Newer drugs are often much more expensive than older, generically available agents, and their routine use can dramatically increase a hospital's pharmacy expenditure.

Finally, the choice of antimicrobial agent must be influenced by a physician's familiarity with the drug. The rapid explosion of penicillin, cephalosporin, and quinolone agents makes it impossible for physicians to be familiar with the doses, pharmacokinetics, and adverse effects of all agents. Errors in selection and administration are more frequent if the physician attempts to use too large an armamentarium of drugs, especially when dealing with critically ill patients with changing hepatic and renal function and when considering the interaction of the drug with other medications. It seems preferable for the physician to be very familiar with the pharmacology of a limited antibiotic armamentarium and to select other agents or newer agents only when clearly indicated, judiciously using specific information from convenient handbooks or calling consultants (3, 46, 58).

REFERENCES

1. Archer GL: Molecular epidemiology of multiresistant *Staphylococcus epidermidis. J. Antimicrob Chemother* 21(suppl):133–138, 1988.
2. Balfour Jr HH, et al: Burroughs Wellcome Collaborative Acyclovir Study Group. Acyclovir halts progression of herpes zoster in immunocompromised patients. *N Engl J Med* 308:1448–1453, 1983.
3. Bartlett JG: *1991 Pocketbook of Infectious Disease Therapy.* Williams & Wilkins, Baltimore, 1991.
4. Bennett JE, et al: Amphotericin B-flucytosine in cryptococcal meningitis. *N Engl J Med* 301:126–131, 1979.
5. Bennett JE: Antifungal agents. In: Mandell GL, Douglas Jr RG, Bennett JE (eds): *Principles and Practice of Infectious Diseases,* 3rd ed. New York, Churchill Livingstone, pp 361–370, 1990.
6. Blum RM, Liao SHT, De Miranda P: Overview of acyclovir pharmacokinetic disposition in adults and children. *Am J Med* 73(suppl):186–192, 1982.
7. Bodey GP, Alvarez ME, Jones PG et al: Imipenem/cilistatin as initial therapy for febrile cancer patients. *Antimicrob Agents Chemother* 30:211–214, 1986.
8. Branch RA: Prevention of amphotericin B-induced renal impairment. *Arch Intern Med* 148:2389–2394, 1988.
9. Brewer NS, Hellinger WC: The monobactams. *Mayo Clin Proc* 66:1152–1157, 1991.
10. Brogden RN, Ward A: Ceftriaxone: a reappraisal of its antibacterial activity and pharmacokinetic properties, and an update on its therapeutic use with particular reference to once-daily administration. *Drugs* 35:604–645, 1988.
11. Burks LC, Aisner J, Fortner CL, Wiernik PH: Meperidine for the treatment of shaking chills and fever. *Arch Intern Med* 140:483–484, 1980.
12. Chatis PA, Miller CH, Schrager LE, Crumpacker CS: Successful treatment with foscarnet of an acyclovir-resistant mucocutaneous infection with herpes simplex virus in a patient with acquired immunodeficiency syndrome. *N Engl J Med* 320:297–300, 1989.
13. Cockerill FR, Edson RS: Trimethoprim-sulfamethoxazole. *Mayo Clin Proc* 66:1260–1269, 1991.
14. Coleman DL, Horowitz RI, Andriole VT: Association between serum inhibitory and bactericidal concentrations and therapeutic outcome in bacterial endocarditis. *Am J Med* 73:260–267, 1982.
15. Collaborative DHPG Treatment Study Group: Treatment of serious cytomegalovirus infections with 9-(1,3-dihydroxy-2-propoxymethyl) guanine in patients with AIDS and other immunodeficiencies. *N Engl J Med* 314:801–805, 1986.
16. Collins T, Gerding DN: Aminoglycosides versus betalactams in Gram-negative pneumonia. *Semin Respir Infect* 6:136–146, 1991.
17. Connor JD, Hintz M, Van Dyke R, McCormick JB, McIntosh K: Ribavirin pharmacokinetics in children and adults during therapeutic trials. In Smith RA, Knight V, Smith JAD (eds): *Clinical Applications of Ribavirin.* Orlando, FL, Academic Press, pp 107–123, 1984.
18. Davis RL, Smith AL, Koup JR: The "redman's syndrome" and slow infusion of vancomycin. *Ann Intern Med* 104:285–286, 1986.
19. Doern GV, Jergensen JH, Thornsberry C, et al: National collaborative study of the prevalence of antimicrobial resistance among clinical isolates of *Hemophilus influenzae. Antimicrob Agents Chemother* 32:185, 1988.
20. Donowitz GR, Mandell GL: Beta-lactam antibiotics. *N Engl J Med* 318:419–426, 490–500, 1988.
21. Edson RS, Terrell CL: The aminoglycosides. *Mayo Clin Proc* 66:1158–1164, 1991.

22. Emanuel D, et al: Cytomegalovirus pneumonia after bone marrow transplantation successfully treated with the combination of ganciclovir and high-dose intravenous immune globulin. *Ann Intern Med* 109:777–782, 1988.
23. Erice A, Chou S, Biron KK, Stanat SC, Balfour HH, Jordan MC: Progressive disease due to ganciclovir-resistant cytomegalovirus in immunocompromised patients. *N Engl J Med* 320:289–293, 1989.
24. Erlich KS, Facobson MA, Koehler JE, Follansbee SE, Drennan DP, Gooze L, Safrin S, Mills J: Foscarnet therapy for severe acyclovir-resistant herpes simplex virus type-2 infections in patients with the acquired immunodeficiency syndrome (AIDS): an uncontrolled trial. *Ann Intern Med* 110:710–713, 1989.
25. Farber B, Moellering Jr RC: Retrospective study of the toxicity of preparations of vancomycin from 1974–1981. *Antimicrob Agents Chemother* 23:138–141, 1983.
26. Fischl MA, et al: The efficacy of azidothymidine (AZT) in the treatment of patients with AIDS and AIDS-related complex. *N Engl J Med* 317:185–191, 1987.
27. Grant SM, Clissold SP: Fluconazole—a review of its pharmacologic and pharmacokinetic properties, and therapeutic potential in superficial and systemic mycoses. *Drugs* 39:877–916, 1990.
28. Griffith DL, Novak E, Greenwald CA, Metzler CM, Paxton LM: Clinical experience with cefmetazole sodium in the United States—an overview. *Antimicrob Agents Chemother* 23(suppl D):21–23, 1989.
29. Gustaferro CA, Steckelberg JM: Cephalosporin antimicrobial agents and related compounds. *Mayo Clin Proc* 66:1064–1073, 1991.
30. Hackbarth CJ, Chambers HF, Sande MA: Serum bactericidal titer as a predictor of outcome in endocarditis. *Eur J Clin Microbiol* 5:93–97, 1986.
31. Hall CB, McBride JT, Walsh EE, Bell DM, Gala C, Hildreth S, TenEyck LG, Hall WJ: Aerosolized ribavirin treatment of infants with respiratory syncytial viral infection. *N Engl J Med* 308:1443, 1983.
32. Handwerger S, Perlinar DC, Aharac D, Mc Auliffe V: Concomitant high-level vancomycin and penicillin resistance in clinical isolates of enterococci. *Clin Infect Dis* 14:655–661, 1992.
33. Hellinger WC, Brewer NS; Imipenem. *Mayo Clin Proc* 66:1074–1081, 1991.
34. Hooper DC, Wolfson JS: Fluoroquinolone antimicrobial agents. *N Engl J Med* 324:384–394, 1991.
35. Johnson AP, Uttley AH, Woodford N, George RC: Resistance to vancomycin and teicoplanin: an emerging clinical problem. *Clin Microbiol Rev* 3:280–291, 1990.
36. Karmody CS, Weinstein L: Reversible sensorineural hearing loss with intravenous erythromycin lactobionate. *Ann Otol Rhinol Laryngol* 86:9–11, 1977.
37. Keating MR: Antiviral agents. *Mayo Clin Proc* 66:160–178, 1992.
38. Klastersky J, Hensgens C, Meunier-Carpentier F: Comparative effectiveness of combinations of amikacin with penicillin G and amikacin with carbenicillin in Gram-negative septicemia double blind clinical trial. *J Infect Dis* 134(suppl):433, 1976.
39. Kenny MT, Dulworth JK, Brackman MA: Comparative in vitro activity of teicoplanin and vancomycin against United States clinical trial isolates of Gram-positive cocci. *Diagn Microbiol Infect Dis* 14:29–31, 1991.
40. Knight V, Yu CP, Gilbert BE, Divine GW: Estimating the dosage of ribavirin aerosol according to age and other variables. *J Infect Dis* 158:443–448, 1988.
41. Lepper MH, Dowling HF: Treatment of pneumococcal meningitis with penicillin plus aureomycin: studies including observations on apparent antagonism between penicillin and aureomycin. *Arch Intern Med* 88:489–494, 1951.
42. Lietman PS: Aminoglycosides and spectinomycin: aminocyclitos. In Mandell GL, Douglas Jr RG, Bennett JE (eds): *Principles and Practices of Infectious Diseases*, ed 3. Churchill Livingstone, New York, pp 269–284, 1990.

43. Livornese LL, Dias SC, et al: Hospital acquired infection with vancomycin-resistant enterococcus faecium transmitted by electronic thermometers. *Ann Intern Med* 117:112–116, 1992.
44. Moore RD, Smith CR, Lietman PS: Risk factors for the development of auditory toxicity in patients receiving aminoglycosides. *J Infect Dis* 149:23–30, 1984.
45. Moore RD, Smith CR, Lipsky JJ, Mellits D, Leitman PS: Risk factors for nephrotoxicity in patients with aminoglycosides. *Ann Intern Med* 100:352–357, 1984.
46. Nelson JD: *1991–1992 Pocketbook of Pediatric Antimicrobial Therapy,* ed 9. Williams & Wilkins, Baltimore, 1991.
47. Neu HC: Aztreonam activity, pharmacology, and clinical uses. *Am J Med* 88:25–65, 1990.
48. Neu HC: Synergy and antagonism of combinations with quinolones. *Eur J Clin Microbiol Infect Dis* 10:255–261, 1991.
49. Newfield P, Roizen MF: Hazards of rapid administration of vancomycin. *Ann Intern Med* 91:581, 1979.
50. Peacock JE, Moorman DR, Wenzel RP, et al: Methicillin resistant *Staphylococcus aureus:* microbiologic characteristics, antimicrobial susceptibility, and assessment of virulence of an epidemic strain. *J Infect Dis* 144:575, 1981.
51. Pizzo PA, et al: A randomized trial comparing ceftazidime alone with combination antibiotic therapy in cancer patients with fever and neutropenia. *N Engl J Med* 315:552–558, 1986.
52. Rahal Jr J: Antibiotic combinations: the clinical relevance of synergy and antagonism. *Medicine (Baltimore)* 57:179–195, 1978.
53. Reed EC, Bowden RA, Dandliker PS, Lilleby KE, Meyers JD: Treatment of cytomegalovirus pneumonia and ganciclovir and intravenous cytomegalovirus immunoglobulin in patients with bone marrow transplants. *Ann Intern Med* 109:783–788, 1988.
54. Rhodes KH, Henry NK: Antibiotic therapy for severe infections in infants and children. *Mayo Clin Proc* 66:59–68, 1992.
55. Rodriguez WJ, Kim HW, Brandt CD, Fink RJ, Getson PR, Arrobio J, Murphy TM, McCarthy V, Parrott RH: Aerosolized ribavirin in the treatment of patients with respiratory syncytial virus disease. *Pediatr Infect Dis J* 6:159–163, 1987.
56. Rosenblatt JE: Antiparasitic agents. *Mayo Clin Proc* 66:276–287, 1992.
57. Rosenblatt JE: Laboratory tests used to guide antimicrobial therapy. *Mayo Clin Proc* 66:942–948, 1991.
58. Sanford JP: *Guide to Antimicrobial Therapy 1992.* Antimicrobial Therapy, Dallas, TX, 1992.
59. Sattler FR, Weitekamp MR, Ballard JO: Potential for bleeding with the new beta-lactam antibiotics. *Ann Intern Med* 105:924–931, 1986.
60. Sawyer MH, Webb DE, Balow JE, Straus SE: Acyclovir-induced renal failure: clinical course and histology. *Am J Med* 84:1067–1071, 1988.
61. Saxon A, Beall GN, Rohr AS, Adelman DC: Immediate hypersensitivity reactions to beta-lactam antibiotics. *Ann Intern Med* 107:204–215, 1987.
62. Saxon A, Hassner A, Swabb EA, Wheeler B, Adkinson Jr NF: Lack of cross-reactivity between aztreonam, a monobactam antibiotic, and penicillin in penicillin-allergic subjects. *J Infect Dis* 149:16–22, 1984.
63. Schwalbe RS, Stapleton JT, Gilligan PH: Emergence of vancomycin resistance in coagulase-negative staphylococci. *N Engl J Med* 316:927–931, 1987.
64. Scully BE, Neu HC: Use of aztreonam in the treatment of serious infections due to multiresistant Gram-negative organisms including *Pseudomonas aeruginosa. Am J Med* 78:251–261, 1985.
65. Smilak JD, Wilson WR, Cockerill FR: Tetracyclines, chloramphenicol, erythromycin, clindamycin, and metronidazole. *Mayo Clin Proc* 66:1270–1280, 1991.
66. Smith CR, Baughman KL, Edwards CQ, Rogers JF, Leitman PS: Controlled comparison of amikacin and gentamicin. *N Engl J Med* 296:349–353, 1977.

67. Smith CR, Lietman PS: Effect of furosemide on aminoglycoside-induced nephrotoxicity and auditory toxicity in humans. *Antimicrob Agents Chemother* 23:133–137, 1983.
68. Smith CR, Lipsky JJ, Laskin OL, Hellman DB, Mellits ED, Longstreth J, Lietman PS: Double-blind comparison of the nephrotoxicity and auditory toxicity of gentamicin and tobramycin. *N Engl J Med* 302:1106–1109, 1980.
69. Standiford HC: Tetracyclines and chloramphenicol. In Mandell GL, Douglas Jr RG, Bennett JE (eds): *Principles and Practices of Infectious Diseases,* ed 3. John Wiley & Sons, New York, pp 284–295, 1990.
70. Stern JJ, Hartman BJ, Sharkey P, Rowland V, Squires KE, Murray HW, Graybill JR: Oral fluconazole therapy for patients with acquired immunodeficiency syndrome. *Am J Med* 297:178–179, 1988.
71. Terrell CL, Hughes CE: Antifungal agents used for deep-seated mycotic infections. *Mayo Clin Proc* 66:69–91, 1992.
72. Tucker RM, Williams PL, Arathoon RG, Levine BE, Harstein AL, Hanson LH, Steven DA: Pharmacokinetics of fluconazole in cerebrospinal fluid and serum in human coccidioidal meningitis. *Antimicrob Agents Chemother* 32:369–373, 1988.
73. Van Scoy RE, Wilkowske CJ: Antituberculous agents. *Mayo Clin Proc* 66:179–187, 1992.
74. Van Scoy RE, Wilkowske CJ: Prophylactic use of antimicrobial agents in adult patients. *Mayo Clin Proc* 66:288–292, 1992.
75. Volberding PA, Lagakos SW, Koch MA, et al: Zidovudine in asymptomatic human immunodeficiency virus infection—a controlled trial in persons with less than 500 CD4 positive cells. *N Engl J Med* 322:941, 1990.
76. Walker RC, Wright AJ: The fluoroquinolones. *Mayo Clin Proc* 66:1249–1259, 1991.
77. Weiss ME, Adkinson NF: Beta-lactam allergy. In Mandell GI, Douglas Jr RG, Bennett JE (eds): *Principles and Practice of Infectious Diseases,* ed 3. Churchill Livingstone, New York, pp 264–269, 1990.
78. Whitley RJ, Gnann JW: Drug therapy: acyclovir: a decade later. *N Engl J Med* 327:782–789, 1992.
79. Wilhelm MP: Vancomycin. *Mayo Clin Proc* 66:1165–1170, 1991.
80. Wilkowske CJ: General principles of antimicrobial therapy. *Mayo Clin Proc* 66:931–941, 1991.
81. Wolfson JS, Swartz MN: Serum bactericidal activity as a monitor of antibiotic therapy. *N Engl J Med* 312:968–975, 1985.
82. Woods CA, Kohlhepp SJ, Houghton DC, Gilbert DN: Vancomycin enhancement of experimental tobramycin nephrotoxicity. *Antimicrob Agents Chemother* 30:20–24, 1986.
83. Wright AJ, Wilkowske CJ. The penicillins. *Mayo Clin Proc* 66:1047–1063, 1991.

[illegible] CF [illegible] of nonsteroidal anti-inflammatory [illegible] and [illegible] (1983) [illegible]

[illegible] CR, Lisskv JJ, Lasker [illegible], et al. [illegible] Double-blind comparison of [illegible] and [illegible] for [illegible] in patients [illegible]. *N Engl J Med* 328:[illegible], 1993.

[illegible] Practice [illegible] Wiley, [illegible] New York, pp. [illegible]

[illegible] S [illegible] Murray HW, Craybill [illegible] therapy [illegible] deficiency syndrome [illegible] 1984.

[illegible] Hughes [illegible] *Am J Med* [illegible] 1991.

[illegible] Tucker [illegible] AF [illegible] 124

[illegible] Scott [illegible] in [illegible] 1968.

[illegible] *Eng J Med* [illegible]

[illegible] Van [illegible] Wilkinson [illegible] adult [illegible]

[illegible] Denning [illegible] Lancet [illegible] [illegible] *N Engl J Med* [illegible] 1991.

[illegible] Mandell GL, [illegible] Douglas RG, Bennett JE, eds. Principles and Practice of Infectious Diseases. New York: Churchill Livingstone, 1990.

[illegible] *Ann Intern Med* [illegible] 1992.

[illegible] 133-151, 1991.

[illegible] antimicrobial therapy [illegible] 1992.

[illegible] activity [illegible] *N Engl J Med* [illegible] 1986.

[illegible] Houghton [illegible] *Antimicrob Agents Chemother* [illegible] 1988.

[illegible] *Clin* [illegible] 1991.

CHAPTER

12

Endocrine/Metabolism[a]

As an endocrinologist, I became involved in critical care medicine because hormones mediate the body's response to critical illness, and hormones are among the most valuable group of medications used in the treatment of critically ill patients. In this chapter, the reader is presented with valuable information regarding different hormones that are used in the treatment of acute illness. Certainly as a consequence of the stress hormone response to critical illness, hyperglycemia is common. For this reason, knowledge of the utilization of insulin therapy is requisite for the critical care practitioner. In addition, alterations of water metabolism (the syndrome of inappropriate antidiuretic hormone (ADH) or diabetes insipidus) are important problems that frequently confront the intensivist. For that reason, this chapter also includes information on antidiuretic hormone analogues.

Thyroid glandular dysfunction is common in intensive care unit patients and thus is included in this chapter. Similarly, calcium homeostasis is an issue that frequently arises and hence this important mineral is also discussed. In this chapter, the specific areas of concern addressed are:

[a]The material in this chapter was contributed by the following: Tables 12.1–12.3 were contributed by Gary P. Zaloga, M.D.; Tables 12.4 and 12.5 were contributed by Kenneth D. Burman, M.D., Col., M.C.; Tables 12.6–12.10, 12.12, and 12.13 were contributed by Gary P. Zaloga, M.D., and Bart Chernow, M.D.; Table 12.11 was contributed by John P. Grant, M.D., and Laurence H. Ross, M.D.

1. Relative activity of vasopressin peptides (Table 12.1)
2. Vasopressin analogues (Table 12.2)
3. Glucagon therapy (Table 12.3)
4. Pharmacology of agents used to treat hyperthyroidism (Table 12.4)
5. Pharmacology of agents used to treat hypothyroidism (Table 12.5)
6. Insulin preparations (Table 12.6)
7. Serum changes in the differential diagnosis of diabetic ketoacidosis (Table 12.7)
8. Treatment of diabetic ketoacidosis (Table 12.8)
9. Treatment of hyperglycemic hyperosmolar nonketotic syndrome (Table 12.9)
10. Insulin-drug interactions (Table 12.10)
11. Drug interference with urine glucose determinations (Table 12.11)
12. Calcium preparations (Table 12.12)
13. Magnesium supplements (Table 12.13)

TABLE 12.1. Relative Activity of Vasopressin Peptides

Receptor	*Antidiuretic (V2)*	*Pressor (V1)*
8-Arginine vasopressin	100	100
8-Lysine vasopressin	80	60
1-Desamino-8-*d*-arginine vasopressin (dDAVP)	1200	0.40

TABLE 12.2. Vasopressin Analogues

Agent	*Dose*	*Duration*	*Formulation*
Desmopressin (dDAVP)	10 μg i.n.[a]	12–24 h	2.5 and 5.0 ml for i.n. (100 μg/ml)
	or		
	1–2 μg i.v. or s.c. q12h	12–24 h	1- and 10-ml vials for i.v. or s.c. (4 μg/ml)
Aqueous vasopressin	1.6–2 mIU/kg/h i.v. or 5–10 U s.c. q4–6h; (children 3–5 U s.c.)	3–6 h 4–8 h	Pitressin 0.5- and 1.0-ml ampules; (20 U/ml)
Lysine vasopressin (lypressin)	2–4 U i.n. q4–6h	3–6 h	5-ml bottle (50 U/ml)

[a] i.n., intranasal.

TABLE 12.4. Pharmacology of Agents Used to Treat Hyperthyroidism[a]

Agent	*Maintenance Dose*	*Mechanism of Action*	*Common or Serious Adverse Effects*
Commonly used			
Propylthiouracil (6-propyl-2-thiouracil)	50–300 mg tid, p.o.	Inhibits thyroid hormone synthesis; inhibits T_4 extrathyroidal conversion to T_3[b]	Skin rash, nausea, epigastric distress, agranulocytosis, granulocytopenia, hepatitis, lupus-like syndrome
Methimazole (1-methyl-2-mercaptoimidazole)	5–30 mg tid, p.o.	Inhibits thyroid hormone synthesis	As above
dl-Propranolol or Atenolol[c]	10–80 mg qid, p.o. 50–100 mg, once daily, p.o.	Decreases β-adrenergic-mediated activity and helps ameliorate signs and symptoms of thyrotoxicosis	Cardiovascular, bronchospasm, central nervous system; must be used with care in patients with congestive heart failure or asthma
Nonroutine agents[d]			
Lithium carbonate	600 mg tid, p.o., to produce blood levels between 0.5 and 1.3 mEq/liter	Probably decreases thyroidal secretion and possibly inhibits extrathyroidal T_4 to T_3 conversion	Hand tremor, polyuria, drowsiness, lack of coordination, ataxia, blurred vision; may cause increased thyroid size and in certain subjects may cause either hypothyroidism or, rarely, hyperthyroidism

TABLE 12.4. *(Continued)*

Agent	*Maintenance Dose*	*Mechanism of Action*	*Common or Serious Adverse Effects*
Iodides[e]	5 drops SSKI tid, p.o., or 5 drops Lugol's solution tid, p.o.	Decreases thyroidal secretion	Parotitis or skin rash or serum sickness-like reaction; prolonged use may lead to unabated hypersecretion of thyroid hormone
Ipodate sodium[e]	3 g p.o. every 2–3 days or 1 g daily	Decreases thyroidal secretion and extrathyroidal T_4 to T_3 conversion	Skin rash, agranulocytosis, liver disease; should not be used in patients with history of iodide allergy

[a]The prescribing physician should be very knowledgeable with regard to the mechanism of action and potential warnings and side effects of these agents, and appropriately detailed textbooks or articles should be consulted prior to their use.

[b]T_4, *l*-thyroxine; T_3, triiodothyronine.

[c]Any β-adrenergic blocking agent can be used. *dl*-Propranolol has been utilized for the longest time and thus is preferred in some unusual circumstances (e.g., pregnancy). On the other hand, a cardioselective, long-acting blocker (e.g., atenolol) may have advantages in the routine thyrotoxic patient.

[d]None of these agents has been studied adequately in the prolonged treatment of hyperthyroidism. As a general rule these agents should not be utilized for longer than 1 month, since the potential complications have not been investigated and the likelihood of causing unabated thyrotoxicosis exists, especially with iodide-containing substances.

[e]Saturated solution potassium iodide (SSKI) (1 g/ml) contains 76.4% iodine. Five drops tid (assuming 20 drops/ml) gives about 573 mg iodine. Lugol's solution (125 mg/ml) of total iodine contains 5 g of iodine and 10 g of potassium iodide in each 100 ml. Five drops tid gives about 94 mg of iodine daily. It is assumed at present that the antithyroid action of ipodate is related partly to the release of iodides and partly to the ipodate molecule itself. Contains 61.4% iodine, so one 3-g dose of ipodate has 1842 mg of iodine. For purposes of this chapter, iodide and iodine are used interchangeably.

TABLE 12.5. Pharmacology of Agents Used to Treat Hypothyroidism[a]

Medication	*Maintenance Dose*	*Common or Serious Adverse Effects*
l-Thyroxine	0.075–0.200 mg daily (75–200 μg)	Precipitation or aggravation of cardiac disease, arrhythmias, angina pectoris; may aggravate diabetes mellitus and adrenal insufficiency
l-Triiodothyronine	25 μg tid or qid	As above

[a]These guidelines apply to the routine ambulatory patient with hypothyroidism; consult Chapter 44 in *The Pharmacologic Approach to the Critically Ill Patient*, Third Edition, for information on the treatment of myxedema coma.

TABLE 12.6. Insulin Preparations

Type of Insulin	Action	Protein	Peak s.c. Action (h)	Duration s.c. (hr)	Route	Concentration (U/ml)
Regular (crystalline)[a]	Rapid	None	1–3	5–7	i.v., s.c., i.m.	100
Semilente	Rapid	None	2–4	10–16	s.c.	100
NPH[a]	Intermediate	Protamine	6–14	18–28	s.c.	100
Lente[a]	Intermediate	None	6–14	18–28	s.c.	100
Ultralente[a]	Prolonged	None	18–24	30–40	s.c.	100
PZI	Prolonged	Protamine	18–24	30–40	s.c.	100

[a] Available as human insulin.

TABLE 12.7. Serum Changes in the Differential Diagnosis of Diabetic Ketoacidosis

Diagnosis	Glucose	Ketones	pH	Anion Gap	Sodium	Blood Urea Nitrogen
Diabetic ketoacidosis	3 +[a] (400–800 mg/dl)	3+	3–	2+	N to –	3 + (30–60 mg/dl)
Hyperglycemic hyperosmolar nonketotic syndrome	4 + (>600 mg/dl)	0 to +	–	N	N to 3+	4 + (70–90 mg/dl)
Alcoholic ketoacidosis	– to + (50–250 mg/dl)	+	+ –	+	+	N
Lactic acidosis	N	0 to +	3–	+	N to –	N to 3+
Hypoglycemia	2–	0 to +	N	N	N	N

[a] +, 2+, 3+, 4+: increased; –, 2–, 3–: decreased; N, normal.

TABLE 12.8. Treatment of Diabetic Ketoacidosis

Fluids

Give 1 liter of isotonic saline on admission followed by 1 liter in 1 h, 1 liter in 2 h, then 150–300 ml/h. If serum sodium rises above 150–155 mEq/liter, switch to 0.5 N saline. When plasma glucose falls below 250 mg/dl, switch to D_5W. Central hemodynamic monitoring may be required in elderly or in patients with cardiac or renal disease.

Insulin

Begin with continuous i.v. infusion of 0.5–1.0 U/h of regular insulin for each 100 mg/dl increase in blood glucose above 100 mg/dl (in isotonic saline). Increase infusion rate if glucose does not fall by 10%/h. When plasma glucose drops to 250 mg/dl, decrease i.v. infusion to 1–3 U of regular insulin per hour and continue until acidosis is corrected (glucose "clamp").

Alternative

Use 0.3 U of regular insulin per kg i.m. or s.c. initially, then 5–10 U of regular insulin i.m. or s.c. per hour; when glucose drops to 250 mg/dl, continue i.m. or s.c. injections at 2–4 h intervals using glucose clamp until acidosis clears. Give injections into deltoids.

Potassium

Give 20 mEq/h; if the patient is oliguric, give 5–10 mEq/h; if K^+ above 6 mEq/liter, stop infusion; if K^+ below 4 mEq/liter, increase infusion. Use continuous ECG monitoring.

Phosphorus

Oral: Neutra-Phos 250 mg q6h.

i.v.: potassium phosphate 0.08–0.16 mmol/kg/6 h. Measure serum phosphorous levels.

Bicarbonate

If arterial pH <7.1 or bicarbonate $<5–7$ mEq/liter, give ½ ampule of bicarbonate (22 mEq); if pH <7.0, give 1 ampule of bicarbonate (44 mEq); monitor arterial or venous pH hourly.

Magnesium

If less than 1.2 mg/dl, give:

Oral: Mg oxide 35 mEq q6–24h

i.v.: $MgSO_4$ or $MgCl_2$ 20–80 mEq/day

Monitor serum glucose, electrolytes, arterial blood gas, anion gap, and hemodynamic and mental status.

TABLE 12.9. Treatment of Hyperglycemic Hyperosmolar Nonketotic Syndrome

Fluids

Restore intravascular volume with isotonic saline, then:

Give 2–3 liters of hypotonic saline (0.45%) in first 2 h followed by one-half of the body water deficit (0.25 × total body water (kg) + urinary losses) over the next 12 h; give the remainder of the body water deficit over the next 24 h; central hemodynamic monitoring may be required in elderly or in those with cardiac or renal disease.

Insulin

Begin with i.v. infusion of 0.5–1.0 U of regular insulin for each 100 mg/dl increase in blood glucose above 100 mg/dl (in hypotonic saline). When serum glucose drops to 250 mg/dl, switch fluid to D_5W and decrease infusion rate of regular insulin to 1–3 U/h (glucose clamp technique). Maintain infusion for 24–36 h. Increase infusion rate if glucose does not fall by 10%/h.

Alternative

5–7 U of regular insulin i.m. or s.c. per hour; when glucose drops to 250 mg/dl, continue i.m. or s.c. injections at 2–4 h intervals using glucose clamp.

Potassium

Give 15–20 mEq/h; if the patient is oliguric, give 5–10 mEq/h; if K^+ above 6 mEq/liter, stop infusion of K^+; if K^+ below 4 mEq/liter, increase infusion rate. Use continuous ECG monitoring.

Phosphorus

Oral: Neutra-Phos 250 mg q6h.

i.v.: potassium phosphate 0.08–0.16 mmol/kg/6 h.

Bicarbonate

If arterial pH <7.1 or bicarbonate <5–7 mEq/liter, give ½ ampule of bicarbonate (22 mEq); if pH <7.0, give 1 ampule of bicarbonate (44 mEq); monitor arterial or venous pH hourly.

Magnesium

If less than 1.2 mg/dl, give:

p.o.: Mg oxide 35 mEq q6–24h.

i.v.: $MgSO_4$ or $MgCl_2$ 20–80 mEq/day.

Monitor serum glucose, electrolytes, arterial blood gas, anion gap, and hemodynamic and mental status.

TABLE 12.10. Insulin-Drug Interactions

Inhibit insulin secretion
Prostaglandin E (furosemide)
Thiazides
Phenytoin
Diazoxide
α-Adrenergic agonists
β-Adrenergic antagonists
Pentamidine
Verapamil
Somatostatin
Dopamine
Suppress insulin action or increase insulin requirements
Glucocorticoids
Oral contraceptives
l-Asparaginase
Growth hormone
Obesity
Pregnancy
Infection
Hyperthyroidism
Hyperadrenocorticalism
Stimulate insulin secretion
Sulfonylureas
Salicylates
Phentolamine
Prostaglandin inhibitors
Glucagon
β-Adrenergic agonists
Potentiate insulin action or decrease insulin requirements
Sulfonylureas
Clonidine
Dicumarol
Terramycin
Monoamine oxidase inhibitors
Endotoxin
Weight loss
Exercise
Renal insufficiency
Pentamidine
Hypothyroidism
Hypoadrenocorticalism

TABLE 12.11. Drug Interference with Urine Glucose Determinations[a,b]

Drug	Effect on Copper Reduction (Clinitest)	Effect on Glucose Oxidase (Tes-Tape)	Dealing with Potential Interferences
Cephalosporins Keflin Keflex Kefzol, Ancef Kafocin Loridine	False-positive (black-brown color)	No effect	Use glucose oxidase test
Vitamin C (in large doses)	False-positive	False-negative	Also may monitor blood glucose[b]
Aspirin and other salicylates (in very large doses)	False-positive	False-negative	Also may monitor blood glucose[b]
Aldomet (methyldopa) (in very large doses)	False-positive	No effect	Use glucose oxidase test
Benemid (probenecid)	False-positive	No effect	Use glucose oxidase test
Achromycin (tetracycline, injection only)	False-positive	False-negative	Also may monitor blood glucose[b]
Pyridium (phenazopyridine)	No effect	False-positive and false-negative	Use copper reduction method
Chloromycetin (chloramphenicol)	False-positive (potentially)	No effect	If in doubt, use glucose oxidase test
Levodopa (in large doses)	False-positive	False-negative	Also may monitor blood glucose[b]

[a]Reprinted with permission from Grant JP: *Handbook of Total Parenteral Nutrition.* WB Saunders, Philadelphia, 1980.

[b]*Note:* Potential interferences with glucose oxidase tests (Tes-Tape) can be eliminated by careful testing. While interfering substances will prevent color development in the part of the paper actually dipped into the urine sample, they will not prevent accurate development in a band across the very highest portion of the wetted tape. A true-negative test occurs when the band remains the same color as the rest of the tape, and a true-positive test occurs when the band changes to one of the colors shown on the color chart.)

TABLE 12.12. Calcium Preparations

	Dosage/Form	*Contents*[a]
Parenteral		
Ca^{2+} gluconate (10%)	10 ml	93 mg Ca^{2+} (4.6 mEq)
Ca^{2+} gluceptate	5 ml	90 mg Ca^{2+} (4.5 mEq)
Ca^{2+} chloride (10%)	10 ml	272 mg Ca^{2+} (13.6 mEq)
Oral		
Ca^{2+} carbonate (e.g., Os-cal 500)	Tablets	500 mg Ca^{2+}
Ca^{2+} gluconate	Tablets	500 mg Ca^{2+}
Ca^{2+} lactate	Tablets	650 mg Ca^{2+}
Ca^{2+} glubionate (e.g., Neo-calglucon)	Syrup	115 mg Ca^{2+}/5 ml

[a] Elemental Ca^{2+}.

TABLE 12.13. Magnesium Supplements[a]

Parenteral	
Mg^{2+} chloride	Loading: 1–2 g i.v. over 5–10 min
1 g = 118 mg Mg^{2+} = 9 mEq	Maintenance: 0.5–2 g/h by infusion
Mg^{2+} sulfate	
1 g = 98 mg Mg^{2+} = 8 mEq	
Enteral	
Mg^{2+} oxide tablets	20–80 mEq/day in divided doses
Tablet = 241 mg Mg^{2+} = 20 mEq	
Mg^{2+} gluconate tablets	20–80 mEq/day in divided doses
500-mg tablet = 27 mg Mg^{2+} = 2.3 mEq	

[a] 1 mEq = 0.5 mmol = 12.3 mg Mg^{2+}

INDEX

Page numbers followed by *t* and *f* indicate tables and figures, respectively.

A
Absorption, drug interactions affecting, 16*t*–19*t*
Absorption rate constant, 3*t*
Acebutolol
dosage adjustment
with dialysis, 64*t*–65*t*
in renal failure, 64*t*–65*t*
pharmacodynamics, in renal failure, 64*t*–65*t*
pharmacokinetics, in renal failure, 64*t*–65*t*
properties of, 221*t*, 232*t*–233*t*
Acecainide, secretion by kidney, 28*t*
Aceclidine
clinical uses, 264*t*–265*t*
side effects, 264*t*–265*t*
Acetaminophen
absorption, drug interactions affecting, 17*t*–18*t*
detoxification, in children, 185
disposition, effect of liver disease, 114*t*
dosage adjustment
with dialysis, 74*t*–75*t*
in liver disease, 114*t*
in renal failure, 74*t*–75*t*
drug interactions, 22*t*
fraction of dose excreted unchanged in urine with normal renal function, in children, 190*t*
hepatic/renal elimination, 114*t*
hepatitis, 185
hepatotoxicity, in children versus adults, 184–185
metabolism
induction by other drug(s), 20*t*
inhibition by other drug(s), 25*t*
overdose, 185
pharmacodynamics, 114*t*
in renal failure, 74*t*–75*t*
pharmacokinetics, 114*t*
in renal failure, 74*t*–75*t*
psychiatric side effects, 267*t*
Acetazolamide, secretion by kidney, 28*t*
Acetohexamide
dosage adjustment
with dialysis, 80*t*–81*t*
in renal failure, 80*t*–81*t*
pharmacodynamics, in renal failure, 80*t*–81*t*
pharmacokinetics, in renal failure, 80*t*–81*t*
N-Acetylcysteine
dosage adjustment
with dialysis, 82*t*–83*t*
in renal failure, 82*t*–83*t*
pharmacodynamics, in renal failure, 82*t*–83*t*
pharmacokinetics, in renal failure, 82*t*–83*t*
N-Acetylprocainamide
disposition, effect of liver disease, 120*t*
dosage adjustment
with dialysis, 66*t*–67*t*
in liver disease, 120*t*
in renal failure, 66*t*–67*t*
hepatic/renal elimination, 120*t*
pharmacodynamics, 120*t*
in renal failure, 66*t*–67*t*
pharmacokinetics, 120*t*
in renal failure, 66*t*–67*t*
secretion by kidney, 28*t*
Achromycin, interference with glucose determination, 382*t*
Acid peptic disease, pharmacotherapy for, 279–297
Acids, organic, renal secretion, 28*t*
Acinetobacter, antimicrobial drugs of choice for, 338*t*
Actinomyces, antimicrobial drugs of choice for, 339*t*
Acute hemorrhagic gastritis, 280
Acyclovir, 358–359
adverse effects of, 359
dosage adjustment
with dialysis, 60*t*–61*t*
in renal failure, 50*t*, 60*t*–61*t*, 336*t*
dosage and administration, 336*t*
drug interactions, with cyclosporine, 29*t*
fraction of dose excreted unchanged in urine with normal renal function, in children, 190*t*
half-life
in end-stage renal disease, 50*t*
normal, 50*t*
infusion, in pediatric patients, 188*t*
intraperitoneal administration, bioavailability after, 48*t*
pharmacodynamics, in renal failure, 60*t*–61*t*
pharmacokinetics, 336*t*
in renal failure, 60*t*–61*t*
psychiatric side effects, 268*t*
serum concentration, with dialysis, 336*t*
Acylated streptokinase/plasminogen complexes, doses with acute myocardial infarction, 240*t*
Adalat. *See* Nifedipine
Adenosine
adverse effects of, 232*t*–233*t*
dosage and administration, 232*t*–233*t*
in infants and children, 183
indications for, 232*t*

Adenosine—*continued*
in treatment of supraventricular tachycardia, 228*t*–229*t*
Adenosine arabinoside, 360
Administration
duration of, and effect of liver disease, 104–105
route of, and effect of liver disease, 104–105
β_2-Adrenergic agents, aerosol preparations and dosages, 158t
β-Adrenergic agents, route of administration, 156*t*
α_1-Adrenergic agonist, in treatment of supraventricular tachycardia, 228*t*–229*t*
β-Adrenergic agonists
clinical use, in asthma, 139–140
dosage, 157*t*
dosage adjustment
with dialysis, 64*t*–65*t*
in renal failure, 64*t*–65*t*
duration of action, 156*t*
pharmacodynamics
in critical illness, 8*t*–9*t*
in renal failure, 64*t*–65*t*
pharmacokinetics, in renal failure, 64*t*–65*t*
preparation, 157*t*
properties, 220*t*–221*t*, 232*t*–233*t*
psychiatric side effects, 270*t*
receptor, 156*t*
route of administration, 157*t*
in treatment of supraventricular tachycardia, 228*t*–229*t*
use, clinical settings that influence, 220*t*–221*t*
β_2-Adrenergic agonists, in treatment of hyperkalemia, 86*t*–87*t*
Adrenocorticosteroids, psychiatric side effects, 269*t*
Adrenocorticotropic hormone, antiemetic effects, 318
Adriamycin
disposition, effect of liver disease, 115*t*
dosage adjustment, in liver disease, 115*t*
hepatic/renal elimination, 115*t*
pharmacodynamics, 115*t*
pharmacokinetics, 115*t*
Adult respiratory distress syndrome, pharmacologic approach to patient with, 141–144
Adverse effects. *See also specific drug*
in pediatric patients, 182–187
Albuterol
dosage, 157*t*
dosage adjustment
with dialysis, 78*t*–79*t*
in renal failure, 78*t*–79*t*
duration of action, 156*t*
pharmacodynamics, in renal failure, 78*t*–79*t*
pharmacokinetics, in renal failure, 78*t*–79*t*
preparation, 157*t*
receptor, 156*t*
route of administration, 156*t*–157*t*
Alcoholic myopathy, interactions with muscle relaxants, 208*t*–209*t*
Aldomet, interference with glucose determination, 382*t*
Alfentanil
cost, 201*t*
disposition, effect of liver disease, 124*t*
dosage, in mechanically ventilated patients, 201*t*
dosage adjustment
with dialysis, 74*t*–75*t*, 82*t*–83*t*
in liver disease, 124*t*
in renal failure, 74*t*–75*t*, 82*t*–83*t*
hepatic/renal elimination, 124*t*
metabolism, inhibition by other drug(s), 23*t*
pharmacodynamics, 124*t*
in renal failure, 74*t*–75*t*, 82*t*–83*t*
pharmacokinetics, 124*t*
in renal failure, 74*t*–75*t*, 82*t*–83*t*
use, in adult ICU patients, 204*t*–205*t*
Allopurinol
dosage adjustment
with dialysis, 78*t*–79*t*
in renal failure, 78*t*–79*t*
drug interactions, 22*t*
pharmacodynamics, in renal failure, 78*t*–79*t*
pharmacokinetics, in renal failure, 78*t*–79*t*
Alprazolam
dosage adjustment
with dialysis, 70*t*–71*t*
in renal failure, 70*t*–71*t*
metabolism, inhibition by other drug(s), 24*t*
pharmacodynamics, in renal failure, 70*t*–71*t*
pharmacokinetics, in renal failure, 70*t*–71*t*
Altace. *See* Ramipril
Aluminum hydroxide, 281–283
Amantadine
disposition, effect of liver disease, 110*t*
dosage adjustment
in liver disease, 110*t*
in renal failure, 336*t*
dosage and administration, 336*t*
hepatic/renal elimination, 110*t*
pharmacodynamics, 110*t*
pharmacokinetics, 110*t*, 336*t*
psychiatric side effects, 269*t*
secretion by kidney, 28*t*

serum concentration, with dialysis, 336*t*
Amikacin, 345–347, 355
disposition, effect of liver disease, 110*t*
dosage adjustment
with dialysis, 52*t*–53*t*
in liver disease, 110*t*
in renal failure, 52*t*–53*t*, 335*t*
dosage and administration, 335*t*
hepatic/renal elimination, 110*t*
infusion, in pediatric patients, 188*t*
intraperitoneal administration, bioavailability after, 48*t*
pharmacodynamics, 110*t*
in renal failure, 52*t*–53*t*
pharmacokinetics, 110*t*, 335*t*
in renal failure, 52*t*–53*t*
serum concentration, with dialysis, 335*t*
volume of distribution, in renal failure, 47*t*
Amiloride
dosage adjustment
with dialysis, 68*t*–69*t*
in renal failure, 68*t*–69*t*
dosage and administration, 84*t*
half-life, 84*t*
pharmacodynamics, in renal failure, 68*t*–69*t*
pharmacokinetics, in renal failure, 68*t*–69*t*
secretion by kidney, 28*t*
site of action, 84*t*
Aminocaproic acid, psychiatric side effects, 269*t*
Aminoglutethimide, psychiatric side effects, 268*t*
Aminoglycosides, 345–347
absorption, drug interactions affecting, 18*t*
adverse effects of, 346–347
distribution, 346
dosage adjustment
with dialysis, 52*t*–53*t*
in renal failure, 50*t*, 52*t*–53*t*, 335*t*
dosage and administration, 335*t*
drug interactions
with cyclosporine, 29*t*
with nondepolarizing muscle relaxants, 207*t*
elimination, 346
fraction of dose excreted unchanged in urine with normal renal function, in children, 190*t*
half-life
in end-stage renal disease, 50*t*
normal, 50*t*
intraperitoneal administration, bioavailability after, 48*t*
monitoring guidelines, 7*t*
nephrotoxicity, 346–347
ototoxicity, 346
pharmacodynamics, in renal failure, 52*t*–53*t*
pharmacokinetic parameters, 6*t*
pharmacokinetics, 335*t*
in renal failure, 52*t*–53*t*
psychiatric side effects, 268*t*
serum concentration, with dialysis, 335*t*
serum level, 347
toxicity, protection against, in children, 186
p-Aminohippurate, secretion by kidney, 28*t*
Aminophylline
clinical use, in asthma, 140
infusion, in pediatric patients, 188*t*
Aminosalicylates, 318–321
5-Aminosalicylic acid, 319–321
Amiodarone
adverse effects of, 232*t*–233*t*
dosage adjustment
with dialysis, 64*t*–65*t*
in renal failure, 64*t*–65*t*
dosage and administration, 232*t*–233*t*
drug interactions, 22*t*
indications for, 232*t*
pharmacodynamics, in renal failure, 64*t*–65*t*
pharmacokinetics, in renal failure, 64*t*–65*t*
psychiatric side effects, 269*t*
Amitriptyline
dosage adjustment
with dialysis, 72*t*–73*t*
in renal failure, 72*t*–73*t*
metabolism, inhibition by other drug(s), 24*t*
pharmacodynamics, in renal failure, 72*t*–73*t*
pharmacokinetics, in renal failure, 72*t*–73*t*
Amlodipine
dosage adjustment
with dialysis, 66*t*–67*t*
in renal failure, 66*t*–67*t*
pharmacodynamics, in renal failure, 66*t*–67*t*
pharmacokinetics, in renal failure, 66*t*–67*t*
Amodiaquine, psychiatric side effects, 268*t*
Amphetamine, elimination, 10*t*
Amphojel, 282*t*
Amphotericin, fraction of dose excreted unchanged in urine with normal renal function, in children, 190*t*
Amphotericin B, 355–357
adverse effects of, 356
dosage adjustment
with dialysis, 60*t*–61*t*

Amphotericin B—*continued*
in renal failure, 60*t*–61*t*, 336*t*
dosage and administration, 336*t*
drug interactions, with cyclosporine, 29*t*
infusion, in pediatric patients, 188*t*
pharmacodynamics, in renal failure, 60*t*–61*t*
pharmacokinetics, 336*t*
in renal failure, 60*t*–61*t*
psychiatric side effects, 268*t*
serum concentration, with dialysis, 336*t*
test dose, 355
Ampicillin, 341
disposition, effect of liver disease, 110*t*
dosage adjustment
with dialysis, 56*t*–57*t*
in liver disease, 110*t*
in renal failure, 56*t*–57*t*, 334*t*
dosage and administration, 334*t*
fraction of dose excreted unchanged in urine with normal renal function, in children, 190*t*
hepatic/renal elimination, 110*t*
pharmacodynamics, 110*t*
in renal failure, 56*t*–57*t*
pharmacokinetics, 110*t*, 334*t*
in renal failure, 56*t*–57*t*
psychiatric side effects, 267*t*
serum concentration, with dialysis, 334*t*
Ampicillin/sulbactam, 333
dosage adjustment, in renal failure, 334*t*
dosage and administration, 334*t*
intraperitoneal administration, bioavailability after, 48*t*
pharmacokinetics, 334*t*
serum concentration, with dialysis, 334*t*
Amrinone
dosage adjustment
with dialysis, 70*t*–71*t*
in renal failure, 70*t*–71*t*
infusion (Inocor), 238*t*–239*t*
in children, 192*t*
pharmacodynamics, in renal failure, 70*t*–71*t*
pharmacokinetics, in renal failure, 70*t*–71*t*
Amylobarbital
disposition, effect of liver disease, 122*t*
dosage adjustment, in liver disease, 122*t*
hepatic/renal elimination, 122*t*
pharmacodynamics, 122*t*
pharmacokinetics, 122*t*
Amyotrophic lateral sclerosis, interactions with muscle relaxants, 208*t*–209*t*
Anabolic steroids, psychiatric side effects, 269*t*
Anaerobes, antimicrobial drugs of choice for, 339*t*
Analgesics
disposition, effect of liver disease, 114*t*–115*t*
dosage adjustment, in liver disease, 114*t*–115*t*
hepatic/renal elimination, 114*t*–115*t*
monitoring guidelines, 7*t*
pharmacodynamics, 114*t*–115*t*
pharmacokinetic parameters, 6*t*
pharmacokinetics, 114*t*–115*t*
psychiatric side effects, 267*t*
Ancef, interference with glucose determination, 382*t*
Angiotensin-converting enzyme inhibitors
dosage adjustment
with dialysis, 62*t*–63*t*
in renal failure, 62*t*–63*t*
oral, properties of, 223*t*
pharmacodynamics
in critical illness, 10*t*–11*t*
in renal failure, 62*t*–63*t*
pharmacokinetics, in renal failure, 62*t*–63*t*
Antacids, 280–284
aluminum compounds, 281–283
adverse effects, 281–283
calcium compounds, 283–284
composition, 282*t*
dosage and administration, 280–281
drug interactions, 281
magnesium compounds, 283
mechanisms of action, 280
neutralizing capacity, 282*t*
route of administration, 280
Anthelminthics, psychiatric side effects, 267*t*
Anthraquinone derivatives, laxative effect, 316
Antiarrhythmic agents, 230*t*–233*t*
dosage adjustment
with dialysis, 64*t*–67*t*
in renal failure, 64*t*–67*t*
monitoring guidelines, 7*t*
pharmacodynamics
in critical illness, 8*t*–9*t*
in renal failure, 64*t*–67*t*
pharmacokinetics, 6*t*
in renal failure, 64*t*–67*t*
psychiatric side effects, 269*t*
Antiasthmatics
monitoring guidelines, 7*t*
pharmacokinetic parameters, 6*t*
Antibacterial agents, 332–353
Antibiotics
cost, 365
disposition, effect of liver disease, 110*t*

dosage adjustment, in liver disease, 110t–114t
hepatic/renal elimination, 110t
infusion, in pediatric patients, 188t
pharmacodynamics, 110t
pharmacokinetics, 110t
psychiatric side effects, 267t
Anticancer drugs
disposition, effect of liver disease, 115t–116t
dosage adjustment, in liver disease, 115t–116t
hepatic/renal elimination, 115t–116t
pharmacodynamics, 115t–116t
pharmacokinetics, 115t–116t
Anticholinergics, 261t
psychiatric side effects, 268t–269t
Anticholinesterases
clinical uses, 264t–265t
side effects, 264t–265t
in treatment of supraventricular tachycardia, 228t–229t
Anticonvulsants
dosage adjustment
with dialysis, 76t–77t
in renal failure, 76t–77t
drug interactions, 20t–21t
monitoring guidelines, 7t
pharmacodynamics, in renal failure, 76t–77t
pharmacokinetics, 6t
in renal failure, 76t–77t
psychiatric side effects, 267t
Antidiarrheal agents, 297–302
Antiemetics, 316–318
Antiepileptic agents
disposition, in liver disease, 116t
dosage adjustment
effect of liver disease, 116t
in liver disease, 116t
hepatic/renal elimination, 116t
pharmacodynamics, 116t
pharmacokinetics, 116t
Antifungal agents, 355–358
disposition, effect of liver disease, 110t
dosage adjustment
with dialysis, 60t–61t
in liver disease, 110t–114t
in renal failure, 60t–61t, 336t
dosage and administration, 336t
hepatic/renal elimination, 110t
pharmacodynamics, 110t
in renal failure, 60t–61t
pharmacokinetics, 110t, 336t
in renal failure, 60t–61t
psychiatric side effects, 267t
serum concentration, with dialysis, 336t
Antihistamines
antiemetic properties of, 317
dosage adjustment
with dialysis, 78t–79t
in renal failure, 78t–79t
pharmacodynamics, in renal failure, 78t–79t
pharmacokinetics, in renal failure, 78t–79t
psychiatric side effects, 268t
Antihypertensive agents
dosage adjustment
with dialysis, 60t–64t
in renal failure, 60t–64t
monitoring guidelines, 7t
pharmacodynamics, in renal failure, 60t–64t
pharmacokinetics, 6t
in renal failure, 60t–64t
psychiatric side effects, 270t
Antihypertensive therapy, 218t–219t
combination, effects of, 224t
oral angiotensin-converting enzyme inhibitors for, properties of, 223t
oral calcium channel blockers for, properties of, 222t
Antiinflammatory agents
disposition, effect of liver disease, 117t–118t
dosage adjustment, in liver disease, 117t–118t
hepatic/renal elimination, 117t–118t
pharmacodynamics, 117t–118t
pharmacokinetics, 117t–118t
psychiatric side effects, 267t
Antimicrobial agents, 331–369
additive or synergistic drug combinations, 362
bioavailability, in patients with and without peritonitis, 48t–49t
choice, 362–365
epidemiologic and other factors, 364–365
clinical use, in critically ill patients, 361–365
dosage adjustment
with dialysis, 52t–60t
in renal failure, 52t–60t
intraperitoneal administration, bioavailability after, 48t–49t
mechanism of action, 362
monitoring, 363
guidelines, 7t
pharmacodynamics, in renal failure, 52t–60t
pharmacokinetics, 6t
in renal failure, 52t–60t
pharmacology, 361
Antimicrobial therapy, empiric, 363–364
Antimuscarinic agents, 263t
clinical uses, 264t–265t
side effects, 264t–265t
Antimycobacterial agents, 353–355
dosage adjustment, in renal failure, 335t

Antimycobacterial agents—*continued*
dosage and administration, 335*t*
pharmacokinetics, 335*t*
serum concentration, with dialysis, 335*t*
Antineoplastics, psychiatric side effects, 268*t*
Antiparkinsonians, psychiatric side effects, 269*t*
Antiprotozoal/antipneumocystis agents, 360–361
dosage adjustment, in renal failure, 335*t*
dosage and administration, 335*t*
pharmacokinetics, 335*t*
serum concentration, with dialysis, 335*t*
Antipyretic agents
disposition, effect of liver disease, 117*t*–118*t*
dosage adjustment, in liver disease, 117*t*–118*t*
hepatic/renal elimination, 117*t*–118*t*
pharmacodynamics, 117*t*–118*t*
pharmacokinetics, 117*t*–118*t*
Antipyrine
disposition, effect of liver disease, 117*t*
dosage adjustment, in liver disease, 117*t*
hepatic/renal elimination, 117*t*
metabolism, inhibition by other drug(s), 22*t*
pharmacodynamics, 117*t*
pharmacokinetics, 117*t*
Antithrombotic agents
dosage adjustment
with dialysis, 76*t*–77*t*
in renal failure, 76*t*–77*t*
pharmacodynamics, in renal failure, 76*t*–77*t*
pharmacokinetics, in renal failure, 76*t*–77*t*
Antitubercular agents, 353–355
dosage adjustment
with dialysis, 52*t*–53*t*
in renal failure, 52*t*–53*t*
pharmacodynamics, in renal failure, 52*t*–53*t*
pharmacokinetics, in renal failure, 52*t*–53*t*
Antiulcer agents
dosage adjustment
with dialysis, 78*t*–79*t*
in renal failure, 78*t*–79*t*
monitoring guidelines, 7*t*
pharmacodynamics, in renal failure, 78*t*–79*t*
pharmacokinetics, 6*t*
in renal failure, 78*t*–79*t*
Antiviral agents, 358–360
disposition, effect of liver disease, 110*t*
dosage adjustment
with dialysis, 60*t*–61*t*
in liver disease, 110*t*–114*t*
in renal failure, 60*t*–61*t*, 336*t*
dosage and administration, 336*t*
hepatic/renal elimination, 110*t*
pharmacodynamics, 110*t*
in renal failure, 60*t*–61*t*
pharmacokinetics, 110*t*, 336*t*
in renal failure, 60*t*–61*t*
psychiatric side effects, 268*t*
serum concentration, with dialysis, 336*t*
Anxiety, drugs causing, 267*t*–270*t*
Anxiolytics
cost, 201*t*
dosage, in mechanically ventilated patients, 201*t*
Apparent volume of distribution, 96
Aqueous crystalline penicillin G
dosage adjustment, in renal failure, 334*t*
dosage and administration, 334*t*
pharmacokinetics, 334*t*
serum concentration, with dialysis, 334*t*
Arachnia, antimicrobial drugs of choice for, 339*t*
8-Arginine vasopressin, activity, 372*t*
Arterial disease, causing acute ischemic event, management of, 257*f*
Arthritis and gout agents
dosage adjustment
with dialysis, 78*t*–79*t*
in renal failure, 78*t*–79*t*
pharmacodynamics, in renal failure, 78*t*–79*t*
pharmacokinetics, in renal failure, 78*t*–79*t*
Asparaginase, psychiatric side effects, 268*t*
Aspirin
dosage adjustment
with dialysis, 76*t*–77*t*
in renal failure, 76*t*–77*t*
interference with glucose determination, 382*t*
pharmacodynamics, in renal failure, 76*t*–77*t*
pharmacokinetics, in renal failure, 76*t*–77*t*
Asthma, pharmacologic approach to patient with, 139–140
Atenolol
absorption, drug interactions affecting, 16*t*
disposition, effect of liver disease, 118*t*
dosage adjustment
with dialysis, 64*t*–65*t*
in liver disease, 118*t*
in renal failure, 64*t*–65*t*

fraction of dose excreted unchanged in urine with normal renal function, in children, 190*t*
hepatic/renal elimination, 118*t*
pharmacodynamics, 118*t*
in renal failure, 64*t*–65*t*
pharmacokinetics, 118*t*
in renal failure, 64*t*–65*t*
pharmacology of, 375*t*
properties of, 220*t*, 232*t*–233*t*
Atracurium
characteristics of, 210*t*–211*t*
clearance, 213*t*
clinical pharmacology of, 206*t*–207*t*
cost, 201*t*
disposition, effect of liver disease, 124*t*
dosage
in children, 193*t*
in mechanically ventilated patients, 201*t*
dosage adjustment
with dialysis, 82*t*–83*t*
in liver disease, 124*t*
in renal failure, 82*t*–83*t*
duration of clinical effect, 206*t*
fraction of dose excreted unchanged in urine with normal renal function, in children, 190*t*
hepatic/renal elimination, 124*t*
infusion, in pediatric patients, 188*t*
intubating dose, 206*t*
metabolism, 213*t*
pharmacodynamics, 124*t*
in renal failure, 82*t*–83*t*
pharmacokinetics, 124*t*
in renal failure, 82*t*–83*t*
side effects and adverse reactions to, 210*t*–211*t*
use during mechanical ventilation, 203*t*
Atropine
clinical uses, 264*t*–265*t*
effects of, 263*t*
indications for, 263*t*
side effects, 264*t*–265*t*
in treatment of bradycardia, 230*t*–231*t*
Autoregulation, cerebral, coexistent cerebral vasodilatory stimuli and, 272*f*
Azacitidine, psychiatric side effects, 268*t*
Azathioprine, psychiatric side effects, 268*t*
Azidothymidine, 360
dosage adjustment, in renal failure, 336*t*
dosage and administration, 336*t*
pharmacokinetics, 336*t*
psychiatric side effects, 268*t*
serum concentration, with dialysis, 336*t*
Azithromycin, 355
dosage adjustment
with dialysis, 56*t*–57*t*
in renal failure, 56*t*–57*t*
pharmacodynamics, in renal failure, 56*t*–57*t*
pharmacokinetics, in renal failure, 56*t*–57*t*
Azlocillin, 341
volume of distribution, in renal failure, 47*t*
AZT. *See* Azidothymidine
Aztreonam, 344–345
disposition, effect of liver disease, 110*t*
dosage adjustment
with dialysis, 54*t*–55*t*
in liver disease, 110*t*
in renal failure, 54*t*–55*t*, 334*t*
dosage and administration, 334*t*
hepatic/renal elimination, 110*t*
intraperitoneal administration, bioavailability after, 48*t*
pharmacodynamics, 110*t*
in renal failure, 54*t*–55*t*
pharmacokinetics, 110*t*, 334*t*
in renal failure, 54*t*–55*t*
serum concentration, with dialysis, 334*t*

B
Baclofen, psychiatric side effects, 269*t*
Bacteria, antimicrobial drugs of choice for, 338*t*–339*t*
Bacterial agents, 362–363
Bacteroides, antimicrobial drugs of choice for, 339*t*
Barbiturates
adverse effects of, in pediatric patients, 183
dosage adjustment
with dialysis, 70*t*–71*t*
in renal failure, 70*t*–71*t*
pharmacodynamics, in renal failure, 70*t*–71*t*
pharmacokinetics, in renal failure, 70*t*–71*t*
psychiatric side effects, 267*t*
removal, by resin hemoperfusion, 11*t*
Bases, organic, renal secretion, 28*t*
Benazepril
dosage adjustment
with dialysis, 62*t*–63*t*
in renal failure, 62*t*–63*t*
pharmacodynamics, in renal failure, 62*t*–63*t*
pharmacokinetics, in renal failure, 62*t*–63*t*
properties of, 223*t*
Bendroflumethiazide, dosage and administration, 85*t*
Benemid, interference with glucose determination, 382*t*
Benzamide, 318

Benzodiazepines
absorption, drug interactions affecting, 18*t*
dosage adjustment
with dialysis, 70*t*–73*t*
in renal failure, 70*t*–73*t*
dosage and administration, 247*t*–248*t*
intravenous, characteristics of, 202*t*–203*t*
metabolism, inhibition by other drug(s), 23*t*–24*t*
pharmacodynamics, in renal failure, 70*t*–73*t*
pharmacokinetics, in renal failure, 70*t*–73*t*
pharmacology of, 247*t*–248*t*
properties of, 247*t*–248*t*
Benzthiazide, dosage and administration, 85*t*
Betamethasone
dosage adjustment
with dialysis, 80*t*–81*t*
in renal failure, 80*t*–81*t*
pharmacodynamics, in renal failure, 80*t*–81*t*
pharmacokinetics, in renal failure, 80*t*–81*t*
Betaxolol, properties of, 221*t*
Bethanechol, 303–305
clinical uses, 264*t*–265*t*
contraindications, 304–305
dosage, 304
pharmacokinetics, 304
side effects, 264*t*–265*t*, 304
Bioavailability, of enzyme-limited drugs, 105
Bisacodyl, 316
suppository, properties of, 313*t*
tablets, properties of, 313*t*
Bishydroxycoumarin
absorption, drug interactions affecting, 16*t*, 18*t*
drug interactions, 22*t*
Bismuth salicylates, 299–300
Bitolterol
duration of action, 156*t*
receptor, 156*t*
route of administration, 156*t*
Bleomycin
disposition, effect of liver disease, 115*t*
dosage adjustment, in liver disease, 115*t*
hepatic/renal elimination, 115*t*
pharmacodynamics, 115*t*
pharmacokinetics, 115*t*
psychiatric side effects, 268*t*
Blocadren. *See* Timolol
Blood
drug concentration, 1–2
free fraction of drug in, 101
Bradycardia, drugs used to treat, 230*t*–231*t*
Bretylium
adverse effects of, 232*t*–233*t*
dosage adjustment
with dialysis, 66*t*–67*t*
in renal failure, 66*t*–67*t*
dosage and administration, 232*t*–233*t*
indications for, 232*t*
infusion, in pediatric patients, 188*t*
pharmacodynamics, in renal failure, 66*t*–67*t*
pharmacokinetics, in renal failure, 66*t*–67*t*
volume of distribution, in renal failure, 47*t*
Bromocriptine
absorption, drug interactions affecting, 19*t*
psychiatric side effects, 269*t*
Bulk laxatives, 312
Bumetanide
disposition, effect of liver disease, 121*t*
dosage adjustment
with dialysis, 68*t*–69*t*
in liver disease, 121*t*
in renal failure, 68*t*–69*t*
dosage and administration, 84*t*
half-life, 84*t*
hepatic/renal elimination, 121*t*
pharmacodynamics, 121*t*
in renal failure, 68*t*–69*t*
pharmacokinetics, 121*t*
in renal failure, 68*t*–69*t*
site of action, 84*t*
Bupropion, psychiatric side effects, 269*t*
Burn, interactions with muscle relaxants, 208*t*–209*t*
Buspirone
dosage adjustment
with dialysis, 72*t*–73*t*
in renal failure, 72*t*–73*t*
pharmacodynamics, in renal failure, 72*t*–73*t*
pharmacokinetics, in renal failure, 72*t*–73*t*
Butorphanol
dosage adjustment
with dialysis, 74*t*–75*t*
in renal failure, 74*t*–75*t*
pharmacodynamics, in renal failure, 74*t*–75*t*
pharmacokinetics, in renal failure, 74*t*–75*t*

C
Caffeine
disposition, effect of liver disease, 125*t*
dosage adjustment, in liver disease, 125*t*
hepatic/renal elimination, 125*t*
metabolism, inhibition by other drug(s), 27*t*

pharmacodynamics, 125*t*
pharmacokinetics, 125*t*
Calan. *See* Verapamil
Calcium
homeostasis, 371
preparations, 383*t*
Calcium carbonate, 283–284
Calcium channel blockers
dosage adjustment
with dialysis, 66*t*–69*t*
in renal failure, 66*t*–69*t*
drug interactions, 22*t*
pharmacodynamics
in critical illness, 8*t*–9*t*
in renal failure, 66*t*–69*t*
pharmacokinetics, in renal failure, 66*t*–69*t*
properties of, 222*t*
psychiatric side effects, 270*t*
in treatment of supraventricular tachycardia, 228*t*–229*t*
Calcium gluconate, in treatment of hyperkalemia, 86*t*–87*t*
Calcium polycarbophil, 312
Campylobacter, antimicrobial drugs of choice for, 338*t*
Cannabinols, 318
Capoten. *See* Captopril
Captopril
absorption, drug interactions affecting, 16*t*
disposition, effect of liver disease, 118*t*
dosage adjustment
with dialysis, 62*t*–63*t*
in liver disease, 118*t*
in renal failure, 62*t*–63*t*
hepatic/renal elimination, 118*t*
for hypertensive urgencies, 228*t*–229*t*
pharmacodynamics, 118*t*
in renal failure, 62*t*–63*t*
pharmacokinetics, 118*t*
in renal failure, 62*t*–63*t*
properties of, 223*t*
psychiatric side effects, 270*t*
secretion by kidney, 28*t*
Carbachol
clinical uses, 264*t*–265*t*
side effects, 264*t*–265*t*
Carbamazepine
absorption, drug interactions affecting, 16*t*
disposition, in liver disease, 116*t*
dosage adjustment
with dialysis, 76*t*–77*t*
effect of liver disease, 116*t*
in renal failure, 76*t*–77*t*
drug interactions, 21*t*, 249*t*–250*t*
with cyclosporine, 29*t*
hepatic/renal elimination, 116*t*
metabolism
induction by other drug(s), 20*t*
inhibition by other drug(s), 22*t*–25*t*, 27*t*
pharmacodynamics, 116*t*
in renal failure, 76*t*–77*t*
pharmacokinetics, 116*t*
in renal failure, 76*t*–77*t*
Carbapenem, 344
dosage adjustment
with dialysis, 54*t*–55*t*
in renal failure, 54*t*–55*t*
pharmacodynamics, in renal failure, 54*t*–55*t*
pharmacokinetics, in renal failure, 54*t*–55*t*
Carbenicillin
disposition, effect of liver disease, 110*t*
dosage adjustment
in liver disease, 110*t*
in renal failure, 334*t*
dosage and administration, 334*t*
hepatic/renal elimination, 110*t*
pharmacodynamics, 110*t*
pharmacokinetics, 110*t*, 334*t*
serum concentration, with dialysis, 334*t*
Carbidopa, psychiatric side effects, 269*t*
Carbomethylcellulose sodium, 312
Carbonic anhydrase inhibitors
dosage and administration, 84*t*
half-life, 84*t*
psychiatric side effects, 270*t*
site of action, 84*t*
Cardene. *See* Nicardipine
Cardiac glycosides
dosage adjustment
with dialysis, 68*t*–69*t*
in renal failure, 68*t*–69*t*
pharmacodynamics, in renal failure, 68*t*–69*t*
pharmacokinetics, in renal failure, 68*t*–69*t*
Cardiac pacemakers, implantation, guidelines for, 234*t*
Cardiac pacing, temporary, indications for, 234*t*
Cardiovascular agents, 215–239
disposition, effect of liver disease, 118*t*–121*t*
dosage adjustment
with dialysis, 64*t*–70*t*
in liver disease, 118*t*–121*t*
in renal failure, 64*t*–70*t*
hepatic/renal elimination, 118*t*–121*t*
pharmacodynamics, 118*t*–121*t*
in renal failure, 64*t*–70*t*
pharmacokinetics, 118*t*–121*t*
in renal failure, 64*t*–70*t*
psychiatric side effects, 269*t*
Cardizem. *See* Diltiazem
Carprofen, metabolism, inhibition by other drug(s), 26*t*

Carteolol
dosage adjustment
with dialysis, 64*t*–65*t*
in renal failure, 64*t*–65*t*
pharmacodynamics, in renal failure, 64*t*–65*t*
pharmacokinetics, in renal failure, 64*t*–65*t*
properties of, 221*t*
Cartrol. *See* Carteolol
Castor oil, 316
properties of, 313*t*
Catecholamines
concentration, and effect, 237*f*
duration of action, 156*t*
receptor, 156*t*
route of administration, 156*t*
Cefaclor
disposition, effect of liver disease, 110*t*
dosage adjustment, in liver disease, 110*t*
hepatic/renal elimination, 110*t*
pharmacodynamics, 110*t*
pharmacokinetics, 110*t*
Cefamandole, 342–343
disposition, effect of liver disease, 110*t*
dosage adjustment
with dialysis, 54*t*–55*t*
in liver disease, 110*t*
in renal failure, 54*t*–55*t*, 334*t*
dosage and administration, 334*t*
hepatic/renal elimination, 110*t*
intraperitoneal administration, bioavailability after, 48*t*
pharmacodynamics, 110*t*
in renal failure, 54*t*–55*t*
pharmacokinetics, 110*t*, 334*t*
in renal failure, 54*t*–55*t*
serum concentration, with dialysis, 334*t*
Cefazolin, 342–343
disposition, effect of liver disease, 110*t*
dosage adjustment
with dialysis, 54*t*–55*t*
in liver disease, 110*t*
in renal failure, 54*t*–55*t*, 334*t*
dosage and administration, 334*t*
fraction of dose excreted unchanged in urine with normal renal function, in children, 190*t*
hepatic/renal elimination, 110*t*
intraperitoneal administration, bioavailability after, 48*t*
pharmacodynamics, 110*t*
in renal failure, 54*t*–55*t*
pharmacokinetics, 110*t*, 334*t*
in renal failure, 54*t*–55*t*
serum concentration, with dialysis, 334*t*
volume of distribution, in renal failure, 47*t*
Cefmenoxime
dosage adjustment
with dialysis, 54*t*–55*t*
in renal failure, 54*t*–55*t*
pharmacodynamics, in renal failure, 54*t*–55*t*
pharmacokinetics, in renal failure, 54*t*–55*t*
Cefmetazole, 342
dosage adjustment
with dialysis, 54*t*–55*t*
in renal failure, 54*t*–55*t*
pharmacodynamics, in renal failure, 54*t*–55*t*
pharmacokinetics, in renal failure, 54*t*–55*t*
Cefonicid
dosage adjustment
with dialysis, 54*t*–55*t*
in renal failure, 54*t*–55*t*
pharmacodynamics, in renal failure, 54*t*–55*t*
pharmacokinetics, in renal failure, 54*t*–55*t*
volume of distribution, in renal failure, 47*t*
Cefoperazone, 343
disposition, effect of liver disease, 111*t*
dosage adjustment
with dialysis, 54*t*–55*t*
in liver disease, 111*t*
in renal failure, 50*t*, 54*t*–55*t*
fraction of dose excreted unchanged in urine with normal renal function, in children, 190*t*
half-life
in end-stage renal disease, 50*t*
normal, 50*t*
hepatic/renal elimination, 111*t*
intraperitoneal administration, bioavailability after, 48*t*
pharmacodynamics, 111*t*
in renal failure, 54*t*–55*t*
pharmacokinetics, 111*t*
in renal failure, 54*t*–55*t*
Cefoperazone-sulbactam
dosage adjustment, in renal failure, 334*t*
dosage and administration, 334*t*
pharmacokinetics, 334*t*
serum concentration, with dialysis, 334*t*
Cefotaxime, 342–343
disposition, effect of liver disease, 111*t*
dosage adjustment
with dialysis, 54*t*–55*t*
in liver disease, 111*t*
in renal failure, 54*t*–55*t*, 334*t*
dosage and administration, 334*t*
fraction of dose excreted unchanged in urine with normal renal function, in children, 190*t*

hepatic/renal elimination, 111*t*
intraperitoneal administration, bioavailability after, 48*t*
pharmacodynamics, 111*t*
in renal failure, 54*t*–55*t*
pharmacokinetics, 111*t*, 334*t*
in renal failure, 54*t*–55*t*
serum concentration, with dialysis, 334*t*
Cefotetan, 342
disposition, effect of liver disease, 111*t*
dosage adjustment
with dialysis, 54*t*–55*t*
in liver disease, 111*t*
in renal failure, 54*t*–55*t*
hepatic/renal elimination, 111*t*
pharmacodynamics, 111*t*
in renal failure, 54*t*–55*t*
pharmacokinetics, 111*t*
in renal failure, 54*t*–55*t*
Cefoxitin, 342–343
disposition, effect of liver disease, 111*t*
dosage adjustment
with dialysis, 54*t*–55*t*
in liver disease, 111*t*
in renal failure, 54*t*–55*t*, 334*t*
dosage and administration, 334*t*
fraction of dose excreted unchanged in urine with normal renal function, in children, 190*t*
hepatic/renal elimination, 111*t*
intraperitoneal administration, bioavailability after, 48*t*
pharmacodynamics, 111*t*
in renal failure, 54*t*–55*t*
pharmacokinetics, 111*t*, 334*t*
in renal failure, 54*t*–55*t*
serum concentration, with dialysis, 334*t*
volume of distribution, in renal failure, 47*t*
Ceftazidime, 343
disposition, effect of liver disease, 111*t*
dosage adjustment
with dialysis, 54*t*–55*t*
in liver disease, 111*t*
in renal failure, 54*t*–55*t*, 334*t*
dosage and administration, 334*t*
fraction of dose excreted unchanged in urine with normal renal function, in children, 190*t*
hepatic/renal elimination, 111*t*
pharmacodynamics, 111*t*
in renal failure, 54*t*–55*t*
pharmacokinetics, 111*t*, 334*t*
in renal failure, 54*t*–55*t*
serum concentration, with dialysis, 334*t*
Ceftizoxime, 343
dosage adjustment
with dialysis, 54*t*–55*t*
in renal failure, 54*t*–55*t*
intraperitoneal administration, bioavailability after, 48*t*
pharmacodynamics, in renal failure, 54*t*–55*t*
pharmacokinetics, in renal failure, 54*t*–55*t*
Ceftriaxone, 343
disposition, effect of liver disease, 111*t*
dosage adjustment
with dialysis, 54*t*–55*t*
in liver disease, 111*t*
in renal failure, 50*t*, 54*t*–55*t*, 334*t*
dosage and administration, 334*t*
fraction of dose excreted unchanged in urine with normal renal function, in children, 190*t*
half-life
in end-stage renal disease, 50*t*
normal, 50*t*
hepatic/renal elimination, 111*t*
intraperitoneal administration, bioavailability after, 48*t*
pharmacodynamics, 111*t*
in renal failure, 54*t*–55*t*
pharmacokinetics, 111*t*, 334*t*
in renal failure, 54*t*–55*t*
serum concentration, with dialysis, 334*t*
Cefuroxime, 342
disposition, effect of liver disease, 111*t*
dosage adjustment
with dialysis, 54*t*–55*t*
in liver disease, 111*t*
in renal failure, 54*t*–55*t*
fraction of dose excreted unchanged in urine with normal renal function, in children, 190*t*
hepatic/renal elimination, 111*t*
intraperitoneal administration, bioavailability after, 48*t*
pharmacodynamics, 111*t*
in renal failure, 54*t*–55*t*
pharmacokinetics, 111*t*
in renal failure, 54*t*–55*t*
volume of distribution, in renal failure, 47*t*
Cephalexin, absorption, drug interactions affecting, 16*t*
Cephalosporins, 341–344
adverse effects of, 343–344
distribution, 343
dosage adjustment
with dialysis, 54*t*–55*t*
in renal failure, 50*t*, 54*t*–55*t*, 334*t*
dosage and administration, 334*t*
elimination, 343
half-life
in end-stage renal disease, 50*t*
normal, 50*t*
interference with glucose determination, 382*t*

Cephalosporins—*continued*
intraperitoneal administration, bioavailability after, 48*t*
pharmacodynamics, in renal failure, 54*t*–55*t*
pharmacokinetics, 334*t*
in renal failure, 54*t*–55*t*
psychiatric side effects, 267*t*
secretion by kidney, 28*t*
serum concentration, with dialysis, 334*t*
Cephalothin, 342–343
disposition, effect of liver disease, 111*t*
dosage adjustment
with dialysis, 54*t*–55*t*
in liver disease, 111*t*
in renal failure, 54*t*–55*t*, 334*t*
dosage and administration, 334*t*
hepatic/renal elimination, 111*t*
pharmacodynamics, 111*t*
in renal failure, 54*t*–55*t*
pharmacokinetics, 111*t*, 334*t*
in renal failure, 54*t*–55*t*
serum concentration, with dialysis, 334*t*
Cephamycins, 341–344
adverse effects of, 343–344
dosage adjustment, in renal failure, 334*t*
dosage and administration, 334*t*
pharmacokinetics, 334*t*
serum concentration, with dialysis, 334*t*
Cerebral blood flow, response of
to changes in mean arterial pressure, 271*f*
to changes on $PaCO_2$, 271*f*
Children, unique drug effects in, 180–182
Chlamydia psittaci, antimicrobial drugs of choice for, 340*t*
Chlamydia trachomatis, antimicrobial drugs of choice for, 340*t*
Chloral hydrate
dosage adjustment
with dialysis, 72*t*–73*t*
in renal failure, 72*t*–73*t*
drug interactions, 20*t*
pharmacodynamics, in renal failure, 72*t*–73*t*
pharmacokinetics, in renal failure, 72*t*–73*t*
removal, by resin hemoperfusion, 11*t*
Chlorambucil, psychiatric side effects, 268*t*
Chloramphenicol
disposition, effect of liver disease, 111*t*
dosage adjustment
in liver disease, 111*t*
in renal failure, 335*t*
dosage and administration, 335*t*
drug interactions, 23*t*
fraction of dose excreted unchanged in urine with normal renal function, in children, 190*t*
hepatic/renal elimination, 111*t*
infusion, in pediatric patients, 188*t*
metabolism, induction by other drug(s), 20*t*
pharmacodynamics, 111*t*
pharmacokinetics, 111*t*, 335*t*
psychiatric side effects, 268*t*
serum concentration, with dialysis, 335*t*
volume of distribution, in renal failure, 47*t*
Chloramphenicol succinate
dosage adjustment
with dialysis, 58*t*–59*t*
in renal failure, 58*t*–59*t*
pharmacodynamics, in renal failure, 58*t*–59*t*
pharmacokinetics, in renal failure, 58*t*–59*t*
Chlordiazepoxide
disposition, effect of liver disease, 122*t*
dosage adjustment, in liver disease, 122*t*
hepatic/renal elimination, 122*t*
metabolism, inhibition by other drug(s), 26*t*
pharmacodynamics, 122*t*
pharmacokinetics, 122*t*
Chlormethiazole
disposition, effect of liver disease, 125*t*
dosage adjustment, in liver disease, 125*t*
hepatic/renal elimination, 125*t*
pharmacodynamics, 125*t*
pharmacokinetics, 125*t*
Chloromycetin, interference with glucose determination, 382*t*
Chloroquine
metabolism, inhibition by other drug(s), 24*t*
psychiatric side effects, 267*t*
removal, by resin hemoperfusion, 11*t*
Chlorothiazide
absorption, drug interactions affecting, 16*t*–18*t*
dosage adjustment
with dialysis, 68*t*–69*t*
in renal failure, 68*t*–69*t*
dosage and administration, 85*t*
pharmacodynamics, in renal failure, 68*t*–69*t*
pharmacokinetics, in renal failure, 68*t*–69*t*
Chlorpromazine
absorption, drug interactions affecting, 16*t*
adverse effects of, in children, 182–183
dosage adjustment

with dialysis, 72*t*–73*t*
in renal failure, 72*t*–73*t*
drug interactions, 23*t*
metabolism, induction by other drug(s), 20*t*
pharmacodynamics, in renal failure, 72*t*–73*t*
pharmacokinetics, in renal failure, 72*t*–73*t*
properties of, 317
Chlorpropamide
dosage adjustment
with dialysis, 80*t*–81*t*
in renal failure, 80*t*–81*t*
metabolism, inhibition by other drug(s), 23*t*–24*t*
pharmacodynamics, in renal failure, 80*t*–81*t*
pharmacokinetics, in renal failure, 80*t*–81*t*
Chlorthalidone
dosage adjustment
with dialysis, 68*t*–69*t*
in renal failure, 68*t*–69*t*
dosage and administration, 85*t*
pharmacodynamics, in renal failure, 68*t*–69*t*
pharmacokinetics, in renal failure, 68*t*–69*t*
Choline alkaloids
clinical uses, 264*t*–265*t*
side effects, 264*t*–265*t*
Choline esters
clinical uses, 264*t*–265*t*
side effects, 264*t*–265*t*
Cholinergic agents
clinical uses, 264*t*–265*t*
side effects, 264*t*–265*t*
Cholinergic stimulation, end-organ responses to, 260*t*
Cholinesterase inhibitors, clinical uses of, 262*t*
Cholinomimetics, 261*t*
Chronic obstructive pulmonary disease
pharmacologic approach to patient with, 141
pulmonary hypertension in, pharmacologic approach to patient with, 145–147
Cigarette smoking, drug interactions, 21*t*
Cilastatin, 344
dosage adjustment
with dialysis, 58*t*–59*t*
in renal failure, 58*t*–59*t*
pharmacodynamics, in renal failure, 58*t*–59*t*
pharmacokinetics, in renal failure, 58*t*–59*t*
Cimetidine, 289–292
absorption, drug interactions affecting, 17*t*
adverse effects, 291
contraindications, 291
disposition, effect of liver disease, 125*t*
dosage adjustment
with dialysis, 78*t*–79*t*
in liver disease, 125*t*
in renal failure, 50*t*, 78*t*–79*t*
drug interactions, 24*t*, 292
fraction of dose excreted unchanged in urine with normal renal function, in children, 190*t*
half-life
in end-stage renal disease, 50*t*
normal, 50*t*
hepatic/renal elimination, 125*t*
infusion, in pediatric patients, 188*t*
metabolism, induction by other drug(s), 20*t*
overdosage, 292
pharmacodynamics, 125*t*
in critical illness, 10*t*–11*t*
in renal failure, 78*t*–79*t*
pharmacokinetics, 125*t*, 289–291
in renal failure, 78*t*–79*t*
properties of, 290*t*
psychiatric side effects, 268*t*
secretion by kidney, 28*t*
special considerations, 292
Ciprofloxacin, 347–348
adverse effects of, in pediatric patients, 181
disposition, effect of liver disease, 111*t*
dosage adjustment
with dialysis, 56*t*–57*t*
in liver disease, 111*t*
in renal failure, 56*t*–57*t*
hepatic/renal elimination, 111*t*
intraperitoneal administration, bioavailability after, 48*t*
pharmacodynamics, 111*t*
in renal failure, 56*t*–57*t*
pharmacokinetics, 111*t*
in renal failure, 56*t*–57*t*
psychiatric side effects, 267*t*
secretion by kidney, 28*t*
Cisapride, 306
Cl. *See* Clearance
Clarithromycin, 355
dosage adjustment
with dialysis, 56*t*–57*t*
in renal failure, 56*t*–57*t*
pharmacodynamics, in renal failure, 56*t*–57*t*
pharmacokinetics, in renal failure, 56*t*–57*t*
Clavulanic acid
dosage adjustment
with dialysis, 52*t*–53*t*
in renal failure, 52*t*–53*t*
pharmacodynamics, in renal failure, 52*t*–53*t*

Clavulanic acid—*continued*
pharmacokinetics, in renal failure, 52*t*–53*t*
Clearance, 3*t*, 99–100
free intrinsic, 101
hepatic, 99–101
total or systemic, 99–100
Clindamycin, 349–350
adverse effects of, 350
antimicrobial spectrum, 349–350
disposition, effect of liver disease, 112*t*
distribution, 350
dosage adjustment
with dialysis, 58*t*–59*t*
in liver disease, 112*t*
in renal failure, 58*t*–59*t*, 335*t*
dosage and administration, 335*t*
drug interactions, with nondepolarizing muscle relaxants, 207*t*
elimination, 350
fraction of dose excreted unchanged in urine with normal renal function, in children, 190*t*
hepatic/renal elimination, 112*t*
infusion, in pediatric patients, 188*t*
mechanism of action, 350
pharmacodynamics, 112*t*
in renal failure, 58*t*–59*t*
pharmacokinetics, 112*t*, 335*t*
in renal failure, 58*t*–59*t*
serum concentration, with dialysis, 335*t*
Cl_{nr}, 3*t*
Clofazimine, 355
Clofibrate
disposition, effect of liver disease, 125*t*
dosage adjustment, in liver disease, 125*t*
drug interactions, 20*t*
hepatic/renal elimination, 125*t*
metabolism, induction by other drug(s), 20*t*
pharmacodynamics, 125*t*
pharmacokinetics, 125*t*
volume of distribution, in renal failure, 47*t*
Clomiphene, psychiatric side effects, 269*t*
Clonazepam
dosage adjustment
with dialysis, 70*t*–71*t*
in renal failure, 70*t*–71*t*
metabolism, induction by other drug(s), 20*t*
pharmacodynamics, in renal failure, 70*t*–71*t*
pharmacokinetics, in renal failure, 70*t*–71*t*
Clonidine
for diarrhea, 300
dosage adjustment
with dialysis, 62*t*–63*t*
in renal failure, 62*t*–63*t*
for hypertensive urgencies, 228*t*–229*t*
pharmacodynamics, in renal failure, 62*t*–63*t*
pharmacokinetics, in renal failure, 62*t*–63*t*
psychiatric side effects, 270*t*
Clostridium, antimicrobial drugs of choice for, 339*t*
Clostridium difficile, antimicrobial drugs of choice for, 339*t*
Clotrimazole, psychiatric side effects, 267*t*
Cloxacillin, volume of distribution, in renal failure, 47*t*
Clozapine, metabolism
induction by other drug(s), 20*t*
inhibition by other drug(s), 24*t*
Cl_r, 3*t*
Codeine
comparative narcotic potency, 204*t*–205*t*
dosage adjustment
with dialysis, 74*t*–75*t*
in renal failure, 74*t*–75*t*
dosage and administration, 204*t*–205*t*
pharmacodynamics, in renal failure, 74*t*–75*t*
pharmacokinetics, in renal failure, 74*t*–75*t*
Colchicine
dosage adjustment
with dialysis, 78*t*–79*t*
in renal failure, 78*t*–79*t*
pharmacodynamics, in renal failure, 78*t*–79*t*
pharmacokinetics, in renal failure, 78*t*–79*t*
Colistin sulfate, psychiatric side effects, 268*t*
Colonic inertia, pharmacotherapy for, 302–307
Compazine. *See* Prochlorperazine
Congenital myopathies, interactions with muscle relaxants, 208*t*–209*t*
Constipation, pharmacotherapy for, 311–316
Corgard. *See* Nadolol
Corticosteroids
adverse effects, in pediatric patients, 181
dosage adjustment
with dialysis, 80*t*–81*t*
in renal failure, 80*t*–81*t*
pharmacodynamics, in renal failure, 80*t*–81*t*
pharmacokinetics, in renal failure, 80*t*–81*t*
Cortisone
dosage adjustment
with dialysis, 80*t*–81*t*

in renal failure, 80t–81t
pharmacodynamics, in renal failure, 80t–81t
pharmacokinetics, in renal failure, 80t–81t
Corynebacterium JK, antimicrobial drugs of choice for, 338t
Co-Trimoxazole, intravenous infusion, in pediatric patients, 188t
Coumarin
displacement from protein-binding sites, drug interactions due to, 20t
psychiatric side effects, 269t
Cp_{max}, 3t
Cp_{min}, 3t
Cp_{ss}, 3t
Creatinine clearance
calculation, 189t
estimation, 46, 47t
Crohn's disease, pharmacotherapy for, 318–321
Cryptococcus neoformans, antimicrobial drugs of choice for, 340t
Cyclobenzaprine, psychiatric side effects, 269t
Cyclophosphamide
disposition, effect of liver disease, 115t
dosage adjustment, in liver disease, 115t
hepatic/renal elimination, 115t
pharmacodynamics, 115t
pharmacokinetics, 115t
Cycloserine, psychiatric side effects, 267t
Cyclosporine
absorption, drug interactions affecting, 18t–19t
dosage adjustment
with dialysis, 82t–83t
in renal failure, 82t–83t
drug interactions with, 29t
metabolism
induction by other drug(s), 20t
inhibition by other drug(s), 22t–23t, 25t–26t
pharmacodynamics, in renal failure, 82t–83t
pharmacokinetics, in renal failure, 82t–83t
psychiatric side effects, 268t
Cyclothiazide, dosage and administration, 85t
Cytarabine, psychiatric side effects, 268t
Cytochromes P-450, 92
Cytosine arabinoside
disposition, effect of liver disease, 115t
dosage adjustment, in liver disease, 115t
hepatic/renal elimination, 115t
pharmacodynamics, 115t
pharmacokinetics, 115t

D
Dacarbazine, psychiatric side effects, 268t
Dapsone
metabolism, induction by other drug(s), 20t
psychiatric side effects, 267t
secretion by kidney, 28t
DDAVP. *See* Desmopressin
Debrisoquine, poor and extensive metabolizers of, 103
Delirium, drugs causing, 267t–270t
°, 3t
Demerol. *See* Meperidine
Denervation, interactions with muscle relaxants, 208t–209t
Dermatomyositis, interactions with muscle relaxants, 208t–209t
1-Desamino-8-*d*-arginine vasopressin, activity, 372t
Desipramine
dosage adjustment
with dialysis, 72t–73t
in renal failure, 72t–73t
metabolism, inhibition by other drug(s), 24t, 27t
pharmacodynamics, in renal failure, 72t–73t
pharmacokinetics, in renal failure, 72t–73t
Desmopressin, dosage and administration, 309t, 373t
Despondency, drugs causing, 267t–270t
Dexamethasone
antiemetic effects, 318
disposition, effect of liver disease, 117t
dosage adjustment
with dialysis, 80t–81t
in liver disease, 117t
in renal failure, 80t–81t
hepatic/renal elimination, 117t
pharmacodynamics, 117t
in renal failure, 80t–81t
pharmacokinetics, 117t
in renal failure, 80t–81t
N-Dexmethylmethsuximide, removal, by resin hemoperfusion, 11t
Dextromethorphan, metabolism, inhibition by other drug(s), 23t
Diabetes insipidus, 371
Diabetic ketoacidosis
differential diagnosis of, 378t
treatment of, 379t
Diabetic myopathy, interactions with muscle relaxants, 208t–209t
Dialysis
drug dosage adjustments with, 50t, 52t–83t
in treatment of hyperkalemia, 86t–87t
Diazepam
cost, 201t

Diazepam—*continued*
displacement from protein-binding sites, drug interactions due to, 20*t*
disposition, effect of liver disease, 123*t*
dosage adjustment
with dialysis, 72*t*–73*t*
in liver disease, 123*t*
in renal failure, 72*t*–73*t*
dosage and administration, 247*t*–248*t*
in mechanically ventilated patients, 201*t*
drug interactions, 248*t*
hepatic/renal elimination, 123*t*
intravenous, 202*t*–203*t*
metabolism
induction by other drug(s), 20*t*
inhibition by other drug(s), 23*t*–27*t*
monitoring guidelines, 7*t*
pharmacodynamics, 123*t*
in renal failure, 72*t*–73*t*
pharmacokinetics, 6*t*, 123*t*
in renal failure, 72*t*–73*t*
pharmacology of, 247*t*–248*t*
properties of, 247*t*–248*t*
use during mechanical ventilation, 203*t*
Diazoxide
dosage adjustment
with dialysis, 64*t*–65*t*
in renal failure, 64*t*–65*t*
drug interactions, 20*t*
for hypertensive emergencies, 226*t*–227*t*
pharmacodynamics, in renal failure, 64*t*–65*t*
pharmacokinetics, in renal failure, 64*t*–65*t*
Dicloxacillin, volume of distribution, in renal failure, 47*t*
Didanosine, psychiatric side effects, 269*t*
Dideoxycytidine, 360
Dideoxyinosine
dosage adjustment, in renal failure, 336*t*
dosage and administration, 336*t*
pharmacokinetics, 336*t*
serum concentration, with dialysis, 336*t*
Diethyltoluamide, psychiatric side effects, 269*t*
Diflunisal
absorption, drug interactions affecting, 16*t*
metabolism, induction by other drug(s), 20*t*
Digitalis, psychiatric side effects, 270*t*
Digitalis glycosides, removal, by resin hemoperfusion, 11*t*
Digitoxin
absorption, drug interactions affecting, 16*t*
disposition, effect of liver disease, 118*t*
dosage adjustment
with dialysis, 68*t*–69*t*
in liver disease, 118*t*
in renal failure, 68*t*–69*t*
hepatic/renal elimination, 118*t*
metabolism
induction by other drug(s), 20*t*
inhibition by other drug(s), 22*t*, 27*t*
pharmacodynamics, 118*t*
in renal failure, 68*t*–69*t*
pharmacokinetics, 118*t*
in renal failure, 68*t*–69*t*
Digoxin
absorption, drug interactions affecting, 16*t*–18*t*
adverse effects of, 232*t*–233*t*
dosage adjustment, in renal failure, 50*t*
dosage and administration, 232*t*–233*t*
drug interactions, with cyclosporine, 29*t*
fraction of dose excreted unchanged in urine with normal renal function, in children, 190*t*
half-life
in end-stage renal disease, 50*t*
normal, 50*t*
indications for, 232*t*
metabolism
induction by other drug(s), 20*t*
inhibition by other drug(s), 22*t*, 26*t*–27*t*
monitoring guidelines, 7*t*
pediatric considerations, 186–187
pharmacodynamics, in critical illness, 8*t*–9*t*
pharmacokinetic parameters, 6*t*
in treatment of supraventricular tachycardia, 228*t*–229*t*
volume of distribution, in renal failure, 47*t*
Dihydropyridine, drug interactions, 22*t*
Dilaudid. *See* Hydromorphone
Dilevalol, properties of, 221*t*
Diltiazem
adverse effects of, 232*t*–233*t*
dosage adjustment
with dialysis, 66*t*–67*t*
in renal failure, 66*t*–67*t*
dosage and administration, 232*t*–233*t*
drug interactions, 22*t*
with cyclosporine, 29*t*
indications for, 232*t*
pharmacodynamics, in renal failure, 66*t*–67*t*
pharmacokinetics, in renal failure, 66*t*–67*t*
properties of, 222*t*
psychiatric side effects, 270*t*
in treatment of supraventricular tachycardia, 228*t*–229*t*

Diphenhydramine
  disposition, effect of liver disease, 125*t*
  dosage adjustment
    with dialysis, 78*t*–79*t*
    in liver disease, 125*t*
    in renal failure, 78*t*–79*t*
  hepatic/renal elimination, 125*t*
  infusion, in pediatric patients, 188*t*
  pharmacodynamics, 125*t*
    in renal failure, 78*t*–79*t*
  pharmacokinetics, 125*t*
    in renal failure, 78*t*–79*t*
Diphenoxylate, psychiatric side effects, 269*t*
Diphenoxylate hydrochloride with atropine sulfate, 299
Diphenylhydantoin
  disposition, in liver disease, 116*t*
  dosage adjustment, effect of liver disease, 116*t*
  hepatic/renal elimination, 116*t*
  pharmacodynamics, 116*t*
  pharmacokinetics, 116*t*
Dipyridamole
  dosage adjustment
    with dialysis, 76*t*–77*t*
    in renal failure, 76*t*–77*t*
  pharmacodynamics, in renal failure, 76*t*–77*t*
  pharmacokinetics, in renal failure, 76*t*–77*t*
Disopyramide
  adverse effects of, 230*t*–231*t*
  disposition, effect of liver disease, 119*t*
  dosage adjustment
    with dialysis, 66*t*–67*t*
    in liver disease, 119*t*
    in renal failure, 66*t*–67*t*
  dosage and administration, 230*t*–231*t*
  hepatic/renal elimination, 119*t*
  indications for, 230*t*
  metabolism, induction by other drug(s), 20*t*
  pharmacodynamics, 119*t*
    in renal failure, 66*t*–67*t*
  pharmacokinetics, 119*t*
    in renal failure, 66*t*–67*t*
  psychiatric side effects, 270*t*
  removal, by resin hemoperfusion, 11*t*
Distribution, 96–99
  in liver disease, 97–99
Disulfiram
  drug interactions, 23*t*
  psychiatric side effects, 269*t*
Diuretics. *See also* Potassium-sparing diuretics; Thiazide diuretics
  disposition, effect of liver disease, 121*t*–122*t*
  dosage adjustment
    with dialysis, 68*t*–71*t*
    in liver disease, 121*t*–122*t*
    in renal failure, 68*t*–71*t*
  dosage and administration, 84*t*
  half-life, 84*t*
  hepatic/renal elimination, 121*t*–122*t*
  loop, 84*t*
    secretion by kidney, 28*t*
  metabolism, 84*t*
  pharmacodynamics, 121*t*–122*t*
    in critical illness, 8*t*–9*t*
    in renal failure, 68*t*–71*t*
  pharmacokinetics, 121*t*–122*t*
    in renal failure, 68*t*–71*t*
  pharmacology of, 84*t*
  site of action, 84*t*
Dobutamine
  dosage adjustment
    with dialysis, 70*t*–71*t*
    in renal failure, 70*t*–71*t*
  infusion, 238*t*–239*t*
    in children, 188*t*, 192*t*
  pharmacodynamics
    in critical illness, 8*t*–9*t*
    in renal failure, 70*t*–71*t*
  pharmacokinetics, in renal failure, 70*t*–71*t*
Docusate, 316
  properties of, 313*t*
Dolophine. *See* Methadone
Domperidone, 305
Dopamine
  dosage adjustment
    with dialysis, 70*t*–71*t*
    in renal failure, 70*t*–71*t*
  dosage and administration, in renal failure, 51*t*
  infusion, 238*t*–239*t*
    in children, 188*t*, 192*t*
  pharmacodynamics
    in critical illness, 8*t*–9*t*
    in renal failure, 70*t*–71*t*
  pharmacokinetics, in renal failure, 70*t*–71*t*
Dopamine antagonists, adverse effects of, in children, 182–183
Dosage adjustment, in liver disease, 107–109, 128*t*
Dose-response relationship, 4*f*
Dosing interval, 3*t*
Doxacurium
  characteristics of, 210*t*–211*t*
  clearance, 213*t*
  clinical pharmacology of, 206*t*–207*t*
  disposition, effect of liver disease, 125*t*
  dosage adjustment, in liver disease, 125*t*
  hepatic/renal elimination, 125*t*
  metabolism, 213*t*
  pharmacodynamics, 125*t*
  pharmacokinetics, 125*t*
  side effects and adverse reactions to, 210*t*–211*t*

Doxazosin
dosage adjustment
with dialysis, 62t–63t
in renal failure, 62t–63t
pharmacodynamics, in renal failure, 62t–63t
pharmacokinetics, in renal failure, 62t–63t
Doxepin
dosage adjustment
with dialysis, 72t–73t
in renal failure, 72t–73t
metabolism, inhibition by other drug(s), 27t
pharmacodynamics, in renal failure, 72t–73t
pharmacokinetics, in renal failure, 72t–73t
Doxorubicin
drug interactions, with cyclosporine, 29t
metabolism, inhibition by other drug(s), 22t
Doxycycline
disposition, effect of liver disease, 112t
dosage adjustment
with dialysis, 58t–59t
in liver disease, 112t
in renal failure, 58t–59t
hepatic/renal elimination, 112t
metabolism, induction by other drug(s), 20t
pharmacodynamics, 112t
in renal failure, 58t–59t
pharmacokinetics, 112t
in renal failure, 58t–59t
Drug classification, by dispositional characteristics, 101–103
Drug concentration, and effect, 237f
Drug disposition
characteristics of, 103
and liver disease, 104–107
Drug interactions, 13–15
affecting absorption, 16t–19t
due to displacement from protein-binding sites, 20t
in liver disease, 106–107
types of, 14t
Drug therapy, optimizing, 5f
DynaCirc. *See* Isradipine
Dyphylline
dosage adjustment
with dialysis, 78t–79t
in renal failure, 78t–79t
pharmacodynamics, in renal failure, 78t–79t
pharmacokinetics, in renal failure, 78t–79t
secretion by kidney, 28t

E
Echothiophate
clinical uses, 264t–265t
side effects, 264t–265t
Edrophonium
clinical uses, 262t, 264t–265t
side effects, 264t–265t
in treatment of supraventricular tachycardia, 228t–229t
Elimination, 99–101
dose-dependent, 100
routes of, 103–104
Elimination rate constant, 3t
for nonrenal component, 3t
for renal component, 3t
Enalapril
disposition, effect of liver disease, 119t
dosage adjustment
with dialysis, 62t–63t
in liver disease, 119t
in renal failure, 62t–63t
hepatic/renal elimination, 119t
indications for, 216
pharmacodynamics, 119t
in renal failure, 62t–63t
pharmacokinetics, 119t
in renal failure, 62t–63t
properties of, 223t
Enalaprilat, for hypertensive emergencies, 226t–227t
Encainide
adverse effects of, 230t–231t
dosage adjustment
with dialysis, 66t–67t
in renal failure, 66t–67t
dosage and administration, 230t–231t
indications for, 230t
pharmacodynamics, in renal failure, 66t–67t
pharmacokinetics, in renal failure, 66t–67t
Endocrinology, 371–383
Enterobacter, antimicrobial drugs of choice for, 338t
Enzyme-limited drugs, 102
binding-insensitive, 102
binding-sensitive, 102
bioavailability of, 105
Ephedrine
elimination, 10t
in treatment of bradycardia, 230t–231t
Epinephrine
dosage, 157t
duration of action, 156t
infusion, 238t–239t
in children, 188t, 192t
preparation, 157t
receptor, 156t
route of administration, 156t–157t
Erythromycin, 306–307, 349
adverse effects of, 349

antimicrobial spectrum, 349
disposition, effect of liver disease, 112*t*
distribution, 349
dosage adjustment
with dialysis, 56*t*–57*t*
in liver disease, 112*t*
in renal failure, 56*t*–57*t*
dosage and administration, 307
drug interactions, 23*t*, 307
with cyclosporine, 29*t*
elimination, 349
fraction of dose excreted unchanged in urine with normal renal function, in children, 190*t*
hepatic/renal elimination, 112*t*
indications for, 306
mechanism of action, 306–307, 349
pharmacodynamics, 112*t*
in renal failure, 56*t*–57*t*
pharmacokinetics, 112*t*, 307
in renal failure, 56*t*–57*t*
side effects, 307
volume of distribution, in renal failure, 47*t*
Erythromycin lactobionate
dosage adjustment, in renal failure, 335*t*
dosage and administration, 335*t*
infusion, in pediatric patients, 188*t*
pharmacokinetics, 335*t*
serum concentration, with dialysis, 335*t*
Erythropoietin, psychiatric side effects, 269*t*
Escherichia coli, antimicrobial drugs of choice for, 338*t*
Esmolol
adverse effects of, 230*t*–231*t*
disposition, effect of liver disease, 119*t*
dosage adjustment
with dialysis, 64*t*–65*t*
in liver disease, 119*t*
in renal failure, 64*t*–65*t*
dosage and administration, 230*t*–231*t*
hepatic/renal elimination, 119*t*
indications for, 230*t*
pharmacodynamics, 119*t*
in renal failure, 64*t*–65*t*
pharmacokinetics, 119*t*
in renal failure, 64*t*–65*t*
properties of, 232*t*–233*t*
in treatment of supraventricular tachycardia, 228*t*–229*t*
Esophageal varices, hemorrhage, pharmacotherapy for, 307–311
Estrogens, psychiatric side effects, 269*t*
Ethacrynic acid
dosage adjustment
with dialysis, 68*t*–69*t*
in renal failure, 68*t*–69*t*
dosage and administration, 84*t*
drug interactions, 20*t*
half-life, 84*t*
infusion, in pediatric patients, 188*t*
pharmacodynamics, in renal failure, 68*t*–69*t*
pharmacokinetics, in renal failure, 68*t*–69*t*
psychiatric side effects, 270*t*
site of action, 84*t*
Ethambutol, 354
dosage adjustment
with dialysis, 52*t*–53*t*
in renal failure, 52*t*–53*t*, 335*t*
dosage and administration, 335*t*
pharmacodynamics, in renal failure, 52*t*–53*t*
pharmacokinetics, 335*t*
in renal failure, 52*t*–53*t*
psychiatric side effects, 268*t*
secretion by kidney, 28*t*
serum concentration, with dialysis, 335*t*
volume of distribution, in renal failure, 47*t*
Ethanol
absorption, drug interactions affecting, 18*t*
drug interactions, 21*t*, 23*t*
with cyclosporine, 29*t*
Ethanolamine oleate, 311
Ethchlorvynol, removal, by resin hemoperfusion, 11*t*
Ethionamide, psychiatric side effects, 267*t*
Ethosuximide
dosage adjustment
with dialysis, 76*t*–77*t*
in renal failure, 76*t*–77*t*
pharmacodynamics, in renal failure, 76*t*–77*t*
pharmacokinetics, in renal failure, 76*t*–77*t*
psychiatric side effects, 267*t*
Etintidine, drug interactions, 24*t*
Etomidate
dosage adjustment
with dialysis, 82*t*–83*t*
in renal failure, 82*t*–83*t*
pharmacodynamics, in renal failure, 82*t*–83*t*
pharmacokinetics, in renal failure, 82*t*–83*t*
Etoposide
disposition, effect of liver disease, 115*t*
dosage adjustment, in liver disease, 115*t*
hepatic/renal elimination, 115*t*
pharmacodynamics, 115*t*
pharmacokinetics, 115*t*
psychiatric side effects, 268*t*
Extraction, of drug by liver, 100–101

F
F, 3t
Familial periodic paralysis, interactions with muscle relaxants, 208t–209t
Famotidine, 294–295
disposition, effect of liver disease, 125t
dosage adjustment
with dialysis, 78t–79t
in liver disease, 125t
in renal failure, 78t–79t
dosage and administration, 294
drug interactions, 294–295
hepatic/renal elimination, 125t
overdosage, 295
pharmacodynamics, 125t
in renal failure, 78t–79t
pharmacokinetics, 125t, 294
in renal failure, 78t–79t
properties of, 290t
side effects, 294–295
f_e, 3t
Felodipine
absorption, drug interactions affecting, 18t–19t
dosage adjustment
with dialysis, 66t–67t
in renal failure, 66t–67t
metabolism, inhibition by other drug(s), 23t–24t
pharmacodynamics, in renal failure, 66t–67t
pharmacokinetics, in renal failure, 66t–67t
properties of, 222t
Fenoldopam, metabolism, inhibition by other drug(s), 22t
Fenoprofen
disposition, effect of liver disease, 117t
dosage adjustment, in liver disease, 117t
hepatic/renal elimination, 117t
pharmacodynamics, 117t
pharmacokinetics, 117t
psychiatric side effects, 267t
Fenoterol
duration of action, 156t
receptor, 156t
route of administration, 156t
Fentanyl
adverse effects of, in pediatric patients, 184
comparative narcotic potency, 204t–205t
cost, 201t
disposition, effect of liver disease, 125t
dosage adjustment
with dialysis, 74t–75t
in liver disease, 125t
in renal failure, 74t–75t
dosage and administration, 204t–205t
in mechanically ventilated patients, 201t
hepatic/renal elimination, 125t
pharmacodynamics, 125t
in renal failure, 74t–75t
pharmacokinetics, 125t
in renal failure, 74t–75t
use, in adult ICU patients, 204t–205t
First-order kinetics, 99
Flecainide
adverse effects of, 230t–231t
dosage adjustment
with dialysis, 66t–67t
in renal failure, 66t–67t
dosage and administration, 230t–231t
drug interactions, 23t
indications for, 230t
metabolism, inhibition by other drug(s), 22t, 27t
pharmacodynamics, in renal failure, 66t–67t
pharmacokinetics, in renal failure, 66t–67t
secretion by kidney, 28t
Flow/enzyme-sensitive drugs, 102–103
Flow-limited drugs, 101–102
Fluconazole, 357–358
disposition, effect of liver disease, 112t
dosage adjustment
with dialysis, 60t–61t
in liver disease, 112t
in renal failure, 60t–61t, 336t
dosage and administration, 336t
drug interactions, 24t
with cyclosporine, 29t
hepatic/renal elimination, 112t
intraperitoneal administration, bioavailability after, 49t
metabolism, induction by other drug(s), 20t
pharmacodynamics, 112t
in renal failure, 60t–61t
pharmacokinetics, 112t, 336t
in renal failure, 60t–61t
serum concentration, with dialysis, 336t
Flucytosine, 357
dosage adjustment
with dialysis, 60t–61t
in renal failure, 50t, 60t–61t, 336t
dosage and administration, 336t
half-life
in end-stage renal disease, 50t
normal, 50t
pharmacodynamics, in renal failure, 60t–61t
pharmacokinetics, 336t
in renal failure, 60t–61t
psychiatric side effects, 268t
serum concentration, with dialysis, 336t

Fludrocortisone, metabolism, induction by other drug(s), 20*t*
Fluids, pharmacodynamics, in critical illness, 8*t*–9*t*
Flumazenil
disposition, effect of liver disease, 123*t*
dosage adjustment, in liver disease, 123*t*
hepatic/renal elimination, 123*t*
pharmacodynamics, 123*t*
pharmacokinetics, 123*t*
Fluoroquinolones, 347–348
adverse effects of, in pediatric patients, 181
dosage adjustment
with dialysis, 56*t*–57*t*
in renal failure, 56*t*–57*t*
pharmacodynamics, in renal failure, 56*t*–57*t*
pharmacokinetics, in renal failure, 56*t*–57*t*
5-Fluorouracil
disposition, effect of liver disease, 115*t*
dosage adjustment, in liver disease, 115*t*
hepatic/renal elimination, 115*t*
metabolism, inhibition by other drug(s), 24*t*, 27*t*
pharmacodynamics, 115*t*
pharmacokinetics, 115*t*
psychiatric side effects, 268*t*
Fluoxetine
dosage adjustment
with dialysis, 74*t*–75*t*
in renal failure, 74*t*–75*t*
drug interactions, 24*t*
pharmacodynamics, in renal failure, 74*t*–75*t*
pharmacokinetics, in renal failure, 74*t*–75*t*
Flurazepam
dosage adjustment
with dialysis, 72*t*–73*t*
in renal failure, 72*t*–73*t*
pharmacodynamics, in renal failure, 72*t*–73*t*
pharmacokinetics, in renal failure, 72*t*–73*t*
Folic acid, psychiatric side effects, 269*t*
Foscarnet, 359–360
dosage adjustment, in renal failure, 336*t*
dosage and administration, 336*t*
pharmacokinetics, 336*t*
psychiatric side effects, 269*t*
serum concentration, with dialysis, 336*t*
Fosinopril
dosage adjustment
with dialysis, 62*t*–63*t*
in renal failure, 62*t*–63*t*
pharmacodynamics, in renal failure, 62*t*–63*t*
pharmacokinetics, in renal failure, 62*t*–63*t*
properties of, 223*t*
Fungi, antimicrobial drugs of choice for, 339*t*–340*t*
Furosemide
absorption, drug interactions affecting, 18*t*
disposition, effect of liver disease, 121*t*
dosage adjustment
with dialysis, 68*t*–69*t*
in liver disease, 121*t*
in renal failure, 68*t*–69*t*
dosage and administration, 84*t*
in renal failure, 51*t*
drug interactions, with cyclosporine, 29*t*
half-life, 84*t*
hepatic/renal elimination, 121*t*
pharmacodynamics, 121*t*
in critical illness, 8*t*–9*t*
in renal failure, 68*t*–69*t*
pharmacokinetics, 121*t*
in renal failure, 68*t*–69*t*
psychiatric side effects, 270*t*
site of action, 84*t*
volume of distribution, in renal failure, 47*t*

G
Gallamine
clinical pharmacology of, 206*t*–207*t*
dosage adjustment
with dialysis, 82*t*–83*t*
in renal failure, 82*t*–83*t*
pharmacodynamics, in renal failure, 82*t*–83*t*
pharmacokinetics, in renal failure, 82*t*–83*t*
Ganciclovir, 359
disposition, effect of liver disease, 112*t*
dosage adjustment
with dialysis, 60*t*–61*t*
in liver disease, 112*t*
in renal failure, 60*t*–61*t*, 336*t*
dosage and administration, 336*t*
drug interactions, with cyclosporine, 29*t*
fraction of dose excreted unchanged in urine with normal renal function, in children, 190*t*
hepatic/renal elimination, 112*t*
pharmacodynamics, 112*t*
in renal failure, 60*t*–61*t*
pharmacokinetics, 336*t*, 1076*t*
in renal failure, 60*t*–61*t*
psychiatric side effects, 269*t*
serum concentration, with dialysis, 336*t*

Ganglionic blockers, psychiatric side effects, 270*t*
Gastric pH, 280
Gastroesophageal reflux, pharmacotherapy for, 279–297
Gastrointestinal medications, 279–329
Gastroparesis, pharmacotherapy for, 302–307
Gaviscon, 282*t*
Gelusil, 282*t*
Gentamicin, 345–347
  disposition, effect of liver disease, 112*t*
  dosage adjustment
    with dialysis, 52*t*–53*t*
    in liver disease, 112*t*
    in renal failure, 52*t*–53*t*, 335*t*
  dosage and administration, 335*t*
  hepatic/renal elimination, 112*t*
  infusion, in pediatric patients, 188*t*
  intraperitoneal administration, bioavailability after, 48*t*
  ototoxicity, 346
  pharmacodynamics, 112*t*
    in renal failure, 52*t*–53*t*
  pharmacokinetics, 112*t*, 335*t*
    in renal failure, 52*t*–53*t*
  serum concentration, with dialysis, 335*t*
  toxicity, 347
  volume of distribution, in renal failure, 47*t*
Glipizide
  dosage adjustment
    with dialysis, 80*t*–81*t*
    in renal failure, 80*t*–81*t*
  metabolism, inhibition by other drug(s), 24*t*
  pharmacodynamics, in renal failure, 80*t*–81*t*
  pharmacokinetics, in renal failure, 80*t*–81*t*
Glucagon therapy, 374*t*
Glucocorticoids, metabolism, induction by other drug(s), 20*t*
Glucose/insulin, in treatment of hyperkalemia, 86*t*–87*t*
Glutethimide
  drug interactions, 21*t*
  removal, by resin hemoperfusion, 11*t*
Glyburide
  dosage adjustment
    with dialysis, 80*t*–81*t*
    in renal failure, 80*t*–81*t*
  metabolism, inhibition by other drug(s), 24*t*
  pharmacodynamics, in renal failure, 80*t*–81*t*
  pharmacokinetics, in renal failure, 80*t*–81*t*
Glycerin, 315
Glycerin suppository, properties of, 313*t*
Glycopeptides
  dosage adjustment
    with dialysis, 56*t*–57*t*
    in renal failure, 56*t*–57*t*
  pharmacodynamics, in renal failure, 56*t*–57*t*
  pharmacokinetics, in renal failure, 56*t*–57*t*
Glycopyrrolate
  clinical uses, 264*t*–265*t*
  effects of, 263*t*
  indications for, 263*t*
  side effects, 264*t*–265*t*
Glypressin, 310
Gram-negative bacilli, antimicrobial drugs of choice for, 338*t*–339*t*
Gram-negative cocci, antimicrobial drugs of choice for, 338*t*
Gram-positive bacilli, antimicrobial drugs of choice for, 338*t*
Gram-positive cocci, antimicrobial drugs of choice for, 338*t*
Griseofulvin
  drug interactions, 21*t*
  metabolism, induction by other drug(s), 21*t*
  psychiatric side effects, 267*t*
Guanabenz
  dosage adjustment
    with dialysis, 62*t*–63*t*
    in renal failure, 62*t*–63*t*
  pharmacodynamics, in renal failure, 62*t*–63*t*
  pharmacokinetics, in renal failure, 62*t*–63*t*
Guanethidine, psychiatric side effects, 270*t*

H

Haemophilus influenzae, antimicrobial drugs of choice for, 338*t*
Half-life, 3*t*, 97
  in liver disease, 97
Haloperidol
  adverse effects of, in children, 182–183
  dosage adjustment
    with dialysis, 72*t*–73*t*
    in renal failure, 72*t*–73*t*
  metabolism
    induction by other drug(s), 21*t*
    inhibition by other drug(s), 25*t*
  monitoring guidelines, 7*t*
  pharmacodynamics, in renal failure, 72*t*–73*t*
  pharmacokinetic parameters, 6*t*
  pharmacokinetics, in renal failure, 72*t*–73*t*
Halothane
  hepatotoxicity, in children versus adult, 184–185
  psychiatric side effects, 269*t*

Hematoma, intracerebral
  blood pressure management with, 258*t*
  management of, 258*t*
Heparin
  dosage adjustment
    with dialysis, 76*t*–77*t*
    in renal failure, 76*t*–77*t*
  drug interactions, 20*t*
  pharmacodynamics, in renal failure, 76*t*–77*t*
  pharmacokinetics, in renal failure, 76*t*–77*t*
  secretion by kidney, 28*t*
Hepatic clearance, 99–101
Herpes simplex, antimicrobial drugs of choice for, 340*t*
Herpes zoster, antimicrobial drugs of choice for, 340*t*
Hexobarbital
  disposition, effect of liver disease, 123*t*
  dosage adjustment, in liver disease, 123*t*
  hepatic/renal elimination, 123*t*
  pharmacodynamics, 123*t*
  pharmacokinetics, 123*t*
Histamine H_1-receptor antagonists
  dosage adjustment
    with dialysis, 78*t*–79*t*
    in renal failure, 78*t*–79*t*
  pharmacodynamics, in renal failure, 78*t*–79*t*
  pharmacokinetics, in renal failure, 78*t*–79*t*
Histamine H_2-receptor antagonists, 288–297
  comparison of, 290*t*
  dosage adjustment
    with dialysis, 78*t*–79*t*
    in renal failure, 78*t*–79*t*
  drug interactions, 24*t*
  monitoring guidelines, 7*t*
  pharmacodynamics
    in critical illness, 10*t*–11*t*
    in renal failure, 78*t*–79*t*
  pharmacokinetics, 6*t*
    in renal failure, 78*t*–79*t*
Histoplasma capsulatum, antimicrobial drugs of choice for, 340*t*
Hydantoins, psychiatric side effects, 267*t*
Hydralazine
  dosage adjustment
    with dialysis, 64*t*–65*t*
    in renal failure, 64*t*–65*t*
  for hypertensive emergencies, 226*t*–227*t*
  pharmacodynamics, in renal failure, 64*t*–65*t*
  pharmacokinetics, in renal failure, 64*t*–65*t*
  psychiatric side effects, 270*t*
Hydralazine/isosorbide dinitrate, indications for, 216
Hydrochlorothiazide
  disposition, effect of liver disease, 122*t*
  dosage adjustment
    with dialysis, 68*t*–69*t*
    in liver disease, 122*t*
    in renal failure, 68*t*–69*t*
  dosage and administration, 85*t*
  hepatic/renal elimination, 122*t*
  pharmacodynamics, 122*t*
    in renal failure, 68*t*–69*t*
  pharmacokinetics, 122*t*
    in renal failure, 68*t*–69*t*
  psychiatric side effects, 270*t*
Hydrocortisone
  dosage adjustment
    with dialysis, 80*t*–81*t*
    in renal failure, 80*t*–81*t*
  pharmacodynamics, in renal failure, 80*t*–81*t*
  pharmacokinetics, in renal failure, 80*t*–81*t*
Hydroflumethiazide, dosage and administration, 85*t*
Hydromorphone
  comparative narcotic potency, 204*t*–205*t*
  dosage and administration, 204*t*–205*t*
Hydroxyzine
  dosage adjustment
    with dialysis, 78*t*–79*t*
    in renal failure, 78*t*–79*t*
  pharmacodynamics, in renal failure, 78*t*–79*t*
  pharmacokinetics, in renal failure, 78*t*–79*t*
Hyperglycemic hyperosmolar nonketotic syndrome, treatment of, 380*t*
Hyperkalemia
  interactions with muscle relaxants, 208*t*–209*t*
  treatment of, 86*t*–87*t*
Hypertension, treatment of. *See* Antihypertensive therapy
Hypertensive crises, causes of, 225*t*
Hypertensive emergencies, parenteral drugs for, 226*t*–227*t*
Hypertensive urgencies, oral drugs for, 228*t*–229*t*
Hyperthyroidism, agents used to treat, 375*t*–376*t*
Hypnotic drugs
  disposition, effect of liver disease, 122*t*–124*t*
  dosage adjustment, in liver disease, 122*t*–124*t*
  hepatic/renal elimination, 122*t*–124*t*
  pharmacodynamics, 122*t*–124*t*
  pharmacokinetics, 122*t*–124*t*

Hypoglycemic agents
dosage adjustment
with dialysis, 80t–81t
in renal failure, 80t–81t
pharmacodynamics, in renal failure, 80t–81t
pharmacokinetics, in renal failure, 80t–81t
Hypokalemia, interactions with muscle relaxants, 208t–209t
Hypothyroidism, agents used to treat, 377t

I
Ibuprofen
disposition, effect of liver disease, 117t
dosage adjustment, in liver disease, 117t
hepatic/renal elimination, 117t
pharmacodynamics, 117t
pharmacokinetics, 117t
psychiatric side effects, 267t
Ifosfamide, psychiatric side effects, 268t
Imipenem, 344
disposition, effect of liver disease, 112t
dosage adjustment
with dialysis, 54t–55t
in liver disease, 112t
in renal failure, 54t–55t
hepatic/renal elimination, 112t
pharmacodynamics, 112t
in renal failure, 54t–55t
pharmacokinetics, 112t
in renal failure, 54t–55t
Imipenem/cilastatin
dosage adjustment, in renal failure, 334t
dosage and administration, 334t
drug interactions, with cyclosporine, 29t
fraction of dose excreted unchanged in urine with normal renal function, in children, 190t
infusion, in pediatric patients, 188t
intraperitoneal administration, bioavailability after, 49t
pharmacokinetics, 334t
serum concentration, with dialysis, 334t
Imipramine
absorption, drug interactions affecting, 19t
dosage adjustment
with dialysis, 72t–73t
in renal failure, 72t–73t
metabolism, inhibition by other drug(s), 24t, 26t–27t
pharmacodynamics, in renal failure, 72t–73t
pharmacokinetics, in renal failure, 72t–73t
Indapamide
dosage adjustment
with dialysis, 68t–69t
in renal failure, 68t–69t
dosage and administration, 85t
pharmacodynamics, in renal failure, 68t–69t
pharmacokinetics, in renal failure, 68t–69t
Inderal. *See* Propranolol
Indomethacin
disposition, effect of liver disease, 117t
dosage adjustment, in liver disease, 117t
drug interactions, with cyclosporine, 29t
hepatic/renal elimination, 117t
metabolism, inhibition by other drug(s), 26t
pharmacodynamics, 117t
pharmacokinetics, 117t
psychiatric side effects, 267t
Infectious disease medications, 331–369
Inflammatory bowel disease, pharmacotherapy for, 318–321
Influenza A, antimicrobial drugs of choice for, 340t
Infusion, plasma drug concentration with, 12f
Inotropic agents
indications for, 217
infusions, 238t–239t
preparation, for pediatric patient, 192t
Insulin, 371
dosage adjustment
with dialysis, 80t–81t
in renal failure, 80t–81t
pharmacodynamics
in critical illness, 8t–9t
in renal failure, 80t–81t
pharmacokinetics, in renal failure, 80t–81t
preparations, 378t
Insulin-drug interactions, 381t
Interferon, psychiatric side effects, 268t
Interleukin-2, psychiatric side effects, 268t
Intraaortic balloon pump, indications for, 217
Intracerebral hemorrhage, nontraumatic, causes of, 255t
Intraconazole
dosage adjustment
with dialysis, 60t–61t
in renal failure, 60t–61t
pharmacodynamics, in renal failure, 60t–61t
pharmacokinetics, in renal failure, 60t–61t
Intracranial hypertension, causes of, 273t

Intracranial pressure
  intracranial volume and, 272*f*
  strategies for controlling, 274*t*
  strategies for reducing, 275*f*
Intravenous bolus, plasma drug concentration with, 12*f*
Intravenous infusions, in infants and children, 188*t*
Iodides, pharmacology of, 376*t*
Ipodate sodium, pharmacology of, 376*t*
Ipratropium
  dosage adjustment
    with dialysis, 78*t*–79*t*
    in renal failure, 78*t*–79*t*
  pharmacodynamics, in renal failure, 78*t*–79*t*
  pharmacokinetics, in renal failure, 78*t*–79*t*
Ischemic stroke, conditions associated with, 254*t*
Isoetharine
  duration of action, 156*t*
  receptor, 156*t*
  route of administration, 156*t*
Isoniazid, 353–354
  absorption, drug interactions affecting, 16*t*, 18*t*
  disposition, effect of liver disease, 113*t*
  dosage adjustment
    with dialysis, 52*t*–53*t*
    in liver disease, 112*t*
    in renal failure, 52*t*–53*t*, 335*t*
  dosage and administration, 335*t*
  drug interactions, 25*t*
  fast and show acetylators of, 103
  hepatic/renal elimination, 113*t*
  hepatotoxicity, in children versus adult, 184–185
  pharmacodynamics, 113*t*
    in renal failure, 52*t*–53*t*
  pharmacokinetics, 113*t*, 335*t*
    in renal failure, 52*t*–53*t*
  psychiatric side effects, 267*t*
  serum concentration, with dialysis, 335*t*
  volume of distribution, in renal failure, 47*t*
Isoniazid hepatitis, 184–185
Isoproterenol
  dosage, 157*t*
  duration of action, 156*t*
  infusion, 238*t*–239*t*
    in children, 192*t*
  preparation, 157*t*
  receptor, 156*t*
  route of administration, 156*t*–157*t*
  in treatment of bradycardia, 230*t*–231*t*
Isoptin. *See* Verapamil
Isosorbide
  dosage adjustment
    with dialysis, 64*t*–65*t*
    in renal failure, 64*t*–65*t*
  pharmacodynamics, in renal failure, 64*t*–65*t*
  pharmacokinetics, in renal failure, 64*t*–65*t*
Isradipine
  disposition, effect of liver disease, 119*t*
  dosage adjustment
    with dialysis, 66*t*–67*t*
    in liver disease, 119*t*
    in renal failure, 66*t*–67*t*
  hepatic/renal elimination, 119*t*
  pharmacodynamics, 119*t*
    in renal failure, 66*t*–67*t*
  pharmacokinetics, 119*t*
    in renal failure, 66*t*–67*t*
  properties of, 222*t*

K
k, 3*t*
ka, 3*t*
Kafocin, interference with glucose determination, 382*t*
Kanamycin, 345–347
  disposition, effect of liver disease, 113*t*
  dosage adjustment, in liver disease, 113*t*
  hepatic/renal elimination, 113*t*
  infusion, in pediatric patients, 188*t*
  pharmacodynamics, 113*t*
  pharmacokinetics, 113*t*
Kaolin, for diarrhea, 300
Kaopectate, for diarrhea, 300
ke, 3*t*
Keflex, interference with glucose determination, 382*t*
Keflin, interference with glucose determination, 382*t*
Kefzol, interference with glucose determination, 382*t*
Kerlone. *See* Betaxolol
Ketamine
  dosage adjustment
    with dialysis, 82*t*–83*t*
    in renal failure, 82*t*–83*t*
  pharmacodynamics, in renal failure, 82*t*–83*t*
  pharmacokinetics, in renal failure, 82*t*–83*t*
Ketoconazole, 358
  absorption, drug interactions affecting, 17*t*
  dosage adjustment
    with dialysis, 60*t*–61*t*
    in renal failure, 60*t*–61*t*
  drug interactions, 25*t*
    with cyclosporine, 29*t*
  pharmacodynamics, in renal failure, 60*t*–61*t*
  pharmacokinetics, in renal failure, 60*t*–61*t*

Ketoconazole—*continued*
psychiatric side effects, 268*t*
Ketoprofen, metabolism, inhibition by other drug(s), 26*t*
Ketorolac
dosage adjustment
with dialysis, 76*t*–77*t*
in renal failure, 76*t*–77*t*
pharmacodynamics, in renal failure, 76*t*–77*t*
pharmacokinetics, in renal failure, 76*t*–77*t*
Kidney. *See also* Renal failure
function, with liver disease, 95
organic acids actively secreted by, 28*t*
organic bases actively secreted by, 28*t*
Klebsiella pneumoniae, antimicrobial drugs of choice for, 339*t*
knr, 3*t*
kr, 3*t*

L
Labetalol
absorption, drug interactions affecting, 19*t*
disposition, effect of liver disease, 119*t*
dosage adjustment
with dialysis, 64*t*–65*t*
in liver disease, 119*t*
in renal failure, 64*t*–65*t*
hepatic/renal elimination, 119*t*
for hypertensive emergencies, 226*t*–227*t*
pharmacodynamics, 119*t*
in renal failure, 64*t*–65*t*
pharmacokinetics, 119*t*
in renal failure, 64*t*–65*t*
properties of, 221*t*
β-Lactamase inhibitors
dosage adjustment
with dialysis, 52*t*–53*t*
in renal failure, 52*t*–53*t*
pharmacodynamics, in renal failure, 52*t*–53*t*
pharmacokinetics, in renal failure, 52*t*–53*t*
β-Lactams, intravenous infusion, in pediatric patients, 188*t*
Lactulose, 314–315
properties of, 313*t*
Laxatives, 311–316
classification of, 313*t*
comparison, 313*t*
Legionella, antimicrobial drugs of choice for, 339*t*
Leptospira, antimicrobial drugs of choice for, 340*t*
Levallorphan, dosage and administration, 204*t*–205*t*
Levatol. *See* Penbutolol
Levodopa
absorption, drug interactions affecting, 16*t*
interference with glucose determination, 382*t*
psychiatric side effects, 269*t*
Levonorgestrel, drug interactions, with cyclosporine, 29*t*
Lidocaine
absorption, drug interactions affecting, 19*t*
adverse effects of, 230*t*–231*t*
disposition, effect of liver disease, 119*t*
dosage adjustment
with dialysis, 66*t*–67*t*
in liver disease, 119*t*
in renal failure, 66*t*–67*t*
dosage and administration, 230*t*–231*t*
hepatic/renal elimination, 119*t*
indications for, 230*t*
infusion, in pediatric patients, 188*t*
metabolism, inhibition by other drug(s), 24*t*, 27*t*
monitoring guidelines, 7*t*
pharmacodynamics, 119*t*
in renal failure, 66*t*–67*t*
pharmacokinetics, 6*t*, 119*t*
in renal failure, 66*t*–67*t*
psychiatric side effects, 270*t*
Lincomycin, drug interactions, with nondepolarizing muscle relaxants, 207*t*
Lisinopril
disposition, effect of liver disease, 120*t*
dosage adjustment
with dialysis, 62*t*–63*t*
in liver disease, 120*t*
in renal failure, 62*t*–63*t*
hepatic/renal elimination, 120*t*
pharmacodynamics, 120*t*
in renal failure, 62*t*–63*t*
pharmacokinetics, 120*t*
in renal failure, 62*t*–63*t*
properties of, 223*t*
Lithium
absorption, drug interactions affecting, 18*t*
fraction of dose excreted unchanged in urine with normal renal function, in children, 190*t*
Lithium carbonate
dosage adjustment
with dialysis, 72*t*–73*t*
in renal failure, 72*t*–73*t*
pharmacodynamics, in renal failure, 72*t*–73*t*
pharmacokinetics, in renal failure, 72*t*–73*t*
pharmacology of, 375*t*
Liver
cirrhosis, architecture and blood flow in, 93–95

disease
dosage adjustment in, 107–109, 128*t*
drug interactions in, 106–107
drugs used with caution or not at all in, 109*t*
renal function with, 95
severity, 106
enzymes, 92
extraction of drug by, 100–101
failure, pharmacotherapy in, 91–138
function, 92–93
homeostatic and metabolic functions, 92
reserve and recuperative properties, 93
Loperamide, 298
Lopressor. *See* Metoprolol
Lorazepam
cost, 201*t*
disposition, effect of liver disease, 123*t*
dosage adjustment
with dialysis, 72*t*–73*t*
in liver disease, 123*t*
in renal failure, 72*t*–73*t*
dosage and administration, 247*t*–248*t*
in mechanically ventilated patients, 201*t*
fraction of dose excreted unchanged in urine with normal renal function, in children, 190*t*
hepatic/renal elimination, 123*t*
intravenous, 202*t*–203*t*
monitoring guidelines, 7*t*
pharmacodynamics, 123*t*
in renal failure, 72*t*–73*t*
pharmacokinetic parameters, 6*t*
pharmacokinetics, 123*t*
in renal failure, 72*t*–73*t*
pharmacology of, 247*t*–248*t*
properties of, 247*t*–248*t*
use during mechanical ventilation, 203*t*
Lorcainide
disposition, effect of liver disease, 120*t*
dosage adjustment, in liver disease, 120*t*
hepatic/renal elimination, 120*t*
pharmacodynamics, 120*t*
pharmacokinetics, 120*t*
Lorfan. *See* Levallorphan
Loridine, interference with glucose determination, 382*t*
Lotensin. *See* Benazepril
Lovastatin, metabolism, induction by other drug(s), 21*t*
Lower motor neuron lesions, interactions with muscle relaxants, 208*t*–209*t*
Lypressin. *See* Lysine vasopressin
Lysine vasopressin
activity, 372*t*
dosage and administration, 309*t*, 373*t*

M
Maalox, 282*t*
Macrolides, 348–350
dosage adjustment
with dialysis, 56*t*–57*t*
in renal failure, 56*t*–57*t*
pharmacodynamics, in renal failure, 56*t*–57*t*
pharmacokinetics, in renal failure, 56*t*–57*t*
Magnesium
adverse effects of, 232*t*–233*t*
dosage and administration, 232*t*–233*t*
indications for, 232*t*
infusion, in pediatric patients, 188*t*
supplements, 383*t*
Magnesium citrate, properties of, 313*t*
Magnesium hydroxide, 283
properties of, 313*t*
Magnesium oxide, 283
Magnesium salts, 283, 314–315
Magnesium sulfate, 314
clinical use, in asthma, 140
properties of, 313*t*
Mannitol, dosage and administration, in renal failure, 51*t*
Mecamylamine
psychiatric side effects, 270*t*
secretion by kidney, 28*t*
Mefenamic acid, drug interactions, 20*t*
Mefloquine, psychiatric side effects, 267*t*
Melphalan, drug interactions, with cyclosporine, 29*t*
Mepacrine, secretion by kidney, 28*t*
Meperidine
comparative narcotic potency, 204*t*–205*t*
disposition, effect of liver disease, 114*t*
dosage adjustment
with dialysis, 74*t*–75*t*
in liver disease, 114*t*
in renal failure, 74*t*–75*t*
dosage and administration, 204*t*–205*t*
hepatic/renal elimination, 114*t*
metabolism, inhibition by other drug(s), 24*t*
monitoring guidelines, 7*t*
pharmacodynamics, 114*t*
in renal failure, 74*t*–75*t*
pharmacokinetics, 6*t*, 114*t*
in renal failure, 74*t*–75*t*
psychiatric side effects, 267*t*
use, in adult ICU patients, 204*t*–205*t*
Mephenytoin, poor and extensive metabolizers of, 103
Meprobamate
metabolism
induction by other drug(s), 21*t*
inhibition by other drug(s), 23*t*
removal, by resin hemoperfusion, 11*t*

Mercaptopurine
absorption, drug interactions affecting, 19*t*
metabolism, inhibition by other drug(s), 22*t*
Metabolism, 371–383
route of, and effects of liver disease, 104
Metaproterenol
dosage, 157*t*
duration of action, 156*t*
preparation, 157*t*
receptor, 156*t*
route of administration, 156*t*–157*t*
Metformin, secretion by kidney, 28*t*
Methacholine
clinical uses, 264*t*–265*t*
side effects, 264*t*–265*t*
Methadone
comparative narcotic potency, 204*t*–205*t*
disposition, effect of liver disease, 114*t*
dosage adjustment
with dialysis, 74*t*–75*t*
in liver disease, 114*t*
in renal failure, 74*t*–75*t*
dosage and administration, 204*t*–205*t*
hepatic/renal elimination, 114*t*
metabolism, induction by other drug(s), 21*t*
pharmacodynamics, 114*t*
in renal failure, 74*t*–75*t*
pharmacokinetics, 114*t*
in renal failure, 74*t*–75*t*
Methaqualone, removal, by resin hemoperfusion, 11*t*
Methenamine, psychiatric side effects, 268*t*
Methicillin
dosage adjustment
with dialysis, 56*t*–57*t*
in renal failure, 56*t*–57*t*, 334*t*
dosage and administration, 334*t*
fraction of dose excreted unchanged in urine with normal renal function, in children, 190*t*
pharmacodynamics, in renal failure, 56*t*–57*t*
pharmacokinetics, 334*t*
in renal failure, 56*t*–57*t*
serum concentration, with dialysis, 334*t*
volume of distribution, in renal failure, 47*t*
Methimazole, pharmacology of, 375*t*
Methohexital
disposition, effect of liver disease, 123*t*
dosage adjustment, in liver disease, 123*t*
hepatic/renal elimination, 123*t*
pharmacodynamics, 123*t*
pharmacokinetics, 123*t*
Methotrexate
disposition, effect of liver disease, 116*t*
dosage adjustment, in liver disease, 116*t*
hepatic/renal elimination, 116*t*
pharmacodynamics, 116*t*
pharmacokinetics, 116*t*
psychiatric side effects, 268*t*
secretion by kidney, 28*t*
Methsuximide, psychiatric side effects, 267*t*
Methyclothiazide, dosage and administration, 85*t*
Methylcellulose, 312
properties of, 313*t*
Methyldopa
absorption, drug interactions affecting, 16*t*
dosage adjustment
with dialysis, 62*t*–63*t*
in renal failure, 62*t*–63*t*
for hypertensive emergencies, 226*t*–227*t*
pharmacodynamics, in renal failure, 62*t*–63*t*
pharmacokinetics, in renal failure, 62*t*–63*t*
psychiatric side effects, 270*t*
Methyldopate, intravenous infusion, in pediatric patients, 188*t*
N-Methylnicotinamide, secretion by kidney, 28*t*
Methylphenidate, drug interactions, 25*t*
Methylprednisolone
dosage adjustment
with dialysis, 80*t*–81*t*
in renal failure, 80*t*–81*t*
drug interactions, with cyclosporine, 29*t*
metabolism, inhibition by other drug(s), 25*t*
pharmacodynamics, in renal failure, 80*t*–81*t*
pharmacokinetics, in renal failure, 80*t*–81*t*
Methyltestosterone, drug interactions, with cyclosporine, 29*t*
Metoclopramide, 302–303
adverse effects of, 303
adverse effects of, in children, 182–183
clinical uses, 264*t*–265*t*
dosage, 303
dosage adjustment
with dialysis, 80*t*–81*t*
in renal failure, 80*t*–81*t*
drug interactions, with cyclosporine, 29*t*
mechanism of action, 302–303
pharmacodynamics, in renal failure, 80*t*–81*t*

pharmacokinetics, 303
in renal failure, 80t–81t
psychiatric side effects, 269t
side effects, 264t–265t
special considerations with, 303
Metocurine
characteristics of, 210t–211t
clearance, 213t
clinical pharmacology of, 206t–207t
cost, 201t
dosage, in mechanically ventilated patients, 201t
dosage adjustment
with dialysis, 82t–83t
in renal failure, 82t–83t
duration of clinical effect, 206t
intubating dose, 206t
metabolism, 213t
pharmacodynamics, in renal failure, 82t–83t
pharmacokinetics, in renal failure, 82t–83t
side effects and adverse reactions to, 210t–211t
Metolazone
dosage adjustment
with dialysis, 70t–71t
in renal failure, 70t–71t
dosage and administration, 85t
drug interactions, with cyclosporine, 29t
pharmacodynamics, in renal failure, 70t–71t
pharmacokinetics, in renal failure, 70t–71t
Metoprolol
absorption, drug interactions affecting, 19t
disposition, effect of liver disease, 120t
dosage adjustment
with dialysis, 64t–65t
in liver disease, 120t
in renal failure, 64t–65t
hepatic/renal elimination, 120t
metabolism
induction by other drug(s), 21t
inhibition by other drug(s), 22t, 24t, 26t
pharmacodynamics, 120t
in renal failure, 64t–65t
pharmacokinetics, 120t
in renal failure, 64t–65t
properties of, 220t, 232t–233t
Metrizamide, psychiatric side effects, 269t
Metronidazole, 352–353
disposition, effect of liver disease, 113t
dosage adjustment
with dialysis, 58t–59t
in liver disease, 113t
in renal failure, 58t–59t, 335t
dosage and administration, 335t
fraction of dose excreted unchanged in urine with normal renal function, in children, 190t
hepatic/renal elimination, 113t
infusion, in pediatric patients, 188t
metabolism, inhibition by other drug(s), 24t
pharmacodynamics, 113t
in renal failure, 58t–59t
pharmacokinetics, 113t, 335t
in renal failure, 58t–59t
psychiatric side effects, 267t
serum concentration, with dialysis, 335t
Mexiletine
adverse effects of, 230t–231t
dosage adjustment
with dialysis, 66t–67t
in renal failure, 66t–67t
dosage and administration, 230t–231t
drug interactions, 25t
elimination, 10t
indications for, 230t
metabolism, induction by other drug(s), 21t
pharmacodynamics, in renal failure, 66t–67t
pharmacokinetics, in renal failure, 66t–67t
psychiatric side effects, 270t
Mezlocillin, 341
dosage adjustment
with dialysis, 56t–57t
in renal failure, 56t–57t
pharmacodynamics, in renal failure, 56t–57t
pharmacokinetics, in renal failure, 56t–57t
Miconazole, 358
Midazolam
adverse effects of, in pediatric patients, 184
cost, 201t
disposition, effect of liver disease, 123t
dosage adjustment
with dialysis, 72t–73t
in liver disease, 123t
in renal failure, 72t–73t
dosage and administration, 247t–248t
in mechanically ventilated patients, 201t
fraction of dose excreted unchanged in urine with normal renal function, in children, 190t
hepatic/renal elimination, 123t
intravenous, 202t–203t
monitoring guidelines, 7t
pharmacodynamics, 123t
in renal failure, 72t–73t
pharmacokinetics, 6t, 123t

Midazolam—*continued*
in renal failure, 72*t*–73*t*
pharmacology of, 247*t*–248*t*
properties of, 247*t*–248*t*
use during mechanical ventilation, 203*t*
Milk of Magnesia, 282*t*, 314
Milrinone
dosage adjustment
with dialysis, 70*t*–71*t*
in renal failure, 70*t*–71*t*
pharmacodynamics, in renal failure, 70*t*–71*t*
pharmacokinetics, in renal failure, 70*t*–71*t*
Minocycline
dosage adjustment
with dialysis, 58*t*–59*t*
in renal failure, 58*t*–59*t*
pharmacodynamics, in renal failure, 58*t*–59*t*
pharmacokinetics, in renal failure, 58*t*–59*t*
Minoxidil
dosage adjustment
with dialysis, 64*t*–65*t*
in renal failure, 64*t*–65*t*
for hypertensive urgencies, 228*t*–229*t*
pharmacodynamics, in renal failure, 64*t*–65*t*
pharmacokinetics, in renal failure, 64*t*–65*t*
Misoprostol, 295–296
adverse reactions, 296–297
contraindications, 296
dosage and administration, 296
indications for use, 296
mechanisms of action, 295–296
overdosage, 297
pharmacokinetics, 296
Mithramycin, psychiatric side effects, 268*t*
Mivacurium
characteristics of, 210*t*–211*t*
clearance, 213*t*
clinical pharmacology of, 206*t*–207*t*
duration of clinical effect, 206*t*
intubating dose, 206*t*
metabolism, 213*t*
side effects and adverse reactions to, 210*t*–211*t*
Monobactam, 344–345
dosage adjustment
with dialysis, 54*t*–55*t*
in renal failure, 54*t*–55*t*
pharmacodynamics, in renal failure, 54*t*–55*t*
pharmacokinetics, in renal failure, 54*t*–55*t*
Monopril. *See* Fosinopril
Moricizine
adverse effects of, 203*t*–231*t*
dosage and administration, 203*t*–231*t*
drug interactions, 21*t*
indications for, 203*t*
metabolism, inhibition by other drug(s), 24*t*
Morphine
adverse effects of, in pediatric patients, 183
comparative narcotic potency, 205*t*
cost, 201*t*
disposition, effect of liver disease, 115*t*
dosage adjustment
with dialysis, 74*t*–75*t*
in liver disease, 115*t*
in renal failure, 74*t*–75*t*
dosage and administration, 204*t*–205*t*
in mechanically ventilated patients, 201*t*
hepatic/renal elimination, 115*t*
metabolism, induction by other drug(s), 21*t*
monitoring guidelines, 7*t*
pharmacodynamics, 115*t*
in renal failure, 74*t*–75*t*
pharmacokinetics, 6*t*, 115*t*
in renal failure, 74*t*–75*t*
psychiatric side effects, 267*t*
use, in adult ICU patients, 204*t*–205*t*
use during mechanical ventilation, 203*t*
Moxalactam
dosage adjustment
with dialysis, 54*t*–55*t*
in renal failure, 54*t*–55*t*
intraperitoneal administration, bioavailability after, 48*t*
pharmacodynamics, in renal failure, 54*t*–55*t*
pharmacokinetics, in renal failure, 54*t*–55*t*
volume of distribution, in renal failure, 47*t*
Mucolytics, in pulmonary disease, 147–149
Mucor-Absidia-Rhizopus, antimicrobial drugs of choice for, 340*t*
Multiple sclerosis, interactions with muscle relaxants, 208*t*–209*t*
Muscle disease, interactions with muscle relaxants, 208*t*–209*t*
Muscle relaxants
duration of clinical effect, 206*t*
interactions, with disease, 208*t*–209*t*
intubating dose, 206*t*
Muscle-wasting disease, interactions with muscle relaxants, 208*t*–209*t*
Muscular dystrophy, interactions with muscle relaxants, 208*t*–209*t*

Myasthenia gravis, interactions with muscle relaxants, 208*t*–209*t*
Myasthenic syndrome, interactions with muscle relaxants, 208*t*–209*t*
Mycobacterium tuberculosis, antimicrobial drugs of choice for, 339*t*
Mycoplasma pneumoniae, antimicrobial drugs of choice for, 340*t*
Mylanta, 282*t*
Myotonia congenita, interactions with muscle relaxants, 208*t*–209*t*
Myotonia dystrophica, interactions with muscle relaxants, 208*t*–209*t*
Myotonic syndrome, interactions with muscle relaxants, 208*t*–209*t*
Myxedema myopathy, interactions with muscle relaxants, 208*t*–209*t*

N
Nadolol
  dosage adjustment
    with dialysis, 64*t*–65*t*
    in renal failure, 64*t*–65*t*
  pharmacodynamics, in renal failure, 64*t*–65*t*
  pharmacokinetics, in renal failure, 64*t*–65*t*
  properties of, 232*t*–233*t*
Nafcillin
  disposition, effect of liver disease, 113*t*
  dosage adjustment
    with dialysis, 58*t*–59*t*
    in liver disease, 113*t*
    in renal failure, 50*t*, 58*t*–59*t*, 334*t*
  dosage and administration, 334*t*
  drug interactions, with cyclosporine, 29*t*
  fraction of dose excreted unchanged in urine with normal renal function, in children, 190*t*
  half-life
    in end-stage renal disease, 50*t*
    normal, 50*t*
  hepatic/renal elimination, 113*t*
  pharmacodynamics, 113*t*
    in renal failure, 58*t*–59*t*
  pharmacokinetics, 113*t*, 334*t*
    in renal failure, 58*t*–59*t*
  serum concentration, with dialysis, 334*t*
Nalidixic acid
  adverse effects of, in pediatric patients, 181
  drug interactions, 20*t*
  psychiatric side effects, 267*t*
Nalline. *See* Nalorphine
Nalorphine, dosage and administration, 204*t*–205*t*
Naloxone
  dosage adjustment
    with dialysis, 74*t*–75*t*
    in renal failure, 74*t*–75*t*
  dosage and administration, 204*t*–205*t*
  pharmacodynamics, in renal failure, 74*t*–75*t*
  pharmacokinetics, in renal failure, 74*t*–75*t*
Naproxen
  disposition, effect of liver disease, 117*t*
  dosage adjustment, in liver disease, 117*t*
  hepatic/renal elimination, 117*t*
  pharmacodynamics, 117*t*
  pharmacokinetics, 117*t*
  psychiatric side effects, 267*t*
  volume of distribution, in renal failure, 47*t*
Narcan. *See* Naloxone
Narcotic antagonists
  dosage adjustment
    with dialysis, 74*t*–75*t*
    in renal failure, 74*t*–75*t*
  dosage and administration, 204*t*–205*t*
  pharmacodynamics, in renal failure, 74*t*–75*t*
  pharmacokinetics, in renal failure, 74*t*–75*t*
Narcotics
  dosage adjustment
    with dialysis, 74*t*–75*t*
    in renal failure, 74*t*–75*t*
  pharmacodynamics, in renal failure, 74*t*–75*t*
  pharmacokinetics, in renal failure, 74*t*–75*t*
Nausea and vomiting, pharmacotherapy for, 316–318
Neisseria gonorrhoeae, antimicrobial drugs of choice for, 338*t*
Neisseria meningitidis, antimicrobial drugs of choice for, 338*t*
Neomycin, 345–347
  disposition, effect of liver disease, 113*t*
  dosage adjustment, in liver disease, 113*t*
  hepatic/renal elimination, 113*t*
  pharmacodynamics, 113*t*
  pharmacokinetics, 113*t*
Neostigmine
  clinical uses, 262*t*, 264*t*–265*t*
  dosage adjustment
    with dialysis, 82*t*–83*t*
    in renal failure, 82*t*–83*t*
  pharmacodynamics, in renal failure, 82*t*–83*t*
  pharmacokinetics, in renal failure, 82*t*–83*t*
  side effects, 264*t*–265*t*
Netilmicin, 345–347
  dosage adjustment
    with dialysis, 52*t*–53*t*
    in renal failure, 52*t*–53*t*

Netilmicin—*continued*
pharmacodynamics, in renal failure, 52*t*–53*t*
pharmacokinetics, in renal failure, 52*t*–53*t*
Neuroleptic malignant syndrome, diagnostic criteria for, 266*t*
Neurologic psychiatric medications, 241–279
Neuromuscular agents
dosage adjustment
with dialysis, 82*t*–83*t*
in renal failure, 82*t*–83*t*
monitoring guidelines, 7*t*
pharmacodynamics, in renal failure, 82*t*–83*t*
pharmacokinetics, 6*t*
in renal failure, 82*t*–83*t*
Neuromuscular blocking agents
clinical pharmacology of, 206*t*–207*t*
dosage
in children, 193*t*
in mechanically ventilated patients, 201*t*
infusion, in pediatric patients, 188*t*
responsiveness to
conditions affecting, 212*t*
drugs affecting, 212*t*
Nicardipine
dosage adjustment
with dialysis, 66*t*–67*t*
in renal failure, 66*t*–67*t*
drug interactions, with cyclosporine, 29*t*
for hypertensive emergencies, 226*t*–227*t*
pharmacodynamics, in renal failure, 66*t*–67*t*
pharmacokinetics, in renal failure, 66*t*–67*t*
properties of, 222*t*
Nifedipine
disposition, effect of liver disease, 120*t*
dosage adjustment
with dialysis, 66*t*–67*t*
in liver disease, 120*t*
in renal failure, 66*t*–67*t*
hepatic/renal elimination, 120*t*
for hypertensive urgencies, 228*t*–229*t*
metabolism, inhibition by other drug(s), 25*t*, 27*t*
pharmacodynamics, 120*t*
in renal failure, 66*t*–67*t*
pharmacokinetics, 120*t*
in renal failure, 66*t*–67*t*
properties of, 222*t*
psychiatric side effects, 270*t*
Nimodipine
dosage adjustment
with dialysis, 68*t*–69*t*
in renal failure, 68*t*–69*t*
pharmacodynamics, in renal failure, 68*t*–69*t*
pharmacokinetics, in renal failure, 68*t*–69*t*
Nisoldipine
absorption, drug interactions affecting, 19*t*
metabolism, inhibition by other drug(s), 27*t*
Nitrates, indications for, 217
Nitrazepam
disposition, effect of liver disease, 123*t*
dosage adjustment, in liver disease, 123*t*
hepatic/renal elimination, 123*t*
metabolism, inhibition by other drug(s), 26*t*
pharmacodynamics, 123*t*
pharmacokinetics, 123*t*
Nitrendipine
dosage adjustment
with dialysis, 68*t*–69*t*
in renal failure, 68*t*–69*t*
pharmacodynamics, in renal failure, 68*t*–69*t*
pharmacokinetics, in renal failure, 68*t*–69*t*
Nitrofurantoin, psychiatric side effects, 267*t*
Nitroglycerin
dosage adjustment
with dialysis, 64*t*–65*t*
in renal failure, 64*t*–65*t*
for hypertensive emergencies, 226*t*–227*t*
intravenous, indications for, 217
pharmacodynamics
in critical illness, 8*t*–9*t*
in renal failure, 64*t*–65*t*
pharmacokinetics, in renal failure, 64*t*–65*t*
Nitroprusside
dosage adjustment
with dialysis, 64*t*–65*t*
in renal failure, 64*t*–65*t*
indications for, 217
infusion, in pediatric patients, 188*t*
monitoring guidelines, 7*t*
pharmacodynamics
in critical illness, 8*t*–9*t*
in renal failure, 64*t*–65*t*
pharmacokinetics, 6*t*
in renal failure, 64*t*–65*t*
Nizatidine, 295
overdosage, 295
properties of, 290*t*
side effects and adverse reactions to, 295
Nocardia, antimicrobial drugs of choice for, 339*t*
Nondepolarizing neuromuscular blocking agents

classification, 210t–211t
clearance, 213t
metabolism, 213t
recommended doses, 210t–211t
side effect profiles of, 210t–211t
usual clinical effects, 210t–211t
Nonnarcotic analgesics
dosage adjustment
with dialysis, 74t–77t
in renal failure, 74t–77t
pharmacodynamics, in renal failure, 74t–77t
pharmacokinetics, in renal failure, 74t–77t
Nonsteroidal antiinflammatory agents, secretion by kidney, 28t
Norepinephrine
dosage adjustment
with dialysis, 70t–71t
in renal failure, 70t–71t
infusion, 238t–239t
in children, 188t, 192t
pharmacodynamics
in critical illness, 8t–9t
in renal failure, 70t–71t
pharmacokinetics, in renal failure, 70t–71t
Norfloxacin
adverse effects of, in pediatric patients, 182
drug interactions, with cyclosporine, 29t
Nortriptyline
dosage adjustment
with dialysis, 74t–75t
in renal adjustment, 74t–75t
pharmacodynamics, in renal adjustment, 74t–75t
pharmacokinetics, in renal adjustment, 74t–75t
Numorphan. *See* Oxymorphone
Nutrition, in critical illness, 8t–9t

O
Octreotide, 301–302
dosage and administration, 301
Ofloxacin, 348
dosage adjustment
with dialysis, 56t–57t
in renal failure, 56t–57t, 335t
dosage and administration, 335t
pharmacodynamics, in renal failure, 56t–57t
pharmacokinetics, 335t
in renal failure, 56t–57t
psychiatric side effects, 267t
serum concentration, with dialysis, 335t
Olsalazine, 319
Omeprazole, 287–288
adverse effects, 288
disposition, effect of liver disease, 126t
dosage adjustment
with dialysis, 78t–79t
in liver disease, 126t
in renal failure, 78t–79t
dosage and administration, 288
drug interactions, 25t, 288
hepatic/renal elimination, 126t
pharmacodynamics, 126t
in renal failure, 78t–79t
pharmacokinetics, 126t
in renal failure, 78t–79t
Opiates, antidiarrheal effects, 297–299
Opioids, use, in adult ICU patients, 204t–205t
Oral anticoagulants, metabolism
induction by other drug(s), 21t
inhibition by other drug(s), 23t, 26t
Oral contraceptives
drug interactions, 20t–21t, 26t
metabolism, induction by other drug(s), 21t
Oral hypoglycemics, psychiatric side effects, 269t
Orphenadrine, psychiatric side effects, 269t
Osmotic diuretics (mannitol)
dosage and administration, 84t
half-life, 84t
site of action, 84t
Osmotic laxatives, 314–315
Oxacillin
dosage adjustment
with dialysis, 58t–59t
in renal failure, 58t–59t, 334t
dosage and administration, 334t
fraction of dose excreted unchanged in urine with normal renal function, in children, 190t
pharmacodynamics, in renal failure, 58t–59t
pharmacokinetics, 334t
in renal failure, 58t–59t
serum concentration, with dialysis, 334t
Oxazepam
disposition, effect of liver disease, 124t
dosage adjustment
with dialysis, 72t–73t
in liver disease, 124t
in renal failure, 72t–73t
hepatic/renal elimination, 124t
pharmacodynamics, 124t
in renal failure, 72t–73t
pharmacokinetics, 124t
in renal failure, 72t–73t
Oxidating drugs, plasma half-life, in pediatric patient, 191t
Oxygen therapy, clinical use, in asthma, 140

Oxymorphone
comparative narcotic potency, 204t–205t
dosage and administration, 204t–205t
Oxyphenbutazone, drug interactions, 26t

P
Pancuronium
characteristics of, 210t–211t
clearance, 213t
clinical pharmacology of, 206t–207t
cost, 201t
dosage
in children, 193t
in mechanically ventilated patients, 201t
dosage adjustment
with dialysis, 82t–83t
in renal failure, 82t–83t
duration of clinical effect, 206t
fraction of dose excreted unchanged in urine with normal renal function, in children, 190t
infusion, in pediatric patients, 188t
intubating dose, 206t
metabolism, 213t
induction by other drug(s), 21t
monitoring guidelines, 7t
pharmacodynamics, in renal failure, 82t–83t
pharmacokinetic parameters, 6t
pharmacokinetics, in renal failure, 82t–83t
side effects and adverse reactions to, 210t–211t
use during mechanical ventilation, 203t
Aminosalicylic acid, psychiatric side effects, 267t
Paramyotonia, interactions with muscle relaxants, 208t–209t
Paroxetine
dosage adjustment
with dialysis, 74t–75t
in renal failure, 74t–75t
pharmacodynamics, in renal failure, 74t–75t
pharmacokinetics, in renal failure, 74t–75t
Pectin, for diarrhea, 300
Pediatrics, 179–197
Pefloxacin, metabolism, induction by other drug(s), 21t
Penbutolol
dosage adjustment
with dialysis, 64t–65t
in renal failure, 64t–65t
pharmacodynamics, in renal failure, 64t–65t
pharmacokinetics, in renal failure, 64t–65t
properties of, 221t
Penicillamine, absorption, drug interactions affecting, 16t
Penicillin G
dosage adjustment
with dialysis, 58t–59t
in renal failure, 50t, 58t–59t
half-life
in end-stage renal disease, 50t
normal, 50t
infusion, in pediatric patients, 188t
pharmacodynamics, in renal failure, 58t–59t
pharmacokinetics, in renal failure, 58t–59t
Penicillins, 332–341
acylamino, 341
adverse reactions to, 333–337
antibacterial spectrum, 332–333
classification of, 332–333
clinical use, 341
distribution, 333
dosage adjustment
with dialysis, 56t–57t
in renal failure, 56t–57t, 334t
dosage and administration, 334t
elimination, 333
fraction of dose excreted unchanged in urine with normal renal function, in children, 190t
hypersensitivity reactions, 333–337
pharmacodynamics, in renal failure, 56t–57t
pharmacokinetics, 334t
in renal failure, 56t–57t
properties of, 332
secretion by kidney, 28t
serum concentration, with dialysis, 334t
toxic reactions to, 337
Pentamidine, 360–361
adverse effects of, 361
distribution, 361
dosage adjustment
with dialysis, 58t–59t
in renal failure, 58t–59t, 335t
dosage and administration, 335t
elimination, 361
mechanism of action, 360
pharmacodynamics, in renal failure, 58t–59t
pharmacokinetics, 335t
in renal failure, 58t–59t
serum concentration, with dialysis, 335t
Pentazocine
comparative narcotic potency, 204t–205t
disposition, effect of liver disease, 115t
dosage adjustment, in liver disease, 115t

dosage and administration, 204t–205t
hepatic/renal elimination, 115t
pharmacodynamics, 115t
pharmacokinetics, 115t
psychiatric side effects, 267t

Pentobarbital
cost, 201t
disposition, effect of liver disease, 124t
dosage, in mechanically ventilated patients, 201t
dosage adjustment, in liver disease, 124t
hepatic/renal elimination, 124t
metabolism
induction by other drug(s), 21t
inhibition by other drug(s), 23t
pharmacodynamics, 124t
pharmacokinetics, 124t
use in patients with status epilepticus, 253t, 255t

Pentolinium, psychiatric side effects, 270t

Pentoxifylline
dosage adjustment
with dialysis, 82t–83t
in renal failure, 82t–83t
metabolism, inhibition by other drug(s), 25t
pharmacodynamics, in renal failure, 82t–83t
pharmacokinetics, in renal failure, 82t–83t

Pergolide, psychiatric side effects, 269t

Pharmacodynamics, 4f
age-related differences, 180
definition, 180
in pediatric patients, 180–187

Pharmacokinetics, 1–12, 4f
age-related differences, 180
factors affecting, 4f
principles, clinical illustration of, 5t
terminology, 3t

Phenobarbital
absorption, drug interactions affecting, 16t
adverse effects of, in pediatric patients, 184
cost, 201t
disposition, effect of liver disease, 116t
dosage, in mechanically ventilated patients, 201t
dosage adjustment, in liver disease, 116t
drug interactions, 20t–21t, 246t–247t
with cyclosporine, 29t
elimination, 10t
hepatic/renal elimination, 116t
metabolism, inhibition by other drug(s), 23t, 25t
monitoring guidelines, 7t
pharmacodynamics, 116t
pharmacokinetics, 6t, 116t

Phenolphthalein, 315
properties of, 313t

Phenothiazines
antiemetic, 317
dosage adjustment
with dialysis, 72t–73t
in renal failure, 72t–73t
pharmacodynamics, in renal failure, 72t–73t
pharmacokinetics, in renal failure, 72t–73t

Phensuximide, psychiatric side effects, 267t

Phentolamine, for hypertensive emergencies, 226t–227t

Phenylbutazone
disposition, effect of liver disease, 117t
dosage adjustment, in liver disease, 117t
drug interactions, 20t, 26t
hepatic/renal elimination, 117t
metabolism, induction by other drug(s), 21t
pharmacodynamics, 117t
pharmacokinetics, 117t
psychiatric side effects, 267t
removal, by resin hemoperfusion, 11t

Phenylephrine, in treatment of supraventricular tachycardia, 228t–229t

Phenytoin
absorption, drug interactions affecting, 16t, 18t
displacement from protein-binding sites, drug interactions due to, 20t
dosage adjustment
with dialysis, 76t–79t
in renal failure, 76t–79t
drug interactions, 20t–21t, 244t–245t
with cyclosporine, 29t
metabolism
induction by other drug(s), 21t
inhibition by other drug(s), 22t–27t
monitoring guidelines, 7t
pharmacodynamics, in renal failure, 76t–79t
pharmacokinetics, 6t
in renal failure, 76t–79t
volume of distribution, in renal failure, 47t

Physostigmine
clinical uses, 262t, 264t–265t
side effects, 264t–265t

Pilocarpine
clinical uses, 264t–265t
side effects, 264t–265t

Pindolol
disposition, effect of liver disease, 120t
dosage adjustment
with dialysis, 64t–65t
in liver disease, 120t
in renal failure, 64t–65t

Pindolol—*continued*
hepatic/renal elimination, 120*t*
pharmacodynamics, 120*t*
in renal failure, 64*t*–65*t*
pharmacokinetics, 120*t*
in renal failure, 64*t*–65*t*
properties of, 220*t*, 232*t*–233*t*
volume of distribution, in renal failure, 47*t*
Pipecuronium
characteristics of, 210*t*–211*t*
clearance, 213*t*
clinical pharmacology of, 206*t*–207*t*
metabolism, 213*t*
side effects and adverse reactions to, 210*t*–211*t*
Piperacillin, 341
dosage adjustment
with dialysis, 58*t*–59*t*
in renal failure, 50*t*, 58*t*–59*t*, 334*t*
dosage and administration, 334*t*
half-life
in end-stage renal disease, 50*t*
normal, 50*t*
intraperitoneal administration, bioavailability after, 49*t*
pharmacodynamics, in renal failure, 58*t*–59*t*
pharmacokinetics, 334*t*
in renal failure, 58*t*–59*t*
serum concentration, with dialysis, 334*t*
Pirbuterol
duration of action, 156*t*
receptor, 156*t*
route of administration, 156*t*
Piroxicam
absorption, drug interactions affecting, 16*t*
metabolism, inhibition by other drug(s), 25*t*
Plasma concentration
average, 3*t*
with infusion, 12*f*
with intravenous bolus, 12*f*
maximum (peak), 3*t*
minimum (trough), 3*t*
steady-state, 99
Plasma protein binding, 96–99
Plasminogen activators, doses, for patients with acute myocardial infarction, 240*t*
Plendil. *See* Felodipine
Pneumocystis carinii, antimicrobial drugs of choice for, 340*t*
Poliomyelitis, interactions with muscle relaxants, 208*t*–209*t*
Polyarteritis nodosa, interactions with muscle relaxants, 208*t*–209*t*
Polycarbophil, 312
properties of, 313*t*
Polyethylene glycol (solution), 314–315
Polymyositis, interactions with muscle relaxants, 208*t*–209*t*
Polymyxin, drug interactions, with nondepolarizing muscle relaxants, 207*t*
Polythiazide, dosage and administration, 85*t*
Potassium-sparing diuretics
dosage and administration, 84*t*
half-life, 84*t*
site of action, 84*t*
Pralidoxime
clinical uses, 264*t*–265*t*
side effects, 264*t*–265*t*
Pravastatin
metabolism, induction by other drug(s), 21*t*
psychiatric side effects, 269*t*
Prazosin
disposition, effect of liver disease, 121*t*
dosage adjustment
with dialysis, 62*t*–63*t*
in liver disease, 121*t*
in renal failure, 62*t*–63*t*
hepatic/renal elimination, 121*t*
for hypertensive urgencies, 228*t*–229*t*
metabolism, inhibition by other drug(s), 22*t*
pharmacodynamics, 121*t*
in renal failure, 62*t*–63*t*
pharmacokinetics, 121*t*
in renal failure, 62*t*–63*t*
psychiatric side effects, 270*t*
Prednisolone
disposition, effect of liver disease, 118*t*
dosage adjustment
with dialysis, 80*t*–81*t*
in liver disease, 118*t*
in renal failure, 80*t*–81*t*
drug interactions, with cyclosporine, 29*t*
hepatic/renal elimination, 118*t*
metabolism, inhibition by other drug(s), 25*t*–26*t*
pharmacodynamics, 118*t*
in renal failure, 80*t*–81*t*
pharmacokinetics, 118*t*
in renal failure, 80*t*–81*t*
Preload challenge, pharmacodynamics, in critical illness, 8*t*–9*t*
Primidone
disposition, effect of liver disease, 124*t*
dosage adjustment
with dialysis, 78*t*–79*t*
in liver disease, 124*t*
in renal failure, 78*t*–79*t*
hepatic/renal elimination, 124*t*
metabolism, inhibition by other drug(s), 25*t*
pharmacodynamics, 124*t*
in renal failure, 78*t*–79*t*
pharmacokinetics, 124*t*

in renal failure, 78*t*–79*t*
psychiatric side effects, 267*t*
Prinivil. *See* Lisinopril
Probenecid
drug interactions, 26*t*
secretion by kidney, 28*t*
Procainamide
adverse effects of, 230*t*–231*t*
disposition, effect of liver disease, 121*t*
dosage adjustment
with dialysis, 66*t*–67*t*
in liver disease, 121*t*
in renal failure, 50*t*, 66*t*–67*t*
dosage and administration, 230*t*–231*t*
half-life
in end-stage renal disease, 50*t*
normal, 50*t*
hepatic/renal elimination, 121*t*
indications for, 230*t*
infusion, in pediatric patients, 188*t*
metabolism, inhibition by other drug(s), 22*t*
monitoring guidelines, 7*t*
pharmacodynamics, 121*t*
in renal failure, 66*t*–67*t*
pharmacokinetics, 6*t*, 121*t*
in renal failure, 66*t*–67*t*
psychiatric side effects, 270*t*
secretion by kidney, 28*t*
Procarbazine, psychiatric side effects, 268*t*
Procardia. *See* Nifedipine
Prochlorperazine (Compazine)
adverse effects of, in children, 182–183
properties of, 317
Promethazine
dosage adjustment
with dialysis, 72*t*–73*t*
in renal failure, 72*t*–73*t*
pharmacodynamics, in renal failure, 72*t*–73*t*
pharmacokinetics, in renal failure, 72*t*–73*t*
psychiatric side effects, 268*t*
Propafenone
adverse effects of, 230*t*–231*t*
dosage adjustment
with dialysis, 66*t*–67*t*
in renal failure, 66*t*–67*t*
dosage and administration, 230*t*–231*t*
drug interactions, 26*t*
indications for, 230*t*
metabolism, inhibition by other drug(s), 27*t*
pharmacodynamics, in renal failure, 66*t*–67*t*
pharmacokinetics, in renal failure, 66*t*–67*t*
Propantheline
clinical uses, 264*t*–265*t*
effects of, 263*t*
indications for, 263*t*
side effects, 264*t*–265*t*
Propofol
cost, 201*t*
dosage, in mechanically ventilated patients, 201*t*
monitoring guidelines, 7*t*
pharmacokinetic parameters, 6*t*
Propoxyphene
disposition, effect of liver disease, 115*t*
dosage adjustment
with dialysis, 74*t*–75*t*
in liver disease, 115*t*
in renal failure, 74*t*–75*t*
drug interactions, 27*t*
hepatic/renal elimination, 115*t*
pharmacodynamics, 115*t*
in renal failure, 74*t*–75*t*
pharmacokinetics, 115*t*
in renal failure, 74*t*–75*t*
psychiatric side effects, 267*t*
Propranolol
absorption, drug interactions affecting, 17*t*–19*t*
adverse effects of, 230*t*–231*t*
disposition, effect of liver disease, 121*t*
dosage adjustment
with dialysis, 64*t*–65*t*
in liver disease, 121*t*
in renal failure, 64*t*–65*t*
dosage and administration, 230*t*–231*t*
drug interactions, 21*t*, 27*t*
hepatic/renal elimination, 121*t*
indications for, 230*t*
metabolism, inhibition by other drug(s), 22*t*–23*t*, 25*t*–27*t*
pharmacodynamics, 121*t*
in renal failure, 64*t*–65*t*
pharmacokinetics, 121*t*
in renal failure, 64*t*–65*t*
properties of, 220*t*, 232*t*–233*t*
in treatment of supraventricular tachycardia, 228*t*–229*t*
dl-Propranolol, pharmacology of, 375*t*
Propylthiouracil, pharmacology of, 375*t*
Prostaglandins, 152–154
clinical use
in adult respiratory distress syndrome, 153–154
in chronic obstructive pulmonary disease, 153
in primary pulmonary hypertension, 152–153
Proteus, antimicrobial drugs of choice for, 339*t*
Proteus mirabilis, antimicrobial drugs of choice for, 339*t*
Protozoa, antimicrobial drugs of choice for, 340*t*
Protriptyline
dosage adjustment
with dialysis, 74*t*–75*t*

Protriptyline—*continued*
in renal adjustment, 74*t*–75*t*
in renal failure, 74*t*–75*t*
pharmacodynamics
in renal adjustment, 74*t*–75*t*
in renal failure, 74*t*–75*t*
pharmacokinetics
in renal adjustment, 74*t*–75*t*
in renal failure, 74*t*–75*t*
Providencia, antimicrobial drugs of choice for, 339*t*
Pseudoephedrine
elimination, 10*t*
secretion by kidney, 28*t*
Pseudomonas aeruginosa, antimicrobial drugs of choice for, 339*t*
Psychiatric side effects, drugs with, 267*t*–270*t*
Psychosis, drugs causing, 267*t*–270*t*
Psyllium, 312
properties of, 313*t*
Pulmonary disease, pharmacotherapy in, 139–178
Pulmonary embolism, pharmacologic approach to patient with, 144–145
Pulmonary hypertension, pharmacologic approach to patient with, 145–147
Pyrazinamide, 354
dosage adjustment
with dialysis, 52*t*–53*t*
in renal failure, 52*t*–53*t*, 335*t*
dosage and administration, 335*t*
pharmacodynamics, in renal failure, 52*t*–53*t*
pharmacokinetics, 335*t*
in renal failure, 52*t*–53*t*
serum concentration, with dialysis, 335*t*
Pyridium, interference with glucose determination, 382*t*
Pyridostigmine
clinical uses, 262*t*, 264*t*–265*t*
dosage adjustment
with dialysis, 82*t*–83*t*
in renal failure, 82*t*–83*t*
pharmacodynamics, in renal failure, 82*t*–83*t*
pharmacokinetics, in renal failure, 82*t*–83*t*
side effects, 264*t*–265*t*
Pyrimethamine, 351–352
dosage adjustment, in renal failure, 335*t*
dosage and administration, 335*t*
pharmacokinetics, 335*t*
serum concentration, with dialysis, 335*t*

Q
Quinacrine
psychiatric side effects, 267*t*
secretion by kidney, 28*t*
Quinapril
dosage adjustment
with dialysis, 62*t*–63*t*
in renal failure, 62*t*–63*t*
pharmacodynamics, in renal failure, 62*t*–63*t*
pharmacokinetics, in renal failure, 62*t*–63*t*
Quinethazone, dosage and administration, 85*t*
Quinidine
adverse effects of, 230*t*–231*t*
disposition, effect of liver disease, 121*t*
dosage adjustment, in liver disease, 121*t*
dosage and administration, 230*t*–231*t*
drug interactions, 27*t*
hepatic/renal elimination, 121*t*
indications for, 230*t*
metabolism
induction by other drug(s), 21*t*
inhibition by other drug(s), 22*t*, 25*t*
pharmacodynamics, 121*t*
pharmacokinetics, 121*t*
psychiatric side effects, 270*t*
Quinidine sulfate
dosage adjustment
with dialysis, 66*t*–67*t*
in renal failure, 66*t*–67*t*
pharmacodynamics, in renal failure, 66*t*–67*t*
pharmacokinetics, in renal failure, 66*t*–67*t*
Quinine
absorption, drug interactions affecting, 17*t*
elimination, 10*t*
Quinolones, 347–348
absorption, drug interactions affecting, 17*t*
adverse effects of, in pediatric patients, 182
drug interactions, 27*t*

R
Ramipril
dosage adjustment
with dialysis, 62*t*–63*t*
in renal failure, 62*t*–63*t*
pharmacodynamics, in renal failure, 62*t*–63*t*
pharmacokinetics, in renal failure, 62*t*–63*t*
properties of, 223*t*
Ranitidine, 292–294
absorption, drug interactions affecting, 17*t*
disposition, effect of liver disease, 126*t*
dosage adjustment
with dialysis, 78*t*–79*t*

in liver disease, 126*t*
in renal failure, 50*t*, 78*t*–79*t*
dosage and administration, 293
drug interactions, 24*t*
fraction of dose excreted unchanged in urine with normal renal function, in children, 190*t*
half-life
in end-stage renal disease, 50*t*
normal, 50*t*
hepatic/renal elimination, 126*t*
infusion, in pediatric patients, 188*t*
pharmacodynamics, 126*t*
in renal failure, 78*t*–79*t*
pharmacokinetics, 126*t*, 293
in renal failure, 78*t*–79*t*
properties of, 290*t*
psychiatric side effects, 268*t*
secretion by kidney, 28*t*
side effects, 293–294
Rauwolfia alkaloids, psychiatric side effects, 270*t*
Renal failure
drug dosage adjustment in, 50*t*
effects on volume of distribution, 47*t*
pharmacotherapy in, 45–90
treatment of, agents used in, 51*t*
Resin hemoperfusion, drug removal by, 11*t*
Resorcinols
duration of action, 156*t*
receptor, 156*t*
route of administration, 156*t*
Ribavirin, 358
dosage adjustment, in renal failure, 336*t*
dosage and administration, 336*t*
pharmacokinetics, 336*t*
serum concentration, with dialysis, 336*t*
Rickettsia, antimicrobial drugs of choice for, 340*t*
Rifabutin, 355
Rifampin, 354
disposition, effect of liver disease, 113*t*
dosage adjustment
with dialysis, 52*t*–53*t*
in liver disease, 113*t*
in renal failure, 52*t*–53*t*, 335*t*
dosage and administration, 335*t*
drug interactions, 20*t*–21*t*
with cyclosporine, 29*t*
fraction of dose excreted unchanged in urine with normal renal function, in children, 190*t*
hepatic/renal elimination, 113*t*
pharmacodynamics, 113*t*
in renal failure, 52*t*–53*t*
pharmacokinetics, 113*t*, 335*t*
in renal failure, 52*t*–53*t*
psychiatric side effects, 268*t*
serum concentration, with dialysis, 335*t*
Riopan, 282*t*
Risks, of drug use, in liver disease, 108

S
Salbutamol
duration of action, 156*t*
receptor, 156*t*
route of administration, 156*t*
Salicylates
drug interactions, 20*t*
elimination, 10*t*
interference with glucose determination, 382*t*
metabolism, induction by other drug(s), 21*t*
psychiatric side effects, 267*t*
removal, by resin hemoperfusion, 11*t*
secretion by kidney, 28*t*
Salicylic acid
disposition, effect of liver disease, 118*t*
dosage adjustment, in liver disease, 118*t*
hepatic/renal elimination, 118*t*
pharmacodynamics, 118*t*
pharmacokinetics, 118*t*
Saline laxatives, 314–315
Salmeterol
duration of action, 156*t*
receptor, 156*t*
route of administration, 156*t*
Salmonella, antimicrobial drugs of choice for, 339*t*
Sclerotherapy, of esophageal varices, 310–311
Scopolamine
antiemetic properties of, 317
clinical uses, 264*t*–265*t*
effects of, 263*t*
indications for, 263*t*
side effects, 264*t*–265*t*
Sectral. *See* Acebutolol
Sedation
in ICU patients, scoring system for assessment of, 202*t*
during mechanical ventilation, commonly used drugs and method of administration, 203*t*
Sedative-hypnotics
cost, 201*t*
dosage, in mechanically ventilated patients, 201*t*
dosage adjustment, in liver disease, 122*t*–124*t*
infusion, in children, 184
Sedatives
clinical use, in asthma, 140
disposition, effect of liver disease, 122*t*–124*t*
dosage adjustment, in liver disease, 122*t*–124*t*

Sedatives—*continued*
hepatic/renal elimination, 122*t*–124*t*
monitoring guidelines, 7*t*
pharmacodynamics, 122*t*–124*t*
pharmacokinetics, 6*t*, 122*t*–124*t*
Seizures
causes, in critically ill patients, 243*t*
in critically ill patients, causes of, 243*t*
Senna, properties of, 313*t*
Sensitivity, 180
Serratia marcescens, antimicrobial drugs of choice for, 339*t*
Sertraline
dosage adjustment
with dialysis, 74*t*–75*t*
in renal failure, 74*t*–75*t*
pharmacodynamics, in renal failure, 74*t*–75*t*
pharmacokinetics, in renal failure, 74*t*–75*t*
Shigella, antimicrobial drugs of choice for, 339*t*
Single-chain urokinase-like plasminogen activation, doses, for patients with acute myocardial infarction, 240*t*
Sodium bicarbonate, in treatment of hyperkalemia, 86*t*–87*t*
Sodium morrhuate, 310–311
Sodium nitroprusside, for hypertensive emergencies, 226*t*–227*t*
Sodium phosphate, 314
Sodium phosphate/biphosphate enema, properties of, 313*t*
Sodium polystyrene sulfonate (SPS, Kayexalate), in treatment of hyperkalemia, 86*t*–87*t*
Sodium tetradecyl sulfate, 311
Sodium valproate
dosage adjustment
with dialysis, 78*t*–79*t*
in renal failure, 78*t*–79*t*
pharmacodynamics, in renal failure, 78*t*–79*t*
pharmacokinetics, in renal failure, 78*t*–79*t*
psychiatric side effects, 267*t*
Somatostatin
antisecretory and antimotility effects, 300–302
dosage and administration, 301
mechanism of action, 301
pharmacokinetics, 301
side effects, 301–302
special consideration with, 302
Sorbitol, 315
Sotalol
adverse effects of, 232*t*–233*t*
dosage adjustment
with dialysis, 64*t*–65*t*
in renal failure, 64*t*–65*t*
dosage and administration, 232*t*–233*t*
indications for, 232*t*
pharmacodynamics, in renal failure, 64*t*–65*t*
pharmacokinetics, in renal failure, 64*t*–65*t*
properties of, 232*t*–233*t*
Spinal cord transection, interactions with muscle relaxants, 208*t*–209*t*
Spironolactone
disposition, effect of liver disease, 122*t*
dosage adjustment
with dialysis, 70*t*–71*t*
in liver disease, 122*t*
in renal failure, 70*t*–71*t*
dosage and administration, 84*t*
half-life, 84*t*
hepatic/renal elimination, 122*t*
pharmacodynamics, 122*t*
in renal failure, 70*t*–71*t*
pharmacokinetics, 122*t*
in renal failure, 70*t*–71*t*
psychiatric side effects, 270*t*
site of action, 84*t*
Staphylococcus aureus, antimicrobial drugs of choice for, 338*t*
Status asthmaticus, management of, 140
Status epilepticus
physiologic changes during, 250*t*–251*t*
refractory generalized tonic-clonic, pentobarbital-induced anesthesia in, 253*t*
treatment of, 252*t*
Steroid myopathy, interactions with muscle relaxants, 208*t*–209*t*
Steroids, clinical use, in asthma, 140
Stimulant laxatives, 315–316
Stimulants, in pulmonary disease, 154–155
Streptococcus bovis, antimicrobial drugs of choice for, 338*t*
Streptococcus faecalis, antimicrobial drugs of choice for, 338*t*
Streptococcus pneumoniae, antimicrobial drugs of choice for, 338*t*
Streptokinase
dosage adjustment
with dialysis, 76*t*–77*t*
in renal failure, 76*t*–77*t*
doses, for patients with acute myocardial infarction, 240*t*
pharmacodynamics, in renal failure, 76*t*–77*t*
pharmacokinetics, in renal failure, 76*t*–77*t*
Streptomycin, 345–347, 355
disposition, effect of liver disease, 113*t*
dosage adjustment
with dialysis, 52*t*–53*t*
in liver disease, 113*t*
in renal failure, 52*t*–53*t*
hepatic/renal elimination, 113*t*

intraperitoneal administration, bioavailability after, 48*t*
ototoxicity, 346
pharmacodynamics, 113*t*
in renal failure, 52*t*–53*t*
pharmacokinetics, 113*t*
in renal failure, 52*t*–53*t*
psychiatric side effects, 267*t*
Stress gastritis, 280
Stress ulcers, pharmacotherapy for, 279–297
Stroke
cardiogenic embolic, management of, 256*f*
ischemic, conditions associated with, 254*t*, 256*t*
Subarachnoid hemorrhage
causes of, 258*t*
early management of, 259*t*
Sublimaze. *See* Fentanyl
Succinimides, psychiatric side effects, 267*t*
Succinylcholine
adverse effects of, 210*t*
clinical pharmacology of, 206*t*–207*t*
dosage, in children, 193*t*
dosage adjustment
with dialysis, 82*t*–83*t*
in renal failure, 82*t*–83*t*
duration of clinical effect, 206*t*
intubating dose, 206*t*
pharmacodynamics, in renal failure, 82*t*–83*t*
pharmacokinetics, in renal failure, 82*t*–83*t*
Sucralfate, 284–286
dosage and administration, 286
drug interactions, 285–286
mechanism of action, 284–285
pharmacokinetics, 285
side effects, 286
special considerations with, 286
Sufentanil
cost, 201*t*
dosage, in mechanically ventilated patients, 201*t*
dosage adjustment
with dialysis, 74*t*–75*t*, 82*t*–83*t*
in renal failure, 82*t*–83*t*
pharmacodynamics, in renal failure, 82*t*–83*t*
pharmacokinetics, in renal failure, 82*t*–83*t*
use, in adult ICU patients, 204*t*–205*t*
Sulbactam
dosage adjustment
with dialysis, 52*t*–53*t*
in renal failure, 52*t*–53*t*
pharmacodynamics, in renal failure, 52*t*–53*t*
pharmacokinetics, in renal failure, 52*t*–53*t*
Sulfadiazine
dosage adjustment, in renal failure, 335*t*
dosage and administration, 335*t*
pharmacokinetics, 335*t*
serum concentration, with dialysis, 335*t*
Sulfamethopyrazine, volume of distribution, in renal failure, 47*t*
Sulfamethoxazole
disposition, effect of liver disease, 113*t*
dosage adjustment
with dialysis, 60*t*–61*t*
in liver disease, 113*t*
in renal failure, 60*t*–61*t*
fraction of dose excreted unchanged in urine with normal renal function, in children, 190*t*
hepatic/renal elimination, 113*t*
pharmacodynamics, 113*t*
in renal failure, 60*t*–61*t*
pharmacokinetics, 113*t*
in renal failure, 60*t*–61*t*
Sulfapyridine, dosage and administration, 319
Sulfasalazine
adverse reactions, 320
dosage and administration, 319
indications, 318
mechanism of action, 318–319
pharmacokinetics, 318–319
special considerations with, 320–321
Sulfinpyrazone
disposition, effect of liver disease, 118*t*
dosage adjustment, in liver disease, 118*t*
drug interactions, 27*t*
hepatic/renal elimination, 118*t*
pharmacodynamics, 118*t*
pharmacokinetics, 118*t*
Sulfisoxazole
disposition, effect of liver disease, 126*t*
dosage adjustment, in liver disease, 126*t*
hepatic/renal elimination, 126*t*
pharmacodynamics, 126*t*
pharmacokinetics, 126*t*
Sulfonamides, 351–352
drug interactions, 27*t*
elimination, 10*t*
psychiatric side effects, 267*t*
secretion by kidney, 28*t*
Sulfonylureas, secretion by kidney, 28*t*
Sulindac, psychiatric side effects, 267*t*
Supraventricular tachycardia, drugs used to treat, 228*t*–229*t*
Suramin, psychiatric side effects, 269*t*
Surfactants
in pulmonary disease, 149–151
recommended dose, 194*t*–195*t*
Sympatholytics, psychiatric side effects, 269*t*

Sympathomimetics, psychiatric side effects, 269*t*
Syndrome of inappropriate antidiuretic hormone, 371
Syringomyelia, interactions with muscle relaxants, 208*t*–209*t*
Systemic lupus erythematosus, interactions with muscle relaxants, 208*t*–209*t*

T

$t_{1/2}$, 3*t*
Talwin. *See* Pentazocine
Tamoxifen
  drug interactions, 27*t*
  psychiatric side effects, 268*t*
Teicoplanin, 350–351
Temazepam
  disposition, effect of liver disease, 124*t*
  dosage adjustment
    with dialysis, 72*t*–73*t*
    in liver disease, 124*t*
    in renal failure, 72*t*–73*t*
  hepatic/renal elimination, 124*t*
  metabolism, induction by other drug(s), 21*t*
  pharmacodynamics, 124*t*
    in renal failure, 72*t*–73*t*
  pharmacokinetics, 124*t*
    in renal failure, 72*t*–73*t*
Tenormin. *See* Atenolol
Tenoxicam, absorption, drug interactions affecting, 17*t*
Teratogens, 181
Terazosin
  dosage adjustment
    with dialysis, 62*t*–63*t*
    in renal failure, 62*t*–63*t*
  pharmacodynamics, in renal failure, 62*t*–63*t*
  pharmacokinetics, in renal failure, 62*t*–63*t*
Terbutaline
  dosage, 157*t*
  dosage adjustment
    with dialysis, 80*t*–81*t*
    in renal failure, 80*t*–81*t*
  duration of action, 156*t*
  pharmacodynamics, in renal failure, 80*t*–81*t*
  pharmacokinetics, in renal failure, 80*t*–81*t*
  preparation, 157*t*
  receptor, 156*t*
  route of administration, 156*t*–157*t*
Terfenadine, metabolism, inhibition by other drug(s), 25*t*
Tetanus, interactions with muscle relaxants, 208*t*–209*t*
Tetracyclines
  absorption, drug interactions affecting, 17*t*
  adverse effects, in pediatric patients, 181
  dosage adjustment
    with dialysis, 58*t*–59*t*
    in renal failure, 58*t*–59*t*, 335*t*
  dosage and administration, 335*t*
  pharmacodynamics, in renal failure, 58*t*–59*t*
  pharmacokinetics, 335*t*
    in renal failure, 58*t*–59*t*
  psychiatric side effects, 268*t*
  serum concentration, with dialysis, 335*t*
Tetraethylammonium, secretion by kidney, 28*t*
Tetrahydrocannabinoid, 318
Theophylline
  absorption, drug interactions affecting, 17*t*
  disposition, effect of liver disease, 126*t*
  dosage adjustment
    with dialysis, 80*t*–81*t*
    in liver disease, 126*t*
    in renal failure, 80*t*–81*t*
  hepatic/renal elimination, 126*t*
  metabolism
    induction by other drug(s), 21*t*
    inhibition by other drug(s), 22*t*–23*t*, 25*t*–27*t*
  monitoring guidelines, 7*t*
  pharmacodynamics, 126*t*
    in renal failure, 80*t*–81*t*
  pharmacokinetics, 6*t*, 126*t*
    in renal failure, 80*t*–81*t*
  removal, by resin hemoperfusion, 11*t*
Thiabendazole, psychiatric side effects, 268*t*
Thiazide diuretics
  dosage adjustment
    with dialysis, 68*t*–69*t*
    in renal failure, 68*t*–69*t*
  dosage and administration, 84*t*–85*t*
  half-life, 84*t*
  pharmacodynamics, in renal failure, 68*t*–69*t*
  pharmacokinetics, in renal failure, 68*t*–69*t*
  secretion by kidney, 28*t*
  site of action, 84*t*
Thiopental
  cost, 201*t*
  disposition, effect of liver disease, 126*t*
  dosage, in mechanically ventilated patients, 201*t*
  dosage adjustment
    with dialysis, 70*t*–71*t*
    in liver disease, 126*t*
    in renal failure, 70*t*–71*t*

hepatic/renal elimination, 126*t*
pharmacodynamics, 126*t*
in renal failure, 70*t*–71*t*
pharmacokinetics, 126*t*
in renal failure, 70*t*–71*t*
Thorazine. *See* Chlorpromazine
Thrombolytic therapy, contraindications to, 240*t*
Thymidine, drug interactions, 27*t*
Thyroid dysfunction, 371
Thyroid hormone, psychiatric side effects, 269*t*
Thyrotoxic myopathy, interactions with muscle relaxants, 208*t*–209*t*
l-Thyroxine, pharmacology of, 377*t*
Ticarcillin, 341
dosage adjustment
with dialysis, 58*t*–59*t*
in renal failure, 50*t*, 58*t*–59*t*, 334*t*
dosage and administration, 334*t*
half-life
in end-stage renal disease, 50*t*
normal, 50*t*
pharmacodynamics, in renal failure, 58*t*–59*t*
pharmacokinetics, 334*t*
in renal failure, 58*t*–59*t*
psychiatric side effects, 268*t*
serum concentration, with dialysis, 334*t*
Ticarcillin-clavulanate, 333, 341
dosage adjustment, in renal failure, 334*t*
dosage and administration, 334*t*
pharmacokinetics, 334*t*
serum concentration, with dialysis, 334*t*
Ticlopidine
dosage adjustment
with dialysis, 76*t*–77*t*
in renal failure, 76*t*–77*t*
drug interactions, 27*t*
pharmacodynamics, in renal failure, 76*t*–77*t*
pharmacokinetics, in renal failure, 76*t*–77*t*
Timentin. *See* Ticarcillin-clavulanate
Timolol
dosage adjustment
with dialysis, 64*t*–65*t*
in renal failure, 64*t*–65*t*
pharmacodynamics, in renal failure, 64*t*–65*t*
pharmacokinetics, in renal failure, 64*t*–65*t*
properties of, 221*t*, 232*t*–233*t*
Tissue plasminogen activators, doses, for patients with acute myocardial infarction, 240*t*
Tobramycin, 345–347
disposition, effect of liver disease, 113*t*
dosage adjustment
with dialysis, 52*t*–53*t*
in liver disease, 113*t*
in renal failure, 52*t*–53*t*, 335*t*
dosage and administration, 335*t*
drug interactions, with nondepolarizing muscle relaxants, 207*t*
hepatic/renal elimination, 113*t*
infusion, in pediatric patients, 188*t*
intraperitoneal administration, bioavailability after, 48*t*
ototoxicity, 346
pharmacodynamics, 113*t*
in renal failure, 52*t*–53*t*
pharmacokinetics, 113*t*, 335*t*
in renal failure, 52*t*–53*t*
psychiatric side effects, 268*t*
serum concentration, with dialysis, 335*t*
toxicity, 347
Tocainide
adverse effects of, 230*t*–231*t*
disposition, effect of liver disease, 121*t*
dosage adjustment
with dialysis, 66*t*–67*t*
in liver disease, 121*t*
in renal failure, 66*t*–67*t*
dosage and administration, 230*t*–231*t*
elimination, 10*t*
hepatic/renal elimination, 121*t*
indications for, 230*t*
metabolism, inhibition by other drug(s), 25*t*
pharmacodynamics, 121*t*
in renal failure, 66*t*–67*t*
pharmacokinetics, 121*t*
in renal failure, 66*t*–67*t*
Tolazamide
dosage adjustment
with dialysis, 80*t*–81*t*
in renal failure, 80*t*–81*t*
pharmacodynamics, in renal failure, 80*t*–81*t*
pharmacokinetics, in renal failure, 80*t*–81*t*
Tolbutamide
absorption, drug interactions affecting, 17*t*
displacement from protein-binding sites, drug interactions due to, 20*t*
disposition, effect of liver disease, 126*t*
dosage adjustment
with dialysis, 80*t*–81*t*
in liver disease, 126*t*
in renal failure, 80*t*–81*t*
drug interactions, 20*t*
hepatic/renal elimination, 126*t*
metabolism
induction by other drug(s), 21*t*
inhibition by other drug(s), 22*t*–27*t*
pharmacodynamics, 126*t*

Tolbutamide—*continued*
in renal failure, 80*t*–81*t*
pharmacokinetics, 126*t*
in renal failure, 80*t*–81*t*
Tolmetin sodium, psychiatric side effects, 267*t*
Toxoplasma gondii, antimicrobial drugs of choice for, 340*t*
Trandate. *See* Labetalol
Traumatized patients, interactions with muscle relaxants, 208*t*–209*t*
Triamcinolone
dosage adjustment
with dialysis, 80*t*–81*t*
in renal failure, 80*t*–81*t*
pharmacodynamics, in renal failure, 80*t*–81*t*
pharmacokinetics, in renal failure, 80*t*–81*t*
Triamterene
disposition, effect of liver disease, 122*t*
dosage adjustment
with dialysis, 70*t*–71*t*
in liver disease, 122*t*
in renal failure, 70*t*–71*t*
dosage and administration, 84*t*
half-life, 84*t*
hepatic/renal elimination, 122*t*
metabolism, inhibition by other drug(s), 25*t*
pharmacodynamics, 122*t*
in renal failure, 70*t*–71*t*
pharmacokinetics, 122*t*
in renal failure, 70*t*–71*t*
secretion by kidney, 28*t*
site of action, 84*t*
Triazolam
dosage adjustment
with dialysis, 72*t*–73*t*
in renal failure, 72*t*–73*t*
pharmacodynamics, in renal failure, 72*t*–73*t*
pharmacokinetics, in renal failure, 72*t*–73*t*
Trichlormethiazide, dosage and administration, 85*t*
Tricyclic antidepressants
dosage adjustment
with dialysis, 72*t*–75*t*
in renal failure, 72*t*–75*t*
pharmacodynamics, in renal failure, 72*t*–75*t*
pharmacokinetics, in renal failure, 72*t*–75*t*
removal, by resin hemoperfusion, 11*t*
l-Triiodothyronine, pharmacology of, 377*t*
Trimethaphan
for hypertensive emergencies, 226*t*–227*t*
psychiatric side effects, 270*t*
Trimethoprim, 351–352
disposition, effect of liver disease, 114*t*
dosage adjustment
with dialysis, 60*t*–61*t*
in liver disease, 114*t*
in renal failure, 60*t*–61*t*
drug interactions, with cyclosporine, 29*t*
fraction of dose excreted unchanged in urine with normal renal function, in children, 190*t*
hepatic/renal elimination, 114*t*
pharmacodynamics, 114*t*
in renal failure, 60*t*–61*t*
pharmacokinetics, 114*t*
in renal failure, 60*t*–61*t*
psychiatric side effects, 268*t*
secretion by kidney, 28*t*
volume of distribution, in renal failure, 47*t*
Trimethoprim-sulfamethoxazole
dosage adjustment, in renal failure, 335*t*
dosage and administration, 335*t*
intraperitoneal administration, bioavailability after, 49*t*
pharmacokinetics, 335*t*
psychiatric side effects, 268*t*
serum concentration, with dialysis, 335*t*
Tubocurarine
dosage adjustment
with dialysis, 82*t*–83*t*
in renal failure, 82*t*–83*t*
pharmacodynamics, in renal failure, 82*t*–83*t*
pharmacokinetics, in renal failure, 82*t*–83*t*
d-Tubocurarine
characteristics of, 210*t*–211*t*
clearance, 213*t*
clinical pharmacology of, 206*t*–207*t*
cost, 201*t*
dosage, in mechanically ventilated patients, 201*t*
duration of clinical effect, 206*t*
intubating dose, 206*t*
metabolism, 213*t*
side effects and adverse reactions to, 210*t*–211*t*

U
Ulcerative colitis, pharmacotherapy for, 318–321
Unasyn, 341. *See* Ampicillin/sulbactam
Unicard. *See* Dilevalol
Urapidil, metabolism, inhibition by other drug(s), 25*t*
Ureido penicillins
dosage adjustment
with dialysis, 56*t*–57*t*
in renal failure, 56*t*–57*t*

pharmacodynamics, in renal failure, 56t–57t
pharmacokinetics, in renal failure, 56t–57t
Urine, glucose determinations, drug interference with, 382t
Urine pH-dependent elimination, clinically important drugs with, 10t
Urokinase, doses, for patients with acute myocardial infarction, 240t

V
Valproic acid
absorption, drug interactions affecting, 17t
adverse effects of, in pediatric patients, 183
displacement from protein-binding sites, drug interactions due to, 20t
disposition, effect of liver disease, 116t
dosage adjustment, in liver disease, 116t
drug interactions, 20t, 27t, 250t–251t
with cyclosporine, 29t
hepatic/renal elimination, 116t
metabolism, induction by other drug(s), 21t
monitoring guidelines, 7t
pharmacodynamics, 116t
pharmacokinetics, 6t, 116t
Vancomycin, 350–351
disposition, effect of liver disease, 114t
dosage adjustment
with dialysis, 56t–57t
in liver disease, 114t
in renal failure, 50t, 56t–57t, 335t
dosage and administration, 335t
fraction of dose excreted unchanged in urine with normal renal function, in children, 190t
half-life
in end-stage renal disease, 50t
normal, 50t
hepatic/renal elimination, 114t
infusion, in pediatric patients, 188t
intraperitoneal administration, bioavailability after, 49t
monitoring guidelines, 7t
pharmacodynamics, 114t
in renal failure, 56t–57t
pharmacokinetics, 6t, 114t, 335t
in renal failure, 56t–57t
serum concentration, with dialysis, 335t
volume of distribution, in renal failure, 47t
Variceal hemorrhage, pharmacotherapy for, 307–311
Vasodilators
dosage adjustment
with dialysis, 64t–65t
in renal failure, 64t–65t
effects, on depressed ventricular function, 235f
indications for, 216–217
pharmacodynamics
in critical illness, 8t–9t
in renal failure, 64t–65t
pharmacokinetics, in renal failure, 64t–65t
principal site of action, 236t
Vasopressin, 308–310
analogues, 309t, 373t
aqueous, dosage and administration, 309t, 373t
dosage and administration, 308
mechanism of action, 308
side effects, 308–310
Vasopressin peptides, relative activity of, 372t
Vasopressors, 308–310
pharmacodynamics, in critical illness, 8t–9t
Vasospasm, prophylactic therapies for, 259t
Vasotec. *See* Enalapril
V_d, 3t
Vecuronium
characteristics of, 210t–211t
clearance, 213t
clinical pharmacology of, 206t–207t
cost, 201t
dosage
in children, 193t
in mechanically ventilated patients, 201t
dosage adjustment
with dialysis, 82t–83t
in renal failure, 82t–83t
duration of clinical effect, 206t
fraction of dose excreted unchanged in urine with normal renal function, in children, 190t
infusion, in pediatric patients, 188t
intubating dose, 206t
metabolism, 213t
monitoring guidelines, 7t
pharmacodynamics
age-related changes in, 182
in renal failure, 82t–83t
pharmacokinetics, 6t
in renal failure, 82t–83t
side effects and adverse reactions to, 210t–211t
use during mechanical ventilation, 203t
Verapamil
absorption, drug interactions affecting, 19t
adverse effects of, 232t–233t
in pediatric patients, 183
disposition, effect of liver disease, 121t

Verapamil—*continued*
dosage adjustment
with dialysis, 68*t*–69*t*
in liver disease, 121*t*
in renal failure, 68*t*–69*t*
dosage and administration, 232*t*–233*t*
drug interactions, 22*t*
with cyclosporine, 29*t*
hepatic/renal elimination, 121*t*
indications for, 232*t*
metabolism, induction by other drug(s), 21*t*
pharmacodynamics, 121*t*
in renal failure, 68*t*–69*t*
pharmacokinetics, 121*t*
in renal failure, 68*t*–69*t*
properties of, 222*t*
psychiatric side effects, 270*t*
in treatment of supraventricular tachycardia, 228*t*–229*t*
Vidarabine, 360
infusion, in pediatric patients, 188*t*
Vigabatrin, drug interactions, 21*t*
Vinblastine, psychiatric side effects, 268*t*
Vincristine, psychiatric side effects, 268*t*
Viruses, antimicrobial drugs of choice for, 340*t*
Visken. *See* Pindolol
Vitamin A, psychiatric side effects, 269*t*
Vitamin B complex, psychiatric side effects, 269*t*
Vitamin C, interference with glucose determination, 382*t*
Vitamin D, psychiatric side effects, 269*t*
Volume of distribution, 3*t*, 96
in renal failure, 47*t*
von Recklinghausen's disease, interactions with muscle relaxants, 208*t*–209*t*

W
Warfarin
absorption, drug interactions affecting, 17*t*
disposition, effect of liver disease, 127*t*
dosage adjustment
with dialysis, 76*t*–77*t*
in liver disease, 127*t*
in renal failure, 76*t*–77*t*
drug interactions, with cyclosporine, 29*t*
hepatic/renal elimination, 127*t*
metabolism, inhibition by other drug(s), 22*t*–27*t*
pharmacodynamics, 127*t*
in critical illness, 8*t*–9*t*
in renal failure, 76*t*–77*t*
pharmacokinetics, 127*t*
in renal failure, 76*t*–77*t*
Water metabolism, 371

Z
Zestril. *See* Lisinopril
Zidovudine. *See* Azidothymidine
disposition, effect of liver disease, 114*t*
dosage adjustment, in liver disease, 114*t*
hepatic/renal elimination, 114*t*
metabolism, inhibition by other drug(s), 26*t*
pharmacodynamics, 114*t*
pharmacokinetics, 114*t*
Zomepirac sodium, psychiatric side effects, 267*t*

TABLE 12.3. Glucagon Therapy

Indication	*Dose (mg)*	*Time for Response*	*Duration of Action*	*Comments*[a]
Hypoglycemia	1–5 mg s.c., i.m., or i.v. bolus	<20 min	Depends on liver glycogen	Start i.v. glucose; may repeat dose
Cardiogenic shock or heart failure	1–5 mg i.v. bolus every 30–60 min or 1–10 mg/h i.v. infusion	5–10 min	20–30 min for bolus	Use antiemetic; watch glucose and K^+
β-Blocker overdose	1–5 mg i.v. bolus every 30–60 min or 1–10 mg/h i.v. infusion	5–10 min	20–30 min for bolus	Repeat dose every 30 min as needed; watch glucose and K^+
Esophageal meat impaction	1 mg i.v. bolus	5 min	30 min	Repeat every 30 min; follow with barium
Diverticular disease	1 mg i.v. bolus every 4 h	3–12 h	2–4 h	Repeat as needed
Renal or biliary calculi	1 mg i.v. bolus every 4 h	1–2 h	2–4 h	Repeat as needed

[a] Administer cautiously to patients with suspected pheochromocytoma or insulinoma.